Mycotoxin Contamination Management Tools and Efficient Strategies in Feed Industry

Mycotoxin Contamination Management Tools and Efficient Strategies in Feed Industry

Editor

Federica Cheli

MDPI • Basel • Beijing • Wuhan • Barcelona • Belgrade • Manchester • Tokyo • Cluj • Tianjin

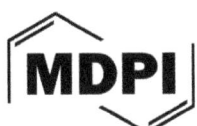

Editor
Federica Cheli
Università degli Studi di Milano
Italy

Editorial Office
MDPI
St. Alban-Anlage 66
4052 Basel, Switzerland

This is a reprint of articles from the Special Issue published online in the open access journal *Toxins* (ISSN 2072-6651) (available at: https://www.mdpi.com/journal/toxins/special_issues/mycotoxin_contamination_feed).

For citation purposes, cite each article independently as indicated on the article page online and as indicated below:

LastName, A.A.; LastName, B.B.; LastName, C.C. Article Title. *Journal Name* **Year**, *Article Number*, Page Range.

ISBN 978-3-03943-010-9 (Hbk)
ISBN 978-3-03943-011-6 (PDF)

© 2020 by the authors. Articles in this book are Open Access and distributed under the Creative Commons Attribution (CC BY) license, which allows users to download, copy and build upon published articles, as long as the author and publisher are properly credited, which ensures maximum dissemination and a wider impact of our publications.

The book as a whole is distributed by MDPI under the terms and conditions of the Creative Commons license CC BY-NC-ND.

Contents

About the Editor vii

Preface to "Mycotoxin Contamination Management Tools and Efficient Strategies in Feed Industry" ix

Federica Cheli
Mycotoxin Contamination Management Tools and Efficient Strategies in Feed Industry
Reprinted from: *Toxins* **2020**, *12*, 480, doi:10.3390/toxins12080480 1

Saowalak Adunphatcharaphon, Awanwee Petchkongkaew, Donato Greco, Vito D'Ascanio, Wonnop Visessanguan and Giuseppina Avantaggiato
The Effectiveness of Durian Peel as a Multi-Mycotoxin Adsorbent
Reprinted from: *Toxins* **2020**, *12*, 108, doi:10.3390/toxins12020108 5

Ibukun Ogunade, Yun Jiang and Andres Pech Cervantes
DI/LC–MS/MS-Based Metabolome Analysis of Plasma Reveals the Effects of Sequestering Agents on the Metabolic Status of Dairy Cows Challenged with Aflatoxin B_1
Reprinted from: *Toxins* **2019**, *11*, 693, doi:10.3390/toxins11120693 23

Oluwatobi Kolawole, Julie Meneely, Brett Greer, Olivier Chevallier, David S. Jones, Lisa Connolly and Christopher Elliott
Comparative In Vitro Assessment of a Range of Commercial Feed Additives with Multiple Mycotoxin Binding Claims
Reprinted from: *Toxins* **2019**, *11*, 659, doi:10.3390/toxins11110659 35

Sung Woo Kim, Débora Muratori Holanda, Xin Gao, Inkyung Park and Alexandros Yiannikouris
Efficacy of a Yeast Cell Wall Extract to Mitigate the Effect of Naturally Co-Occurring Mycotoxins Contaminating Feed Ingredients Fed to Young Pigs: Impact on Gut Health, Microbiome, and Growth
Reprinted from: *Toxins* **2019**, *11*, 633, doi:10.3390/toxins11110633 49

Roua Rejeb, Gunther Antonissen, Marthe De Boevre, Christ'l Detavernier, Mario Van de Velde, Sarah De Saeger, Richard Ducatelle, Madiha Hadj Ayed and Achraf Ghorbal
Calcination Enhances the Aflatoxin and Zearalenone Binding Efficiency of a Tunisian Clay
Reprinted from: *Toxins* **2019**, *11*, 602, doi:10.3390/toxins11100602 79

Mariana Paiva Rodrigues, Andrea Luciana Astoreca, Águida Aparecida de Oliveira, Lauranne Alves Salvato, Gabriela Lago Biscoto, Luiz Antonio Moura Keller, Carlos Alberto da Rocha Rosa, Lilia Renée Cavaglieri, Maria Isabel de Azevedo and Kelly Moura Keller
In Vitro Activity of Neem (*Azadirachta indica*) Oil on Growth and Ochratoxin A Production by *Aspergillus carbonarius* Isolates
Reprinted from: *Toxins* **2019**, *11*, 579, doi:10.3390/toxins11100579 93

Giulia Leni, Martina Cirlini, Johan Jacobs, Stefaan Depraetere, Natasja Gianotten, Stefano Sforza and Chiara Dall'Asta
Impact of Naturally Contaminated Substrates on *Alphitobius diaperinus* and *Hermetia illucens*: Uptake and Excretion of Mycotoxins
Reprinted from: *Toxins* **2019**, *11*, 476, doi:10.3390/toxins11080476 105

Luigi Castaldo, Giulia Graziani, Anna Gaspari, Luana Izzo, Josefa Tolosa, Yelko Rodríguez-Carrasco and Alberto Ritieni
Target Analysis and Retrospective Screening of Multiple Mycotoxins in Pet Food Using UHPLC-Q-Orbitrap HRMS
Reprinted from: *Toxins* **2019**, *11*, 434, doi:10.3390/toxins11080434 . . . . **117**

Lucia Gambacorta, Monica Olsen and Michele Solfrizzo
Pig Urinary Concentration of Mycotoxins and Metabolites Reflects Regional Differences, Mycotoxin Intake and Feed Contaminations
Reprinted from: *Toxins* **2019**, *11*, 378, doi:10.3390/toxins11070378 . . . . **133**

Ran Xu, Niel A. Karrow, Umesh K. Shandilya, Lv-hui Sun and Haruki Kitazawa
In-Vitro Cell Culture for Efficient Assessment of Mycotoxin Exposure, Toxicity and Risk Mitigation
Reprinted from: *Toxins* **2020**, *12*, 146, doi:10.3390/toxins12030146 . . . . **147**

Radmilo Čolović, Nikola Puvača, Federica Cheli, Giuseppina Avantaggiato, Donato Greco, Olivera Đuragić, Jovana Kos and Luciano Pinotti
Decontamination of Mycotoxin-Contaminated Feedstuffs and Compound Feed
Reprinted from: *Toxins* **2019**, *11*, 617, doi:10.3390/toxins11110617 . . . . **179**

About the Editor

Federica Cheli is full professor of Animal Nutrition in the Department of Health, Animal Science and Food Safety at the University of Milan. She is a member of the Coordinating Research Centres (CRC) "Innovation for Well-Being and Environment" (I-WE) of the University of Milan. Her research in the field of animal nutrition is focused on feeding and quality of animal products, mycotoxins in feed and food, quality and safety of feedstuffs (analytical methods, electronic nose and tongue, image analysis, and cell-based bioassays). She has authored and co-authored approximately 80 peer-reviewed journal articles, including review papers and book chapters, and numerous other publications in animal nutrition and feed safety. Professor Cheli is Associate Editor of the *Italian Journal of Animal Science* and member of the International Society for Mycotoxicology, Animal Science and Production Association and The European Federation of Animal Science. She is an expert for FAO/WHO on Hazards Associated with Animal Feed.

Preface to "Mycotoxin Contamination Management Tools and Efficient Strategies in Feed Industry"

Mycotoxins represent a significant issue for the feed industry and the safety of the feed supply chain, with an impact on human health, animal health and production, economies, and international trade. Notifications on the Rapid Alert System for Food and Feed (RASFF) concerning mycotoxins are among the "top 10" hazard categories, with risk decision categorized as "serious". Mycotoxin contamination of feed is a recurring problem in the livestock feed industry in an increasingly competitive marketplace. The globalization of the trade in agricultural commodities and the lack of legislative harmonization have contributed significantly to the discussion about the awareness of mycotoxins entering the feed/food supply chain. The feed industry is a sustainable outlet for food processing industries, converting byproducts into high-quality animal feed. Mycotoxin occurrence in food byproducts from different technological processes is a worldwide topic of interest for the feed industry, aiming to increase the marketability and acceptance of these products as feed ingredients and include them safely in the feed supply chain. Since mycotoxin contamination cannot be completely prevented pre- or post-harvest, precise knowledge of mycotoxin occurrence and repartitioning during technological processes and decontamination strategies is critical and may provide a sound technical basis for feed managers to conform to legislation requirements and reduce the risk of severe adverse health, market, and trade repercussions.

This Special Issue highlights research topics with a high impact for a sustainable and competitive feed industry that focus on new tools for monitoring and managing the risk of mycotoxins at industrial level and strategies to prevent and reduce mycotoxins in compound feed manufacturing.

The editor wishes to thank the contributors, reviewers, and the support of the Toxins editorial staff, whose professionalism and dedication have made this issue possible.

Federica Cheli
Editor

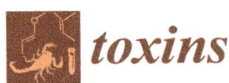

Editorial

Mycotoxin Contamination Management Tools and Efficient Strategies in Feed Industry

Federica Cheli [1,2]

[1] Department of Health, Animal Science and Food Safety, Università degli Studi di Milano, 20134 Milan, Italy; federica.cheli@unimi.it
[2] CRC I-WE (Coordinating Research Centre: Innovation for Well-Being and Environment), Università degli Studi di Milano, 20134 Milan, Italy

Received: 2 June 2020; Accepted: 27 July 2020; Published: 29 July 2020

Mycotoxins represent a risk to the feed supply chain with an impact on animal health, feed industry, economy, and international trade. A high percentage of feed samples have been reported to be contaminated with more than one mycotoxin. Multi-mycotoxin contamination is a topic of great concern, as co-contaminated samples might still exert adverse effects on animals due to additive/synergistic interactions of the mycotoxins. Since mycotoxin contamination cannot be completely prevented pre- or post-harvest, precise knowledge of mycotoxin occurrence, repartitioning during technological processes and decontamination strategies are critical and may provide a sound technical basis for feed managers to conform to legislation requirements and reduce the risk of severe adverse health, market and trade repercussions.

Castaldo et al. [1] developed and validated a quantitative method, using an acetonitrile-based extraction and an ultra-high-performance liquid chromatography coupled to high-resolution mass spectrometry (UHPLC-Q-Orbitrap HRMS), for a multi-mycotoxin screening of 28 mycotoxins and identification of other 45 fungal and bacterial metabolites in dry pet food samples. Results showed mycotoxin contamination in 99% of pet food samples and all positive samples showed co-occurrence of mycotoxins with the simultaneous presence of up to 16 analytes per sample.

Strategies must be developed for mycotoxin reduction in feedstuffs. Čolović et al. [2] reviewed the most recent findings on different processes and strategies for the reduction of toxicity of mycotoxins in animals giving detailed information about the decontamination approaches to mitigate mycotoxin contamination of feedstuffs and compound feed, which could be implemented in practice. Authors conclude that there is increasing business interest in the use of feed additives to avoid mycotoxin absorption and the toxic impacts on farm animals. The efficacy of the additives for the distinct mycotoxins and livestock is a critical point and must be proved. It is recommended that cell lines or in vitro models be used in the simulation instead of living experimental animals. In this scenario, a group of papers deals with in vitro models for assessing mycotoxin toxicity and risk mitigation strategies. Xu et al. [3] reviewed different in vitro intestinal epithelial cells (IECs) or co-culture models that can be used for assessing mycotoxin exposure, toxicity, and risk mitigation. Since ingestion is the most common route of mycotoxin exposure, the intestinal epithelial barrier, comprised of IECs and immune cells such as macrophages, represents ground zero where mycotoxins are absorbed, biotransformed, and elicit toxicity. Several articles investigated the efficacy of feed additives as multi-mycotoxin adsorbent by using in vitro gastro-intestinal models. Adunphatcharaphon et al. [4] characterised and analysed acid-treated durian peel (ATDP), an agricultural waste, for simultaneous adsorption of mycotoxins. Results indicated the potential of ATDP as a multi-mycotoxin biosorbent for aflatoxin B1 (AFB1), ochratoxin A (OTA), zearalenone (ZEN), and fumonisin B1 (FB1), but negligible towards deoxynivalenol (DON). Kolawole et al. [5] carried out a study to assess the efficacy of commercially available feed additives with multi-mycotoxin-binding claims. Their capacity to simultaneously adsorb DON, ZEN, FB1, OTA, AFB1, and T-2 toxin was assessed and compared using an in vitro model designed to simulate the gastrointestinal tract of a monogastric animal. Results showed that only one product (a modified yeast cell wall) effectively adsorbed more than 50% of DON, ZEN, FB1, OTA, T-2 and AFB1. The remaining products were able to moderately bind AFB1 but had less, or in some cases, no effect on ZEN, FB1, OTA and T-2 binding. Rejeb et al. [6] characterized a Tunisian clay, before and after calcination, and investigated the effectiveness of the thermal treatment on the adsorption capacity toward AFG1, AFB2, AFG2, and ZEN using an in vitro gastro-intestinal model. The calcination treatment enhanced mainly the adsorption of aflatoxins. Overall results confirm that mycotoxin binders must undergo rigorous trials under the conditions which best mimic the gastrointestinal environment that they must be active in. Claims on the binding efficiency should only be made when such data has been generated.

A few papers reported results of in vivo studies. Kim et al. [7] evaluated yeast cell wall extract efficacy to reduce multi-mycotoxin (AFs, FUM, and DON) toxicity in pigs and improve performance and gut health in pigs. The yeast cell wall extract effects were more evident in promoting gut health and growth in nursery pigs, which showed higher susceptibility to mycotoxin effects, than in growing pigs. Ogunade et al. [8] applied a targeted metabolomics approach to evaluate the effects of supplementing clay with or without *Saccharomyces cerevisiae* fermentation product on the metabolic status of dairy cows challenged with AFB1. Blood was analysed for metabolomic analysis. The study confirmed the protective effects of sequestering agents in dairy cows challenged with AFB1. Moreover, the combination of arginine, alanine, methylhistidine, and citrulline were found to be excellent potential biomarkers of aflatoxin ingestion in dairy cows fed no sequestering agents. The evaluation of mycotoxin biomarker could be an interesting tool for assessing animal exposure to mycotoxin in feed. Gambacorta et al. [9] measured the urinary mycotoxin and mycotoxin biomarker concentrations to assess pig exposure to mycotoxins in Sweden. They found regional differences that were in good agreement with the occurrence of *Fusarium graminearum* mycotoxins in cereal grains harvested in Sweden. From a safety and risk management perspective, the back-calculated levels of mycotoxins in feeds were low with the exception of a few samples that were higher than the European limits.

Paiva Rodrigues at al. [10] carried out an in vitro study to contribute to the knowledge to develop effective anti-mycotoxigenic natural products for reduction of mycotoxigenic fungi and mycotoxins in foods. Authors evaluated the effects of different concentrations of neem oil on the percentage of growth inhibition of six *Aspergillus carbonarius* strains and OTA production. Results indicated that neem essential oil can be considered as an auxiliary method for the reduction of mycelial growth and OTA production.

One paper deals with an important topic: insects as suitable alternative feed for livestock production. Insects have the ability to grow on a different spectrum of substrates, which could be naturally contaminated by mycotoxins. Studies on insect safety as feed ingredients are mandatory for the feed industry. Leni et al. [11] evaluated the mycotoxin uptake and/or excretion in two different insect species, *Alphitobius diaperinus* (Lesser Mealworm, LM) and *Hermetia illucens* (Black Soldier Fly, BSF), grown on naturally contaminated wheat and/or corn substrates (DON, FB1, FB2, and ZEN). No mycotoxins were detected in BSF larvae, while quantifiable amount of DON and FB1 was found in LM larvae. Mass balance calculations indicated that BSF and LM metabolized mycotoxins in forms not yet known, accumulating them in their body or excreting in the faeces. Results indicate that further studies are required in this direction due to the future employment of insects as feedstuff.

Acknowledgments: We express our gratitude to all contributing authors and reviewers.

Conflicts of Interest: The author declare no conflict of interest.

References

1. Castaldo, L.; Graziani, G.; Gaspari, A.; Izzo, L.; Tolosa, J.; Rodríguez-Carrasco, Y.; Ritieni, A. Target Analysis and Retrospective Screening of Multiple Mycotoxins in Pet Food Using UHPLC-Q-Orbitrap HRMS. *Toxins* **2019**, *11*, 434. [CrossRef] [PubMed]

2. Čolović, R.; Puvača, N.; Cheli, F.; Avantaggiato, G.; Greco, D.; Đuragić, O.; Kos, L.; Pinotti, L. Decontamination of Mycotoxin-Contaminated Feedstuffs and Compound Feed. *Toxins* **2019**, *11*, 617. [CrossRef] [PubMed]
3. Xu, R.; Karrow, N.A.; Shandilya, U.K.; Sun, L.; Kitazawa, H. In-Vitro Cell Culture for Efficient Assessment of Mycotoxin Exposure, Toxicity and Risk Mitigation. *Toxins* **2020**, *12*, 146. [CrossRef] [PubMed]
4. Adunphatcharaphon, S.; Petchkongkaew, A.; Greco, D.; D'Ascanio, V.; Visessanguan, W.; Avantaggiato, G. The Effectiveness of Durian Peel as a Multi-Mycotoxin Adsorbent. *Toxins* **2020**, *12*, 108. [CrossRef]
5. Kolawole, O.; Meneely, J.; Greer, B.; Chevallier, O.; Jones, D.S.; Connolly, L.; Elliott, C. Comparative In Vitro Assessment of a Range of Commercial Feed Additives with Multiple Mycotoxin Binding Claims. *Toxins* **2019**, *11*, 659. [CrossRef]
6. Rejeb, R.; Antonissen, G.; De Boevre, M.; Detavernier, C.; Van de Velde, M.; De Saeger, S.; Ducatelle, R.; Ayed, M.H.; Ghorbal, A. Calcination Enhances the Aflatoxin and Zearalenone Binding Efficiency of a Tunisian Clay. *Toxins* **2019**, *11*, 602. [CrossRef]
7. Kim, S.W.; Muratori Holanda, D.; Gao, X.; Park, I.; Yiannikouris, A. Efficacy of a Yeast Cell Wall Extract to Mitigate the Effect of Naturally Co-Occurring Mycotoxins Contaminating Feed Ingredients Fed to Young Pigs: Impact on Gut Health, Microbiome, and Growth. *Toxins* **2019**, *11*, 633. [CrossRef] [PubMed]
8. Ogunade, D.; Jiang, Y.; Pech Cervantes, A. DI/LC–MS/MS-Based Metabolome Analysis of Plasma Reveals the Effects of Sequestering Agents on the Metabolic Status of Dairy Cows Challenged with Aflatoxin B1. *Toxins* **2019**, *11*, 693. [CrossRef] [PubMed]
9. Gambacorta, L.; Olsen, M.; Solfrizzo, M. Pig Urinary Concentration of Mycotoxins and Metabolites Reflects Regional Differences, Mycotoxin Intake and Feed Contaminations. *Toxins* **2019**, *11*, 378. [CrossRef] [PubMed]
10. Paiva Rodrigues, M.; Astoreca, A.L.; Aparecida de Oliveira, A.; Alves Salvato, L.; Lago Biscoto, G.; Moura Keller, L.A.; Da Rocha Rosa, C.A.; Cavaglieri, L.R.; De Azevedo, K.I.; Keller, K.M. In Vitro Activity of Neem (*Azadirachta indica*) Oil on Growth and Ochratoxin A Production by *Aspergillus carbonarius* Isolates. *Toxins* **2019**, *11*, 579. [CrossRef] [PubMed]
11. Leni, G.; Cirlini, M.; Jacobs, J.; Depraetere, S.; Gianotten, N.; Sforza, S.; Dall'Asta, C. Impact of Naturally Contaminated Substrates on *Alphitobius diaperinus* and *Hermetia illucens*: Uptake and Excretion of Mycotoxins. *Toxins* **2019**, *11*, 476. [CrossRef] [PubMed]

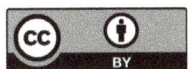

© 2020 by the author. Licensee MDPI, Basel, Switzerland. This article is an open access article distributed under the terms and conditions of the Creative Commons Attribution (CC BY) license (http://creativecommons.org/licenses/by/4.0/).

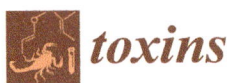

Article

The Effectiveness of Durian Peel as a Multi-Mycotoxin Adsorbent

Saowalak Adunphatcharaphon [1], Awanwee Petchkongkaew [1], Donato Greco [2], Vito D'Ascanio [2], Wonnop Visessanguan [3] and Giuseppina Avantaggiato [2,*]

[1] School of Food Science and Technology, Faculty of Science and Technology, Thammasat University, 99 Mhu 18, Paholyothin road, Khong Luang, Pathum Thani 12120, Thailand; s.adunphatcharaphon@hotmail.com (S.A.); awanwee@tu.ac.th (A.P.)
[2] Institute of Sciences of Food Production (ISPA), National Research Council (CNR), Via Amendola 122/O, 70126 Bari, Italy; donato.greco@ispa.cnr.it (D.G.); vito.dascanio@ispa.cnr.it (V.D.)
[3] Functional Ingredient and Food Innovation Research Group, National Center for Genetic Engineering and Biotechnology (BIOTEC), National Science and Technology Development Agency (NSTDA), 113 Thailand Science Park, Phahonyothin Road, Pathumthani 12120, Thailand; wonnop@biotec.or.th
* Correspondence: giuseppina.avantaggiato@ispa.cnr.it; Tel.: +39-080-592-9348

Received: 16 January 2020; Accepted: 5 February 2020; Published: 8 February 2020

Abstract: Durian peel (DP) is an agricultural waste that is widely used in dyes and for organic and inorganic pollutant adsorption. In this study, durian peel was acid-treated to enhance its mycotoxin adsorption efficacy. The acid-treated durian peel (ATDP) was assessed for simultaneous adsorption of aflatoxin B_1 (AFB$_1$), ochratoxin A (OTA), zearalenone (ZEA), deoxynivalenol (DON), and fumonisin B_1 (FB$_1$). The structure of the ATDP was also characterized by SEM–EDS, FT–IR, a zetasizer, and a surface-area analyzer. The results indicated that ATDP exhibited the highest mycotoxin adsorption towards AFB$_1$ (98.4%), ZEA (98.4%), and OTA (97.3%), followed by FB$_1$ (86.1%) and DON (2.0%). The pH significantly affected OTA and FB$_1$ adsorption, whereas AFB$_1$ and ZEA adsorption was not affected. Toxin adsorption by ATDP was dose-dependent and increased exponentially as the ATDP dosage increased. The maximum adsorption capacity (Q_{max}), determined at pH 3 and pH 7, was 40.7 and 41.6 mmol kg^{-1} for AFB$_1$, 15.4 and 17.3 mmol kg^{-1} for ZEA, 46.6 and 0.6 mmol kg^{-1} for OTA, and 28.9 and 0.1 mmol kg^{-1} for FB$_1$, respectively. Interestingly, ATDP reduced the bioaccessibility of these mycotoxins after gastrointestinal digestion using an in vitro, validated, static model. The ATDP showed a more porous structure, with a larger surface area and a surface charge modification. These structural changes following acid treatment may explain the higher efficacy of ATDP in adsorbing mycotoxins. Hence, ATDP can be considered as a promising waste material for mycotoxin biosorption.

Keywords: mycotoxins; durian peel; agricultural by-products; biosorption; gastrointestinal digestion model; decontamination; equilibrium isotherms

Key Contribution: Acid treatment of durian peel changes the morphological structure of its surface and enhances mycotoxin adsorption efficacy. Acid-treated durian peel is a promising waste material for mycotoxin decontamination.

1. Introduction

Mycotoxins are fungi-derived metabolites capable of causing a dverse effects to both humans and animals. They are produced by toxigenic fungi, including *Aspergillus*, *Penicillium*, *Alternaria*, and *Fusarium* species, under specific temperature and humidity conditions [1–4]. The main mycotoxins occurring in food and feedstuffs are aflatoxins, ochratoxins, zearalenone, deoxynivalenol, and fumonisins [4,5]. Contamination by mycotoxins is common in primary agricultural commodities such as maize, rice, wheat, cereal products, meat, and dried fruits [5–8]. Multi-mycotoxin contamination of food and feedstuffs depends on environmental conditions and type of substrate [9]. A multi-mycotoxin-contaminated diet may induce acute mycotoxicosis with several chronic adverse effects, being mutagenic, carcinogenic, teratogenic, estrogenic, and immunosuppressive [10]. The combined consumption of different mycotoxins may produce synergistic toxic effects [9,11]. Mycotoxin consumption by livestock leads to economic losses for the feed industry and in international trade [12]. Since mycotoxin contamination cannot be completely prevented in pre-harvesting or post-harvesting, it is very difficult to avoid in agricultural commodities [5]. Decontamination strategies therefore play an important role in helping to reduce exposure to mycotoxin-contaminated feed. Strategies that have been developed for mycotoxin reduction in feedstuffs include physical, chemical, and biological methods. However, most have considerable limitations in practical applications [13]. The addition of mycotoxin binders (including activated charcoal, aluminosilicates, and agricultural wastes) to contaminated feed is an innovative and safe approach to counteracting the harmful effects of mycotoxins to livestock [12,14–17]. Mycotoxin adsorbents have several disadvantages, including the adsorption of essential nutrients and trace elements, as well as a rather narrow spectrum of action towards the pool of mycotoxins frequently found in feedstuffs. Therefore, it is very important to find new low-cost and biosustainable mycotoxin adsorbents that are able to simultaneously bind the main mycotoxins of zootechnical interest. Recently, the use of agricultural wastes as mycotoxin biosorbents has been investigated since they have a porous structure and contain a variety of functional groups, including carboxyl and hydroxyl groups, which may be involved in the binding mechanisms of mycotoxins [18,19]. In a recent study, [16] compared the ability of different agricultural by-products to adsorb mycotoxins from liquid media using the isotherm adsorption approach. Grape pomaces, artichoke wastes, and almond hulls were selected as the best mycotoxin biosorbents, being effective in adsorbing AFB_1, ZEA, and OTA. Taking into account these findings, the present study evaluates the efficacy of durian peel waste as an additive for mycotoxin decontamination of feed. Durian Monthong (*Durio zibthinus*) is a popular fruit in Thailand and has many consumers. A large amount of durian peel is thrown away, resulting in social and environmental problems linked to waste disposal. As durian peel contains cellulose (47.2%), hemicellulose (9.63%), lignin (9.89%), and ash (4.20%), it has been extensively studied as a fuel and adsorbent of pollutants and heavy metals [20–23]. To the best of our knowledge, no research has reported reporting the use of durian peel as a multi-mycotoxin binder. The aim of this study is to assess the efficacy of durian peel as a binder, both untreated and acid-treated, in adsorbing the mycotoxins of major concern (aflatoxins, ochratoxins, zearalenone, deoxynivalenol, and fumonisins). The equilibrium isotherm approach was used to study mycotoxin reduction in liquid media at physiological pH values. In addition, the efficacy of these agricultural by-products in reducing mycotoxin bioaccessibility was assessed using a static, validated gastrointestinal model.

2. Results and Discussion

2.1. Characterization of Durian Peel

The surface morphology and elementary composition of DP and ATDP were determined using SEM–EDS. SEM images showed that acid treatment of DP had the effect of modifying its surface (Figure 1). More cavities were recorded on the surface of ATDP than DP. The study of Lazim et al. [22] reported more pores on a DP surface after treatment with sulfuric acid, providing a higher capacity in the removal of bisphenol A. These findings suggest that a change in the morphological structure of the DP surface following acid treatment may affect mycotoxin adsorption.

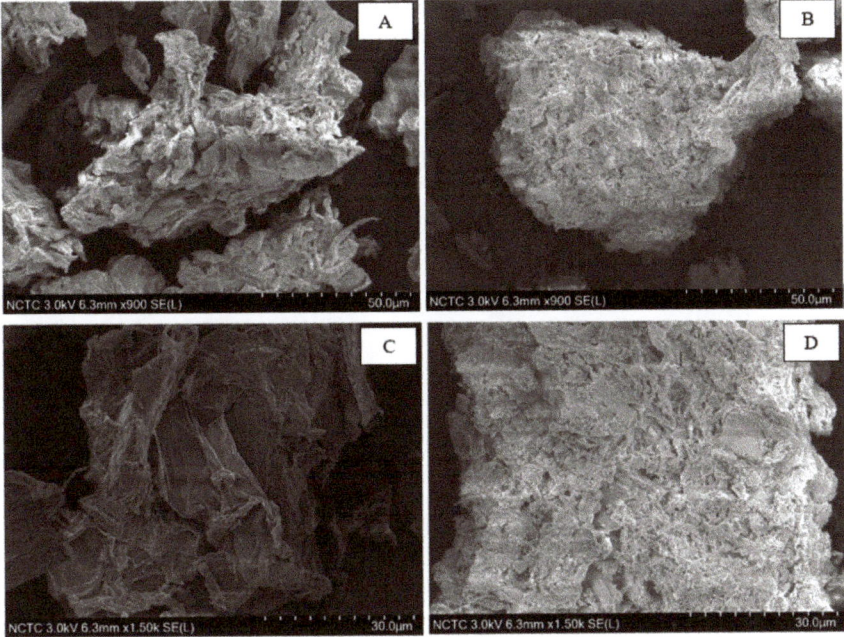

Figure 1. SEM images of durian peel (DP) and acid-treated durian peel (ATDP) at 900× and 1500× magnification. (**A,B**): DP and ATDP at 900×; (**C,D**): DP and ATDP at 1500×.

EDS spectra analysis showed that C and O constitute the major elements of the materials, with C as the dominant component (data not shown). These results are in accordance with the study of Charoenvai [21], which classified the major components of DP as cellulose (47%), hemicellulose (10%), lignin (10%), and ash (4%). Acid treatment affects the elemental composition of the DP surface, thus increasing the proportion of C. The functional groups present on the DP and ATDP surfaces were identified by FTIR (Figure 2). The FTIR spectra of DP obtained were similar to those reported by Lazim et al. [19]. A first intense spectrum band was observed at 3330 cm^{-1}, corresponding to O–H stretching vibrations and H bonding of cellulose, pectin, and lignin, which are the major fiber components of fruit peel [24,25]. A second peak was observed at 2917 cm^{-1}, corresponding to C–H stretching vibrations of the methyl or methylene groups. Interestingly, no peak vibrations were found in the range at 2800–2300 cm^{-1}, which represent N–H or C=O stretching vibrations of the amine and ketone functional groups. The peak at 1730 cm^{-1} corresponded to C=O stretching vibrations of the carbonyl group, while the peaks at 1622 cm^{-1} were related to the amide band (-CONH$_2$). Peaks in the range 1500–1200 cm^{-1} were assigned to strong asymmetric carboxylic groups, methyl groups (bending vibration), aromatic amines, and C–O stretching vibrations of carboxylic acids [25]. Interestingly, a shift in all peak vibrations was observed in the FTIR spectra of ATDP and DP. In addition, ATDP produced no peaks in the range 1450–1250 cm^{-1}. This suggests that modification by acid treatment affected the amine and methyl groups in the DP structure, resulting in a change in adsorption features. Ngabura et al. [25] observed that acidic groups, carboxyl, hydroxyl, and amides are involved in biosorption by DP. Zeta potential values for ATDP and DP differed substantially, with ATDP higher than DP. At pH 3, these values were −23.20 mV for ATDP and −2.55 mV for DP. This difference in zeta potential can be explained by modification of the DP structure, induced by acid treatment. In a previous study [25], acid treatment of DP affected the physical properties of the material. In our study, ATDP had greater BET pore volumes, pore diameters, and surface area (Table 1). These physical properties create greater adsorption at the surfaces. Ngabura et al. [25] found that hydrochloric acid-modified DP (HAMDP) had a more porous structure with a larger surface area than the pristine peel. The BET surface area is negatively correlated with the nanoparticle size, and the nanoparticle size of ATDP was 21-fold less than that of DP (Table 1). The same ratio was observed when comparing the surface areas of the ATDP and DP, with the surface area of ATDP being 21-fold higher than that of DP. This structural modification of the adsorbing surface following acid treatment was confirmed by the SEM–EDS images, which showed a more porous surface on the ATDP. The physico-chemical characterization suggested that the materials have different characteristics and are expected to differently in mycotoxin adsorption.

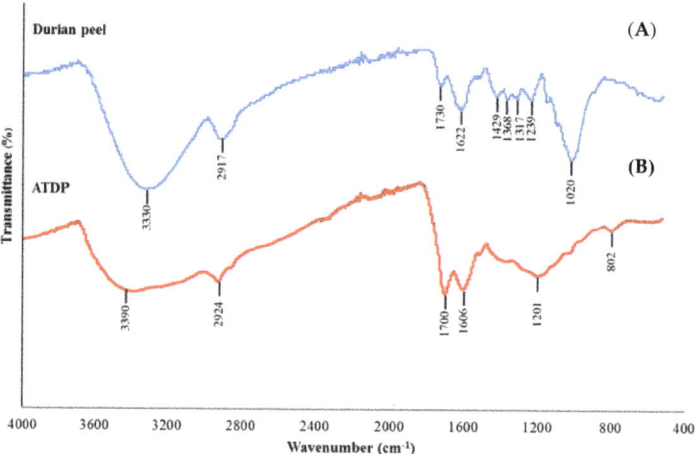

Figure 2. FT-IR spectra of DP (**A**) and ATDP (**B**).

Table 1. BET single point method surface area analysis of DP and ATDP.

Adsorbent	Nanoparticle (nm)	Pore Volume (cm^3/g)	Pore Diameter (nm)	Surface Area (m^2/g)
DP	3032.45	0.004	7.22	1.98
ATDP	142.95	0.162	15.46	41.97

2.2. Screening of DP and ATDP as Multi-Mycotoxin Adsorbing Agents

DP and ATDP at 5 mg/mL dosage (0.5% w/v) were preliminarily tested for their ability to bind the mixture of five mycotoxins. Adsorption experiments were performed at a constant temperature of 37 °C and media of pH 3 and 7, using 1 mM citrate or 100 mM phosphate buffer. To measure mycotoxin adsorption by ATDP at pH 7, a 100-fold concentrated phosphate buffer was required since the ATDP suspension acidified the 1 mM phosphate buffer. As shown in Table 2, adsorption by DP and ATDP depended on the type of mycotoxin and pH of the medium. Maximum mycotoxin adsorption by DP was 53% for ZEA (pH 3), 46% for AFB$_1$ (pH 3), and 18% for OTA (pH 3). AFB$_1$ and ZEA adsorption was not affected by pH. OTA adsorption occurred mainly at pH 3, while FB$_1$ and DON adsorption was negligible (≤2%). Interestingly, treatment with sulfuric acid significantly increased adsorption of most mycotoxins assayed in the study. The ATDP reduced AFB$_1$ and ZEA by more than 98% in media at pH 3 and 7. OTA adsorption by ATDP at pH 3 and 7 was significantly higher than adsorption by DP, being 97% at acid pH and 42% at neutral pH. Acid treatment of DP also increased FB$_1$ adsorption, but at acidic pH only. At pH 3, FB$_1$ adsorption was 86%, while no adsorption was observed at pH 7. Acid treatment did not improve DON adsorption, which in all cases was less than 13%. As previously reported [19], treatment of DP with sulfuric acid modified the physico-chemical properties of the DP adsorption surface, increasing the binding sites available for mycotoxin adsorption.

Table 2. Mycotoxin adsorptions by DP and ATDP tested at different pH values (7 and 3) and at 5 mg/mL of dosage towards a multi-mycotoxin solution containing 1 μg/mL of each toxin. Values are means of triplicate experiments ± standard deviations.

Toxin	DP		ATDP	
	pH 3	pH 7	pH 3	pH 7
AFB_1	46 ± 4	37 ± 2	98.4 ± 0.1	98.4 ± 0.1
ZEA	53 ± 2	52 ± 4	98.4 ± 0.4	99.6 ± 0.2
OTA	18 ± 1	0.7 ± 0.6	97.3 ± 0.1	42.2 ± 0.2
FB_1	0	2.3 ± 0.7	86 ± 3	0
DON	0	2 ± 1	2.0 ± 0.8	13 ± 2

2.3. Effect of Medium pH on Mycotoxin Adsorption and Desorption

Medium pH is an important parameter that affects the binding of mycotoxins by adsorbent materials, by affecting both the charge distribution on the surface of the adsorbents and the degree of ionization of the adsorbates. This is more important for adsorption processes in which electrostatic interactions are involved. An effective multi-mycotoxin adsorbent should sequester a large spectrum of mycotoxins with high efficacy, regardless of the medium pH, and should keep these contaminants bound along the compartments of a GI tract, where pH values ranging from 1.5–7.5 can be encountered. The results for pH (Figure 3) confirmed that AFB_1 and ZEA adsorption by ATDP was stable within the GI tract of monogastric animals since 100% of the toxins were adsorbed at pH values ranging from 3 to 9. A desorption study was performed to assess whether a change of pH caused a release of the sequestered toxins. Mycotoxins were first adsorbed onto ATDP at pH 3, and then the pellet containing the adsorbed mycotoxins was washed first with a buffer at pH 7 and then with methanol. Washing solutions were analyzed for mycotoxin release. As shown in Table 3, AFB_1 and ZEA adsorption was 100% at pH 3. No release was observed in the pH range from 3 to 7. The organic solvent (methanol) extracted 34% of the AFB_1 and 85% of the ZEA, suggesting stronger binding of AFB_1 by ATDP than by ZEA. OTA or FB_1 adsorption and pH were inversely correlated. The adsorption efficacy of ATDP decreased as the pH increased (Figure 3). As OTA and FB_1 hold acid groups in their structure, the pH of the medium is expected to affect the extent of mycotoxin adsorption [26]. OTA adsorption decreased from 97% to 28% as the pH was increased from 3 to 9. Similarly, FB_1 was adsorbed mainly at pH 3, falling to 5% at pH above 6. However, despite the strong pH effect observed for OTA and FB_1, ATDP was effective in retaining the adsorbed fractions after the medium pH was changed from 3 to 7 (Table 3). The organic solvent extracted half of the adsorbed OTA, while FB_1 was poorly desorbed (7%). Overall, our study suggests that ATDP is highly efficacious in retaining FB_1, AFB_1, and OTA when a strong solvent is used. DP is an agricultural waste fiber. In addition to cellulose, hemicellulose, and lignin, it contains phenolic compounds with important biological properties [21]. The specific combination of these chemical components, and the increased adsorption surface obtained by acid treatment, explains the mycotoxin adsorption properties of ATDP.

Table 3. Mycotoxin adsorption and desorption from ATDP. Values are means ± standard deviations of triplicate independent experiments.

Toxin	Adsorption (%)	Desorption (%)	
	pH 3	pH 7	Methanol
AFB_1	100	0	34 ± 3
ZEA	98.9 ± 0.4	0.8 ± 0.2	85 ± 4
OTA	99.0 ± 0.3	2.0 ± 0.5	48 ± 3
FB_1	91 ± 3	1.6 ± 0.3	6.5 ± 0.5

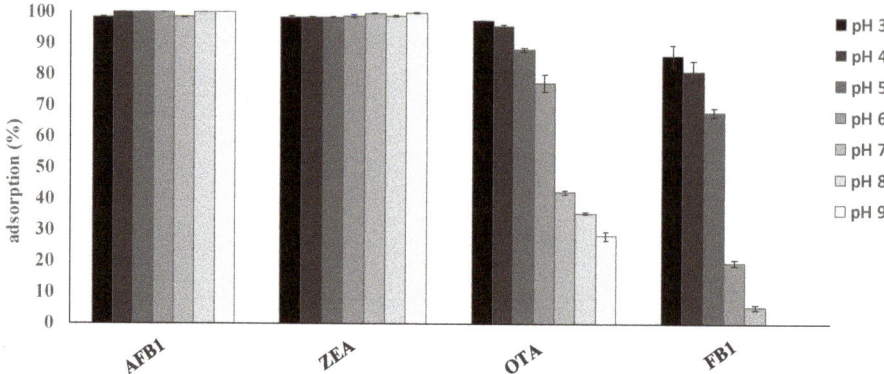

Figure 3. Effect of pH on AFB_1, ZEA, OTA, and FB_1 adsorption by ATDP tested at 5 mg/mL dosage towards a multi-mycotoxin solution containing 1 µg/mL of each toxin. Values are means of triplicate experiments.

2.4. Effect of ATDP Dosage

The effect of ATDP dosage on mycotoxin adsorption was investigated using equilibrium adsorption isotherms. The goal was to calculate the optimal adsorbent dosage for further adsorption tests and to compare the efficacy of ATDP in simultaneously binding different mycotoxins. As shown in Figure 4, AFB_1, ZEA, and OTA removal from a neutral medium increased as the dosage increased. Experimental values adsorption onto ATDP were in the ranges of 48–100% for AFB_1, 31–100% for ZEA, and 0–69% for OTA. No significant FB_1 adsorption was observed at pH 7. The adsorption plots for all toxins showed a characteristic L-shape (Figure 4) and were well fitted by the Langmuir model ($R^2 > 0.99$). This model allowed calculation of both the theoretically estimated maximum adsorption Ads_{max} and the C_{50}, which is the theoretically-estimated adsorbent dosage to achieve a 50% reduction of the absorbable toxin [26]. Predicted Ads_{max} values were $101 \pm 1\%$ for AFB_1, $104 \pm 1\%$ for ZEA, and $103 \pm 1\%$ for OTA (Table 4). Additionally, C_{50} values listed in Table 4 suggest a higher efficacy of ATDP adsorption of AFB_1 and ZEA than of OTA. It should not therefore be useful to increase the dosage of ATDP beyond 6 mg/mL when sequestering AFB_1, ZEA, and OTA from a 1 µg/mL solution (Table 4). In the following equilibrium isotherm studies, the optimal adsorbent dosages were fixed in the range of 0.5 to 5 mg/mL depending on the toxin.

2.5. Equilibrium Adsorption Isotherm

Isotherms are an effective approach to the study of surface adsorption mechanisms, surface properties, and an adsorbent affinity [16]. Nonlinear regression was used to assess the goodness of fit and to calculate the parameters involved in the adsorption mechanism (Ads_{max}, K_L). The mathematical models, including the Freundlich, Langmuir, and Sips equations, were used to predict the amount of AFB_1, ZEA, OTA, and FB_1 adsorbed by ATDP. The model that met regression analysis requirements (homogeneity of variance and normality assumptions), providing a lower statistical error, was used to fit the experimental data (Table 5). The amount of AFB_1, ZEA, OTA, and FB_1 adsorbed per unit mass of ATDP increased gradually as the mycotoxin concentration in the working solution increased. Isotherms showed an exponential relationship and a typical L (Langmuir) shape. In all cases, regardless of medium pH, the Langmuir model was found to best fit the experimental adsorption data. This model assumes that adsorption occurs at definite localized sites, which are identical and equivalent [27]. This implies that the adsorption of AFB_1, ZEA, OTA, and FB_1 by ATDP is homogeneous. As shown in Table 5, AFB_1 adsorption by ATDP produced isotherms showing similar Ads_{max} values at pH 3 and 7. However, affinity was affected by the pH of the medium. The K_L Langmuir constant, which is related to adsorbent affinity, was 2.5-fold higher at pH 7 than pH 3

(Table 5). The increase of pH from 3 to 7 induced an increase in the K_L value from 0.4 ± 0.1 L/mg (125 000 ± 31.250 L/mol) to 1.0 ± 0.1 L/mg (312.500 ± 31 250 L/mol). This resulted in an increase in AFB_1 adsorption affinity. Experimental values for AFB_1 adsorption in percent varied in the ranges of 50–84% at pH 3 and 76–100% at pH 7. The predicted values for maximum adsorption capacity were 12.7 ± 0.9 µg/mg (40.7 ± 2.9 mmol/kg) at pH 3 and 13.0 ± 0.4 µg/mg (41.6 ± 1.3 mmol/kg) at pH 7 (Table 5). These values were in agreement with experimental results obtained at both pH values and were consistent with previous reports that AFB_1 adsorption by agricultural by-products is not dependent on medium pH [16,26]. Compared with previous studies of agricultural by-products, ATDP showed higher AFB_1 adsorption. The Langmuir isotherm was also found to be the best model when studying ZEA adsorption by ATDP (Figure 5 and Table 5). ZEA adsorption was not affected by the change in medium pH from 3 and 7). The experimental values for ZEA adsorption ranged from 70% to 86% at pH 3 and 54% to 100% at pH 7. The predicted maximum adsorption capacity was 5.5 ± 0.3 µg/mg (17.3 ± 0.9 mmol/kg) at pH 3 and 4.9 ± 0.3 µg/mg (15.4 ± 0.9 mmol/kg) at pH 7. The Langmuir K_L parameters were 2.2 ± 0.2 L/mg (700.637 ± 63.694 L/mol) at pH3 and 2.9 ± 0.6 L/mg (923.567 ± 191.082 L/mol) at pH 7. ZEA is a resorcyclic acid lactone and a hydrophobic compound [28]. It is a weak acid due to the presence of the diphenolic moiety and has a pKa of 7.62 [28]. At the pH values considered in this study (pH ≤ 7), it should be in protonated, nonionic form. ZEA adsorption by ATDP may involve hydrophobic interactions occurring at homogeneous adsorption sites with similar energy, as suggested by the Langmuir K_L parameter values. Unlike AFB_1 and ZEA adsorption, OTA adsorption by ATDP was widely affected by pH. The experimental values for OTA adsorption were 47–96% at pH 3 and 46–65% at pH 7. Maximum adsorption capacities calculated at pH 3 and 7 were 18.8 ± 1.5 µg/mg (46.6 ± 3.7 mmol/kg) and 0.26 ± 0.02 µg/mg (0.64 ± 0.05 mmol/kg), respectively. K_L Langmuir values calculated were 1.90 ± 0.21 L/mg (766.129 ± 84.677 L/mol) at pH 3 and 1.30 ± 0.12 L/mg (524.193 ± 48.387 L/mol) at pH 7. As OTA is an ionizable molecule, a change in pH is expected to affect adsorption. The decrease in both Ads_{max} and K_L values for OTA adsorption at pH 7 may reflect by the presence of an anionic form of the toxin, producing repulsion between the OTA molecules and negative charges on the ATDP surface. In addition, these results suggest that hydrophobicity is implicated in OTA adsorption. Indeed, OTA was preferentially adsorbed at pH 3 when the uncharged form was predominant. At pH 7, OTA hydrophobicity decreased, affecting mycotoxin adsorption. In conclusion, OTA adsorption by ATDP may involve several mechanisms, including electrostatic forces and hydrophobic interactions, whose roles depend on the pH of the medium. As observed for OTA, FB_1 adsorption was dependent first on pH, then on the degree of ionization of the molecules. FB_1 adsorption was achieved at pH 3 only, since no adsorption was recorded at pH 7 (Figure 5). The experimental values for FB_1 adsorption were in the range 67–100%. The predicted maximum adsorption capacity was 20.9 ± 1.2 µg/mg (28.9 ± 1.7 mmol/kg) at pH 3 (Table 5). The Langmuir K_L parameter was 1.7 ± 0.4 L/mg (1223.021 ± 287.769 L/mol). It can be concluded that, in acidic aqueous solutions, FB_1 adsorption by ATDP is favoured and occurs mainly by polar non-covalent interactions. These include electrostatic interactions or hydrogen bonds involving the carboxylic functional groups. The efficacy of ATDP in removing mycotoxins from liquid media was significantly higher than previous reports of biosorbents: lactic acid bacteria, yeasts, moulds, and agricultural by-products [16,29–34].

Table 4. The theoretically estimated maximum adsorption (Ads_{max}) and inclusion rate of ATDP to obtain a 50% reduction of the absorbable toxin (C_{50}). Ads_{max} and C_{50} were calculated by fitting the data from Figure 4 with the Langmuir isotherm model.

Toxin	Ads_{max} (%)	C_{50} (mg/mL)
AFB_1	101 ± 1	0.11
ZEA	104 ± 1	0.19
OTA	103 ± 1	5.77

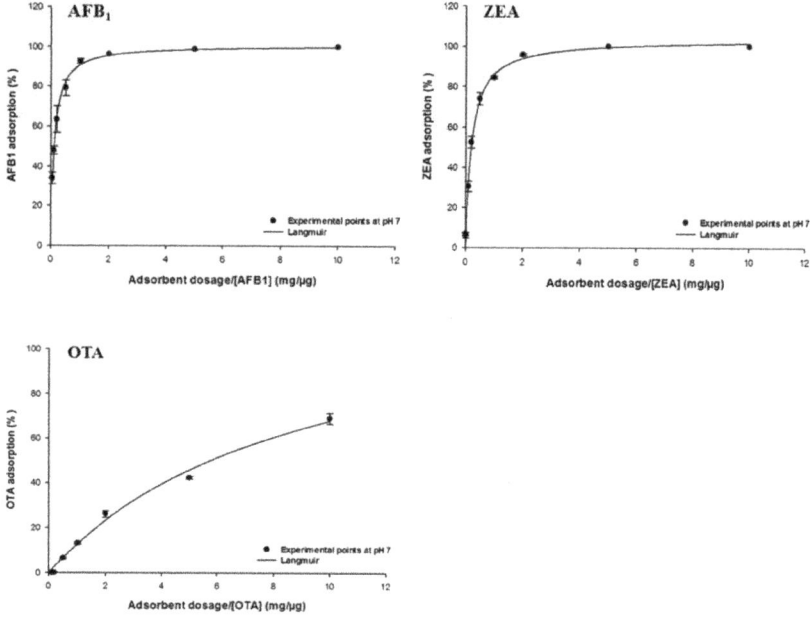

Figure 4. Effect of adsorbent dosage on AFB_1, ZEA, and OTA adsorptions by ATDP. Equilibrium adsorption isotherms were obtained at constant temperature (37 °C) and at pH 7 by testing a fixed amount of toxin (1 µg/mL) with increasing adsorbent dosages (0.1–10 mg/mL).

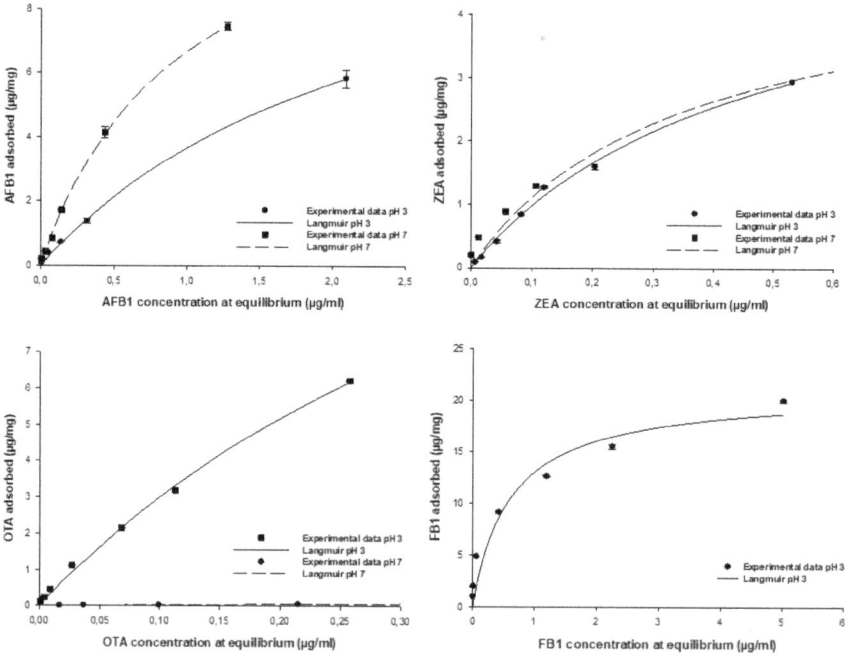

Figure 5. Effect of mycotoxin concentration on AFB_1, ZEA, OTA, and FB_1 adsorption by ATDP. Equilibrium adsorption isotherms were obtained at constant temperature (37 °C) and pH (3 and 7) by testing a fixed amount of ATDP with increasing toxin concentrations (0.025–7.5 µg/mL).

Table 5. The isotherm model parameters of mycotoxin adsorption by ATDP calculated at different pH values.

	Parameters	AFB$_1$		ZEA		OTA		FB1
		pH 3	pH 7	pH 3	pH 7	pH 3	pH 7	pH 3
Freundlich	K$_f$ (±SE)	3.32 ± 0.05	6.43 ± 0.12	4.66 ± 0.17	3.33 ± 0.04	18.09 ± 0.17	0.17 ± 0.00	11.86 ± 0.14
	1/n (±SE)	0.76 ± 0.02	0.67 ± 0.03	0.69 ± 0.02	0.45 ± 0.01	0.79 ± 0.01	0.77 ± 0.02	0.33 ± 0.00
	R^2	0.9977	0.9892	0.9850	0.9948	0.9997	0.9966	0.9976
	SS$_{res}$	0.1705	1.2987	0.0120	0.1517	0.0272	0.0001	4.3605
	S$_{y|x}$	0.1032	0.2849	0.1097	0.1041	0.0379	0.0022	0.4922
	PRESS	0.3656	1.6869	0.2661	0.1668	0.0336	0.0001	4.6588
	Normality	failed	failed	failed	passed	passed	passed	failed
	Constant Variance Test	passed	passed	passed	passed	passed	passed	failed
Langmuir	Ads$_{max}$ (±SE)	12.69 ± 0.93	13.02 ± 0.40	5.47 ± 0.28	4.90 ± 0.34	18.82 ± 1.49	0.26 ± 0.02	20.89 ± 1.20
	K$_L$ (±SE)	0.41 ± 0.05	1.05 ± 0.06	2.17 ± 0.18	2.91 ± 0.61	1.90 ± 0.21	1.30 ± 0.12	1.66 ± 0.35
	R^2	0.9966	0.9980	0.9938	0.9566	0.9970	0.9974	0.9754
	SS$_{res}$	0.2456	0.2394	0.0896	1.2691	0.2609	0.0001	43.4700
	S$_{y|x}$	0.1239	0.1223	0.0706	0.3011	0.1170	0.0019	1.5540
	PRESS	0.4548	0.3329	0.111	1.9306	0.2996	0.0001	50.6400
	Normality	passed	passed	passed	passed	passed	passed	passed
	Constant Variance Test	passed	passed	passed	passed	passed	passed	passed
Sips	q$_m$ (±SE)	-	11.67 ± 0.75	5.28 ± 0.73	-	-	-	91.70 ± 52.45
	A$_s$ (±SE)	-	1.35 ± 0.90	2.38 ± 0.81	-	-	-	0.15 ± 0.10
	1/n = nH (±SE)	-	1.08 ± 0.97	1.02 ± 0.08	-	-	-	0.37 ± 0.03
	R^2	-	0.9983	0.9938	-	-	-	0.9979
	SS$_{res}$	-	0.206	0.0892	-	-	-	3.8247
	S$_{y|x}$	-	0.1172	0.0724	-	-	-	0.4743
	PRESS	-	0.3403	0.1242	-	-	-	4.2181
	Normality	-	failed	passed	-	-	-	failed
	Constant Variance Test	-	passed	failed	-	-	-	failed

2.6. Multi-Mycotoxin Adsorption in Simulated Gastrointestinal Fluid

The aim of this study is to assess whether ATDP, acting as a wide spectrum mycotoxin adsorbent, shows the same adsorption pattern after simulated gastrointestinal digestion. In vitro digestion models are successfully used as tools for assessing the bioaccessibility of nutrients and non-nutrients or the digestibility of macronutrients (e.g., lipids, proteins, and carbohydrates) in food matrices. These methods mimic physiological conditions in the gastrointestinal tract, taking into account the presence of digestive enzymes and their concentrations, pH, digestion time, and salt concentration, among other factors. In vitro assessment of mycotoxin bioaccessibility has been done through a number of approaches including static and dynamic digestion models, simulating the gastro-intestinal tract of monogastric animals and humans [35–38]. In the current study, the standardized digestion model described by Minekus et al. [39], comprising oral, gastric and small intestinal digestion phases, was used to assess the ability of ATDP to reduce the fraction of mycotoxins in the chyme available for absorption. For this purpose, a pool of mycotoxins containing AFB_1, OTA, ZEA, and FB_1 was subjected to gastro-intestinal digestion processes in the presence/absence of ATDP and, subsequently, the liquid fraction of the chyme obtained by centrifugation was analyzed for residual mycotoxin content. Mycotoxin bioaccessibility, calculated after gastric or intestinal (complete) digestion, was defined as the ratio between the initial mycotoxin content and the amount determined in the chyme at the end of the digestion phases. Under our experimental conditions, mycotoxin bioaccessibility was in the range 96.5–33.5% after gastric digestion and 96.3–39.7% after intestinal digestion (Table 6). For the mycotoxins tested, bioaccessibility decreased in the following order: AFB_1 > FB_1 > OTA > ZEA. It is worthy to note that the low values of ZEA or OTA bioaccessibility after gastrointestinal digestion were probably due to the formation of aggregates in the complex environment of the gastrointestinal digestive fluids. For the mycotoxins tested here, bioaccessibility at gastric and intestinal levels did not differ substantially. Digestion of ATDP in the presence of mycotoxin significantly reduced the fraction of toxins available for absorption, at both gastric and intestinal levels. Due to the inclusion of ATDP, mycotoxin bioaccessibility ranged from 25.8% to 0.8% at the gastric level, and from 78.9% to 4.3% at the intestinal level. These preliminary results suggest that ATDP was more effective in sequestering mycotoxins under the physiological conditions present in the stomach when the pH was low. Gastric digestion of ATDP reduced mycotoxin bioaccessibility by $93.6 \pm 0.1\%$ for AFB_1, $97.6 \pm 0.1\%$ for ZEA, $96.2 \pm 1.0\%$ for OTA, and $67.3 \pm 3.7\%$ for FB_1. At the completion of digestion, including the gastric and intestinal digestion phases, the reduction of AFB_1 bioaccessibility by ATDP persisted ($95.1 \pm 0.1\%$). Smaller mycotoxin reductions were recorded at intestinal levels for ZEA ($68.9 \pm 1.1\%$), OTA ($10.1 \pm 2.6\%$), and FB_1 ($2.6 \pm 2.7\%$). Overall findings suggest that AFB_1, ZEA, OTA, and FB_1 are quickly and efficiently sequestered by ATDP in the stomach. During the transit of the chyme from the stomach to the intestine, AFB_1 and ZEA remained bound by ADTP, whereas some OTA and FB_1 were released. The change in pH of the gastrointestinal fluids occurring during digestion may be the main factor driving OTA and FB_1 release at the intestinal level. The model used in this study is a static one, and cannot simulate meal size, peristaltic movement, gastrointestinal transit, or absorption of digested products or water. However, it is a valid approach to investigating the adsorption/release of mycotoxins in a complex environment such as the stomach or the intestine.

Table 6. Percentages of AFB_1, ZEA, OTA, and FB_1 recovered in the gastrointestinal fluids after simulated gastric or gastro-intestinal digestion processes. Mycotoxins were digested in the absence (control) or presence of ATDP. Values are means ± standard deviations of five independent experiments.

Toxin	Bioaccessibility (%)				Bioaccessibility Reduction (%)	
	Gastric Phase		Intestinal Phase		Gastric Phase	Intestinal Phase
	Control	+ATDP	Control	+ATDP		
AFB_1	96.5 ± 0.9	6.3 ± 0.1	96.3 ± 0.8	4.3 ± 0.2	93.6 ± 0.1	95.1 ± 0.0
ZEA	33.5 ± 0.9	0.8 ± 0.1	39.7 ± 1.4	12.4 ± 0.4	97.6 ± 0.1	68.9 ± 1.1
OTA	49.6 ± 0.7	1.9 ± 0.5	43.6 ± 1.3	39.2 ± 1.1	96.2 ± 1.0	10.1 ± 2.6
FB_1	78.8 ± 1.9	25.8 ± 2.9	81.2 ± 2.9	78.9 ± 1.9	67.3 ± 3.7	2.6 ± 2.7

3. Conclusions

Several studies have shown agricultural by-products to be suitable precursor materials for the effective and suitable removal of contaminants from aqueous media, including mycotoxins. Unfortunately, most of these biomaterials are unsuitable for adsorption in their raw form and must be pre-treated to improve their innate adsorption capacities. These pre-treatments include physical processes (drying, autoclaving, grinding, milling, or sieving) and chemical modification with reagents. Physico-chemical modification can enhance adsorption by reducing particle size and increasing surface area. In the present study, chemical activation of DP by sulfuric acid significantly improved surface area for adsorption, pore size distribution, and total pore volume. Structural characterization showed more cavities to be present on the surface of the ATDP than the untreated material (DP). C and O were the major surface elements. In addition, acid treatment changed the functional groups and charge on the adsorbent surface. These structural changes may explain the higher efficacy of ATDP than pristine DP in adsorbing mycotoxins. This is the first time that DP has been evaluated for its efficacy in sequestering mycotoxins. ATDP was found to be more effective than other mycotoxin biosorbent materials in removing mycotoxins from liquid mediums: lactic acid bacteria, yeasts, molds, or other agricultural by-products. Biosorption of mycotoxins was investigated by batch adsorption. Adsorption isotherms indicated that the process is dependent on key operating parameters, including medium pH, adsorbent dose, and initial mycotoxin concentration. Maximum adsorption capacities were described by the Langmuir isotherm. Values of Q_{max} determined at pH 3 and pH 7 were 40.7 and 41.6 mmol kg^{-1} for AFB_1, 15.4 and 17.3 mmol/kg for ZEA, 46.6 and 0.6 mmol/kg for OTA, and 28.9 and 0.1 mmol/kg for FB_1. DON was not sequestered by the raw or pre-treated agricultural by-product. The pH of the medium significantly affected OTA and FB_1 adsorption, whereas AFB_1 and ZEA adsorptions were not pH-dependent. As a consequence, digestion of ATDP (at 0.5% w/v dosage) in the presence of a multi-mycotoxin solution containing 1 µg/mL of each toxin (AFB_1, OTA, ZEA, and FB_1) by a static, validated gastrointestinal model, significantly reduced the bioaccessibility of all mycotoxins (>67% reduction) at gastric level. After digestion was completed, including a gastric and an intestinal step, significant reductions in mycotoxin bioaccessibility were recorded for AFB_1 (94%) and ZEA (69%). These findings suggest that, during transit through the gastro-intestinal tract of a monogastric, most ingested AFB_1 and ZEA can be adsorbed by ATDP and excreted in feces. In contrast, FB_1 and OTA may be adsorbed in the stomach and released into the lumen of the intestine. Taking into account that most mycotoxins are quickly absorbed at the gastric level or in the upper part of the small intestine, the results of this study show the potential of ATDP as a multi-mycotoxin biosorbent. Further research is required to clarify the components of ATDP that are involved in the biosorption of mycotoxins and to confirm its efficacy in vivo.

4. Materials and Methods

4.1. Reagents and Samples

Solid mycotoxin standards (purity >98%), including aflatoxin B_1 (AFB_1), ochratoxin A (OTA), zearalenone (ZEA), deoxynivalenol (DON), and fumonisin B_1 (FB_1) were supplied by Sigma-Aldrich (Milan, Italy). All chemical reagents were purchased from Carlo Erba (Rouen, France), except for sodium chloride (NaCl) and potassium chloride (KCl), which were purchased from VWR (Leuven, Belgium). All solvents (HPLC grade) were purchased from J.T. Baker (Deventer, the Netherlands). Water was of Milli-Q quality (Millipore, Bedford, MA, USA). Digestive enzymes including α-amylase (from human saliva type IX-A, 1000–3000 U/mg), pepsin (from porcine gastric mucosa, 3200–4500 U/mg), pancreatin (from porcine pancreas, 4× USP), and bile bovine were supplied by Sigma-Aldrich (Milan, Italy). Mycotoxin adsorption studies were performed using different media (1 or 100 mmol/L) of different pH: citrate buffer at pH 3 (1 mM), acetate buffers at pH 4 and 5 (100 mM), and phosphate buffers at pH 6–9 (100 mM). Stock solutions of AFB_1, OTA, ZEA, and DON (1 mg/mL) were prepared by dissolving solid commercial toxins in acetonitrile. FB_1 was prepared in acetonitrile–water (50:50, v/v). Stock solutions were stored in the dark at 4 °C. A multi-mycotoxin stock solution containing 200 µg/mL of each toxin was prepared by mixing equal volumes of mycotoxin stock solutions. This was diluted with buffered solutions to prepare the mycotoxin working solutions for adsorption experiments. The Monthong durian peel (DP) used in the study was obtained from a local fruit shop in Bangkok, Thailand. The DP was washed with water to remove surface-adhered dirt and then cut into small pieces. These were oven-dried overnight, then, ground into fine powder using a mechanical grinder and passed through 35-mesh (0.5 mm) sieves. Particles smaller than 0.5 mm were collected and treated with sulfuric acid. The acid-treated material (ATDP) was heated overnight. It was then washed with distilled water to neutralize any acid residues and heated again. Untreated DP and ATDP, of the same particle size, were kept in a desiccator until use.

4.2. Physico-Chemical Characterization of DP and ATDP

The surface morphology and elementary composition of the DP and ATDP were investigated using scanning electron microscopy coupled with energy dispersive X-ray spectroscopy (SEM–EDS) (SU-5000, HITASHI, Tokyo, Japan). For identification of the chemical functional groups present on the DP and ATDP surfaces, a Fourier transform infrared spectroscopy (FTIR) (Nicolet 6700 FT-IR Spectrometer, Thermo Scientific, Waltham, MA, USA) analysis was performed in the spectral range from 4000 to 400 cm^{-1}. The particle size and surface charge were measured using mastersizer and zetasizer instruments (Nano ZS, Malvern, UK). Brunauer–Emmett–Teller (BET) specific surface area, pore size distribution, and total pore volume were obtained from N_2 adsorption–desorption isotherms using a surface area analyzer (Autosorb-1C, Quantachrome Corporation, Boynton Beach, FL, USA). Adsorption isotherms were obtained by measuring the amount of N_2 adsorbed to the surface of both biosorbents at 77.26 K. Desorption isotherms were derived by removing the N_2 adsorbed through a gradual pressure reduction. The methods used to characterize the DP and ATDP are reported elsewhere [25,40,41].

4.3. Multi-Mycotoxin Adsorption Experiments

DP and ATDP efficacy in adsorbing AFB_1, OTA, ZEA, DON, and FB_1 was evaluated at pH 3 and 7 using 1 mM citrate buffer and 100 mM phosphate buffer, respectively. Adsorption experiments were performed following the method of Avantaggiato et al. [26]. Briefly, DP and ATDP (< 500 µm particle size fraction) were weighed in a 4 mL silanized amber glass vial and suspended with an appropriate volume of multi-mycotoxin working solution buffered at pH 3 or 7. The suspensions were mixed for few seconds by vortex and then shaken for 90 min in a thermostatically-controlled shaker (KS 4000, IKA®-Werke GmbH & Co. KG, Staufen, Germany) at 37 °C and 250 rpm. After incubation, 1 mL of each suspension was transferred into an Eppendorf tube and centrifuged for 20 min at 18,000× g and 25 °C. Supernatant samples were analyzed for residual mycotoxin content following the HPLC and UPLC methods described by Avantaggiato et al. [26]. Adsorption experiments were carried out by adding 5 mg/mL of DP and ATDP to a multi-mycotoxin working solution comprising 1 µg/mL of each mycotoxin. To study the effect of pH on mycotoxin adsorption onto ATDP, independent experiments were performed in triplicate at pH values of 3–9, using a 5 mg/mL dosage (corresponding to 0.5% w/v). To investigate the desorption of mycotoxins from ATDP due to pH change, 5 mg of ATDP were dissolved with 1 mL of working solution at pH 3, containing 1 µg/mL of each toxin. Samples were incubated at 37 °C for 90 min in a rotary shaker (250 rpm). After centrifugation, the supernatants were completely removed and analyzed for residual mycotoxin content to calculate mycotoxin adsorption. The adsorbent pellets were washed with 1 mL of buffer at pH 7 and shaken for 30 min at 37 °C and 250 rpm. They were centrifuged, and the supernatants analyzed to assess mycotoxin desorption. This procedure was repeated by washing the pellet with 1 mL of methanol. Desorption studies were performed in triplicate. Adsorption (pH 3) and desorption (pH 7 and methanol) values were calculated for each toxin and expressed as percentages.

4.4. Equilibrium Adsorption Isotherms

Two sets of equilibrium adsorption isotherms were calculated to study the effect of adsorbent dosage and toxin concentration on simultaneous adsorption of AFB_1, OTA, ZEA, and FB_1. Due to the inefficacy of ATDP in adsorbing DON from all media used in the preliminary adsorption trials, DON was excluded from the study. In addition, since FB_1 was not adsorbed at pH 7, equilibrium adsorption isotherms for FB_1 were derived only at pH 3. Equilibrium adsorption isotherms matched to the experimental conditions (90 min equilibrium time, 37 °C, 250 rpm), as used for the preliminary adsorption experiments. The first set of adsorption isotherms was analyzed in triplicate, at constant pH 7, a fixed amount of toxin (1 µg/mL) with ATDP dosages ranging from 0.005–1% *w/v* (0.05–10 mg/mL) for AFB_1, 0.005–1% *w/v* (0.005–10 mg/mL) for ZEA, and 0.01–1% *w/v* (0.1–10 mg/mL) for OTA. Adsorption data were expressed as a percentage of mycotoxin adsorbed and plotted as a function of ATDP dosage. Mycotoxin adsorption plots were fitted using non-linear regression models. The second set of isotherms was derived by testing a fixed amount of ATDP with buffered solutions at toxin concentrations from 0.025–15 µg/mL. These isotherms were used to calculate the parameters related to the adsorption process, including maximum adsorption capacity (Ads_{max}) and affinity (K_L). Adsorbent dosages were set from the preliminary adsorption experiments, using a 0.05% *w/v* (0.5 mg/mL) adsorbent dosage for AFB_1, ZEA, and FB_1. A 0.02% *w/v* (0.2 mg/mL) and a 0.5% *w/v* (5 mg/mL) dosage were used for OTA adsorption at pH 3 and 7, respectively. Adsorption isotherms were obtained by plotting the amount of mycotoxin adsorbed per unit of mass of adsorbent (Q_{eq}) against the concentration of the toxin in the external phase (C_{eq}) under equilibrium conditions, then fitting using non-linear regression models.

4.5. Simulated Gastrointestinal Digestion

Since the gastrointestinal system is the primary target of mycotoxins, the "protective" effect of ATDP in reducing AFB_1, OTA, ZEA, and FB_1 bioaccessibility (i.e., the amount of mycotoxin that is released from the food matrix and is available for absorption through the gut wall) was determined by simulating a gastro-intestinal digestion process. In particular, mycotoxins in the presence or absence (negative controls) of ATDP were subjected to a simulated gastrointestinal digestion process and, subsequently, the digestive fluids obtained after gastric and/or intestinal digestion were analyzed for residual mycotoxin. The standardized digestion model described by Minekus et al. [39] was used in this study. This model describes a three-step procedure simulating digestive processes in the mouth, stomach, and small intestine (where most mycotoxin absorption takes place). A schematic representation of this model is presented in Figure 6. During simulated digestion, samples were rotated head-over-heels in a thermostatically controlled shaker (BFD53, ©BINDER-GmbH, Tuttlingen, Germany) at 37 °C for 2 min and 2 h to simulate, respectively, the oral phase and gastric or intestinal phases. Physiological and enzymatic solutions were prepared as described by Minekus et al. [39]. Simulated digestion started by mixing 5 mL of physiological solution, containing the multi-mycotoxin solution and ATDP at 5 mg/mL (0.5% *w/v*), with 3.5 mL of simulated salivary fluid (SSF). Next, 0.5 mL of salivary α-amylase SSF solution (1500 U/mL) was added, followed by 25 µL of $CaCl_2$ (0.3 M) and 975 µL of water, and thoroughly mixed. The simulated gastric and intestinal solutions were then added in sequence. After 2 min incubation, simulated gastric juice at pH 3 was added, followed by 7.5 mL of simulated gastric fluid (SGF), 1.6 mL of porcine pepsin SGF solution (25,000 U/mL), 5 µL of $CaCl_2$ (0.3 M), 0.2 mL of HCl (1 M), and 0.695 mL of water. After 2 h of simulated gastric digestion, intestinal fluids were added to the gastric chyme to mimic the digestion in the small intestine. Therefore, 20 mL of gastric chyme was mixed in sequence with 11 mL of simulated intestinal fluid (SIF), 5.0 mL of a pancreatin SIF solution (800 U/mL), 2.5 mL of bile (160 mM), 40 µL of $CaCl_2$ (0.3 M), 0.15 mL of NaOH (1 M), and 1.31 mL of water. Before starting intestinal digestion, the pH was adjusted to 7. Two independent sets of simulated digestion experiments were performed to measure mycotoxin bioaccessibility at gastric and intestinal levels. The first set of trials was stopped after the gastric digestion phase. The second set included the gastric and intestinal phases. All experiments, including negative controls (without ATDP), were performed in quintuplicate. At the completion of digestion, the gastric or intestinal fluids were centrifuged at 4500 rpm for 15 min and analyzed by HPLC/UHPLC for residual mycotoxin content. Prior to LC analyses of AFB_1, OTA, ZEA, and FB_1, supernatant samples were cleaned up using immunoaffinity (IMA) columns provided by VICAM© (Watertown, MA, USA): AflaTest© WB, OchraTest© WB, ZearalaTest© WB, and FumoniTest© WB. Briefly, IMA columns were attached to a vacuum manifold (Visiprep™ SPE, Sigma Aldrich, Milan, Italy). Then, 500 µL of sample supernatants were passed through the columns at a flow rate of approximately one drop per second. Each column was washed with 5 mL of phosphate saline buffer (PBS) followed by 5 mL of water. AFB_1, OTA, or ZEA were eluted by 2 mL of methanol in a 4 mL silanized amber vial. FB_1 was eluted using 2 mL of methanol followed by 2 mL of water. Eluates were dried at 50 °C under an air stream (nitrogen was used for FB_1) and the residues were re-dissolved with 250 µL of methanol/water (20:80, v/v), then vortexed for 1 min and injected into the LC systems. The LC analysis was performed following Greco et al. [16].

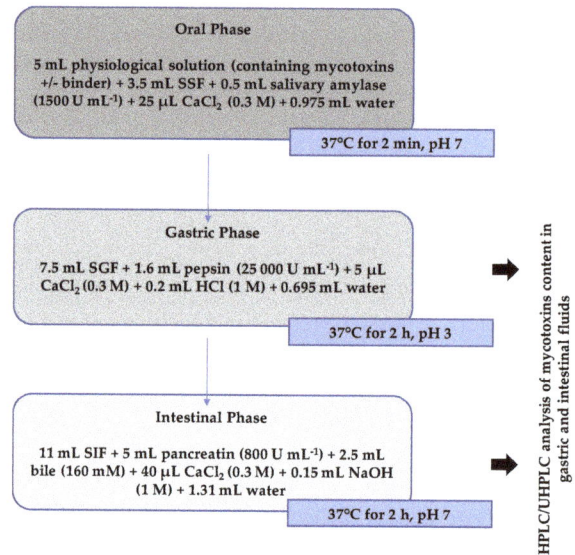

Figure 6. Flow diagram of the simulated digestion model proposed by Minekus et al. [39]. The model consists of a three-step procedure simulating the digestive processes in the mouth, stomach, and small intestine. SSF, SGF, and SIF stand for simulated salivary fluid, simulated gastric fluid, and simulated intestinal fluid, respectively

4.6. Data Calculation and Curve Fitting

Mycotoxin adsorption was measured from the difference between the amount of mycotoxin in the supernatant of the blank tubes and in the supernatant of the experimental tubes. The quantity present in the supernatant of the blank tubes was expressed as percentage of adsorption. ATDP was tested from two sets of equilibrium adsorption isotherms, using the methods reported by Avantaggiato et al. [26]. The first set of equilibrium adsorption isotherms was obtained by plotting the experimental adsorption data, expressed as percentage of mycotoxin adsorbed (Ads%), as a function of product dosage: Ads% = f (dosage). These data were transferred to SigmaPlot software (Systat.com, version 12.3) and fitted using the Langmuir isotherm model. The second set of adsorption isotherms was obtained by plotting the amount of mycotoxin adsorbed per unit of mass of product Q_{eq} against the concentration of the toxin in the external phase C_{eq}, under equilibrium conditions: $Q_{eq} = f(C_{eq})$. These data were transferred to SigmaPlot and fitted using different mathematical isotherm models (i.e., the Langmuir, Freundlich, and Sips models), as described by Avantaggiato et al. [26]. Mycotoxin bioaccessibility, expressed as a percentage, was calculated from the difference between the amount of mycotoxin found in the supernatant of gastric or intestinal fluid after each digestion process and the initial amount of toxin (mycotoxin intake). The efficacy of ATDP in reducing mycotoxin bioaccessibility was calculated as the difference between the bioaccessibility values measured after gastric or intestinal digestion of the control samples (with no ATDP) and experimental samples (containing the mycotoxin binder). Statistical analysis was performed by one-way analysis of variance (ANOVA) using the SigmaPlot software package. The Tukey–Kramer multiple-comparison post-hoc test was used, and differences were considered significant at $p < 0.05$.

Author Contributions: Conceptualization, S.A., A.P., D.G., V.D., G.A.; Methodology, S.A., A.P., D.G., V.D., W.V., G.A.; Software, S.A., D.G., V.D.; Validation, S.A., A.P., D.G., V.D., W.V., G.A.; Formal Analysis, S.A., A.P., D.G., V.D., W.V., G.A.; Investigation, S.A., D.G., V.D.; Resources, A.P., W.V., G.A.; Data Curation, S.A., D.G., V.D.; Writing—Original Draft Preparation, S.A., D.G., V.D.; Writing—Review & Editing, A.P., G.A.; Visualization, S.A., D.G., V.D.; Supervision, A.P., G.A.; Project Administration, A.P., G.A.; Funding Acquisition, A.P., G.A. All authors have read and agreed to the published version of the manuscript.

Funding: This research was funded by Thammasat University Research Fund, Contract No. TUIN 3/2562. The work was also supported by the MycoKey Project (European Union Horizon 2020, Research and Innovation Programme) under Grant Agreement No.678781.

Acknowledgments: The authors would like to thank the National Research Council, Institute of Sciences of Food Production (CNR-ISPA) and the National Center for Genetic Engineering and Biotechnology (BIOTEC), National Science and Technology Development Agency (NSTDA) for instrument support.

Conflicts of Interest: The authors declare no conflict of interest.

References

1. Zain, M.E. Impact of mycotoxins on humans and animals. *J. Saudi Chem. Soc.* **2011**, *15*, 129–144. [CrossRef]
2. Anfossi, L.; Giovannoli, C.; Baggiani, C. Mycotoxin detection. *Curr. Opin. Biotechnol.* **2016**, *37*, 120–126. [CrossRef] [PubMed]
3. Patriarca, A.; Pinto, V.F. Prevalence of mycotoxins in foods and decontamination. *Curr. Opin. Food Sci.* **2017**, *14*, 50–60. [CrossRef]
4. Freire, L.; Sant'Ana, A.S. Modified mycotoxins: An updated review on their formation, detection, occurrence, and toxic effects. *Food Chem. Toxicol.* **2018**, *111*, 189–205. [CrossRef] [PubMed]
5. Zaki, M.M.; El-Midany, S.A.; Shasheen, H.M.; Rizzi, L. Mycotoxins in animals: Occurrence, effects, prevention and management. *J. Toxicol. Environ. Health Sci.* **2012**, *4*, 13–28. [CrossRef]
6. Bennett, J.W.; Klich, M. Mycotoxins. *Clin. Microbiol. Rev.* **2003**, *16*, 497–516. [CrossRef]
7. Zinedine, A.; Soriano, J.M.; Moltó, J.C.; Mañes, J. Review on the toxicity, occurrence, metabolism, detoxification, regulations and intake of zearalenone: An oestrogenic mycotoxin. *Food Chem. Toxicol.* **2007**, *45*, 1–18. [CrossRef]
8. Wei, D.; Wang, Y.; Jiang, D.; Feng, X.; Li, J.; Wang, M. Survey of alternaria toxins and other mycotoxins in dried fruits in China. *Toxins* **2017**, *9*, 200. [CrossRef]
9. Grenier, B.; Oswald, I. Mycotoxin co-contamination of food and feed: Meta-analysis of publications describing toxicological interactions. *World Mycotoxin J.* **2011**, *4*, 285–313. [CrossRef]
10. Paterson, R.R. Toxicology of mycotoxins. *Exp. Suppl.* **2010**, *100*, 31–63.
11. Speijers, G.J.; Speijers, M.H. Combined toxic effects of mycotoxins. *Toxicol. Lett.* **2004**, *153*, 91–98. [CrossRef] [PubMed]
12. Huwig, A.; Freimund, S.; Käppeli, O.; Dutler, H. Mycotoxin detoxication of animal feed by different adsorbents. *Toxicol. Lett.* **2001**, *122*, 179–188. [CrossRef]
13. Kolosova, A.; Stroka, J. Substances for reduction of the contamination of feed by mycotoxins: A review. *World Mycotoxin J.* **2011**, *4*, 225–256. [CrossRef]
14. Pappas, A.C.; Tsiplakou, E.; Georgiadou, M.; Anagnostopoulos, C.; Markoglou, A.N.; Liapis, K.; Zervas, G. Bentonite binders in the presence of mycotoxins: Results of *in vitro* preliminary tests and an *in vivo* broiler trial. *Appl. Clay Sci.* **2014**, *99*, 48–53. [CrossRef]
15. Avantaggiato, G.; Solfrizzo, M.; Visconti, A. Recent advances on the use of adsorbent materials for detoxification of fusarium mycotoxins. *Food Addit. Contam.* **2005**, *22*, 379–388. [CrossRef]

16. Greco, D.; D'Ascanio, V.; Santovito, E.; Logrieco, A.F.; Avantaggiato, G. Comparative efficacy of agricultural by-products in sequestering mycotoxins. *J. Sci. Food Agric.* **2018**, *99*, 1623–1634. [CrossRef]
17. Li, Y.; Tian, G.; Dong, G.; Bai, S.; Han, X.; Liang, J.; Meng, J.; Zhang, H. Research progress on the raw and modified montmorillonites as adsorbents for mycotoxins: A review. *Appl. Clay Sci.* **2018**, *163*, 299–311. [CrossRef]
18. Dai, Y.; Sun, Q.; Wang, W.; Lu, L.; Liu, M.; Li, J.; Yang, S.; Sun, Y.; Zhang, K.; Xu, J.; et al. Utilizations of agricultural waste as adsorbent for the removal of contaminants: A review. *Chemosphere* **2018**, *211*, 235–253. [CrossRef]
19. Lazim, Z.M.; Hadibarata, T.; Puteh, M.H.; Yusop, Z. Adsorption characteristics of bisphenol A onto low-cost modified phyto-waste material in aqueous solution. *Water Air Soil Pollut.* **2015**, *226*, 34. [CrossRef]
20. Nuithitikul, K.; Srikhun, S.; Hirunpraditkoon, S. Influences of pyrolysis condition and acid treatment on properties of durian peel-based activated carbon. *Bioresour. Technol.* **2010**, *101*, 426–429. [CrossRef]
21. Charoenvai, S. Durian peels fiber and recycled HDPE composites obtained by extrusion. *Energy Procedia* **2014**, *56*, 539–546. [CrossRef]
22. Lazim, Z.M.; Hadibarata, T.; Puteh, M.H.; Yusop, Z.; Wirasnita, R.; Nor, N.M. Utilization of durian peel as potential adsorbent for biphenol A removal in aqoues solution. *J. Teknol.* **2015**, *74*, 109–115.
23. Mitan, N.M.M.; Ramlan, M.S.; Nawawi, M.Z.H.; Gazali, M.H.M. Performance of binders in briquetting of durian peel as a solid biofuel. *Mater. Today Proc.* **2018**, *5*, 21753–21758. [CrossRef]
24. Feng, N.; Guo, X.; Liang, S.; Zhu, Y.; Liu, J. Biosorption of heavy metals from aqueous solutions by chemically modified orange peel. *J. Hazard. Mater.* **2011**, *185*, 49–54. [CrossRef]
25. Ngabura, M.; Hussain, S.A.; Ghani, W.A.W.A.; Jami, M.S.; Tan, Y.P. Utilization of renewable durian peels for biosorption of zinc from wastewater. *J. Environ. Chem. Eng.* **2018**, *6*, 2528–2539. [CrossRef]
26. Avantaggiato, G.; Greco, D.; Damascelli, A.; Solfrizzo, M.; Visconti, A. Assessment of multi-mycotoxin adsorption efficacy of grape pomace. *J. Agric. Food Chem.* **2014**, *62*, 497–507. [CrossRef]
27. Foo, K.Y.; Hameed, B.H. Insights into the modeling of adsorption isotherm systems. *Chem. Eng. J.* **2010**, *156*, 2–10. [CrossRef]
28. Lemke, S.L.; Grant, P.G.; Phillips, T.D. Adsorption of zearalenone by organophilic montmorillonite clay. *J. Agric. Food Chem.* **1998**, *46*, 3789–3796. [CrossRef]
29. Niderkorn, V.; Morgavi, D.P.; Aboab, B.; Lemaire, M.; Boudra, V. Cell wall component and mycotoxin moieties involved in the binding of fumonisin B1 and B2 by lactic acid bacteria. *J. Appl. Microbiol.* **2009**, *106*, 977–985. [CrossRef]
30. Sangsila, A.; Faucet-Marquis, V.; Pfohl-Leszkowicz, A.; Itsaranuwat, P. Detoxification of zearalenone by *Lactobacillus pentosus* strains. *Food Control* **2016**, *62*, 187–192. [CrossRef]
31. Armando, M.R.; Pizzolitto, R.P.; Dogi, C.A.; Cristofolini, A.; Merkis, C.; Poloni, V.; Dalcero, A.M.; Cavaglieri, L.R. Adsorption of ochratoxin A and zearalenone by potential probiotic *Saccharomyces cerevisiae* strains and its relation with cell wall thickness. *J. Appl. Microbiol.* **2012**, *113*, 256–264. [CrossRef] [PubMed]
32. Bejaoui, H.; Mathieu, F.; Taillandier, P.; Lebrihi, A. Biodegradation of ochratoxin A by *Aspergillus* section Nigri species isolated from French grapes: A potential means of ochratoxin A decontamination in grape juices and musts. *FEMS Microbiol. Lett.* **2006**, *255*, 203–208. [CrossRef] [PubMed]
33. Solís-Cruz, B.; Hernández-Patlán, D.; Beyssac, E.; Latorre, J.D.; Hernandez-Velasco, X.; Merino-Guzman, R.; Tellez, G.; López-Arellano, R. Evaluation of chitosan and cellulosic polymers as binding adsorbent materials to prevent aflatoxin B1, fumonisin B1, ochratoxin, trichothecene, deoxynivalenol, and zearalenone mycotoxicoses through an *in vitro* gastrointestinal model for poultry. *Polymers* **2017**, *9*, 529. [CrossRef] [PubMed]
34. Vila-Donat, P.; Marín, S.; Sanchis, V.; Ramos, A.J. A review of the mycotoxin adsorbing agents, with an emphasis on their multi-binding capacity, for animal feed decontamination. *Food Chem. Toxicol.* **2018**, *114*, 246–259. [CrossRef]
35. Versantvoort, C.H.; Oomen, A.G.; Van de Kamp, E.; Rompelberg, C.J.; Sips, A.J. Applicability of an *in vitro* digestion model in assessing the bioaccessibility of mycotoxins from food. *Food Chem. Toxicol.* **2005**, *43*, 31–40. [CrossRef]
36. Avantaggiato, G.; Havenaar, R.; Visconti, A. Assessing the zearalenone-binding activity of adsorbent materials during passage through a dynamic in vitro gastrointestinal model. *Food Chem. Toxicol.* **2003**, *41*, 1283–1290. [CrossRef]

37. Avantaggiato, G.; Havenaar, R.; Visconti, A. Evaluation of the intestinal absorption of deoxynivalenol and nivalenol by an in vitro gastrointestinal model, and the binding efficacy of activated carbon and other adsorbent materials. *Food Chem. Toxicol.* **2004**, *42*, 817–824. [CrossRef]
38. Hur, S.J.; Beong, O.L.; Decker, E.A.; Mcclements, D.J. In vitro human digestion models for food applications. *Food Chem.* **2011**, *125*, 1–12. [CrossRef]
39. Minekus, M.; Alminger, M.; Alvito, P.; Balance, S.; Bohn, T.; Bourlieu, C.; Carrière, F.; Boutrou, R.; Corredig, M.; Dupont, D.; et al. A standardised static in vitro digestion method suitable for food—An international consensus. *Food Funct.* **2014**, *5*, 1113–1124. [CrossRef]
40. Cochrane, E.L.; Lu, S.; Gibb, S.W.; Villaescusa, I. A comparison of low-cost biosorbents and commercial sorbents for the removal of copper from aqueous media. *J. Hazard. Mater.* **2006**, *137*, 198–206. [CrossRef]
41. Ismail, A.; Sudrajat, H.; Jumbianti, D. Activated carbon from durian seed by H_3PO_4 activation: Preparation and pore structure characterization. *Indones. J. Chem.* **2010**, *10*, 36–40. [CrossRef]

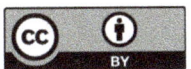

© 2020 by the authors. Licensee MDPI, Basel, Switzerland. This article is an open access article distributed under the terms and conditions of the Creative Commons Attribution (CC BY) license (http://creativecommons.org/licenses/by/4.0/).

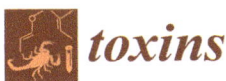

Article

DI/LC–MS/MS-Based Metabolome Analysis of Plasma Reveals the Effects of Sequestering Agents on the Metabolic Status of Dairy Cows Challenged with Aflatoxin B_1

Ibukun Ogunade [1,*], Yun Jiang [2] and Andres Pech Cervantes [3]

1. College of Agriculture, Communities, and the Environment, Kentucky State University, Frankfort, KY 40601, USA
2. Department of Animal Sciences, University of Florida, Gainesville, FL 32611, USA; ogunadeibukun@gmail.com
3. Agricultural Research Station, Fort Valley State University, Fort Valley, GA 31030, USA; xtiemira@gmail.com
* Correspondence: ibukun.ogunade@kysu.edu

Received: 4 November 2019; Accepted: 23 November 2019; Published: 26 November 2019

Abstract: The study applied a targeted metabolomics approach that uses a direct injection and tandem mass spectrometry (DI–MS/MS) coupled with a liquid chromatography–tandem mass spectrometry (LC–MS/MS)-based metabolomics of plasma to evaluate the effects of supplementing clay with or without *Saccharomyces cerevisiae* fermentation product (SCFP) on the metabolic status of dairy cows challenged with aflatoxin B_1. Eight healthy, lactating, multiparous Holstein cows in early lactation (64 ± 11 DIM) were randomly assigned to one of four treatments in a balanced 4 × 4 duplicated Latin square design with four 33 d periods. Treatments were control, toxin (T; 1725 µg aflatoxin B_1 (AFB$_1$)/head/day), T with clay (CL; 200 g/head/day), and CL with SCFP (YEA; 35 g of SCFP/head/day). Cows in T, CL, and YEA were dosed with aflatoxin B_1 (AFB$_1$) from days 26 to 30. The sequestering agents were top-dressed from day 1 to 33. On day 30 of each period, 15 mL of blood was taken from the coccygeal vessels and plasma samples were obtained from blood by centrifugation and analyzed for metabolites using a kit that combines DI–MS/MS with LC–MS/MS-based metabolomics. The data were analyzed using the GLIMMIX procedure of SAS. The model included the effects of treatment, period, and random effects of cow and square. Significance was declared at $p \leq 0.05$. Biomarker profiles for aflatoxin ingestion in dairy cows fed no sequestering agents were determined using receiver–operator characteristic (ROC) curves, as calculated by the ROCCET web server. A total of 127 metabolites such as amino acids, biogenic amines, acylcarnitines, glycerophospholipids, and organic acids were quantified. Compared with the control, T decreased ($p < 0.05$) plasma concentrations of alanine, leucine, and arginine and tended to decrease that of citrulline. Treatment with CL had no effects on any of the metabolites relative to the control but increased ($p \leq 0.05$) concentrations of alanine, leucine, arginine, and that of citrulline ($p = 0.07$) relative to T. Treatment with YEA resulted in greater ($p \leq 0.05$) concentrations of aspartic acid and lysine relative to the control and the highest ($p \leq 0.05$) plasma concentrations of alanine, valine, proline, threonine, leucine, isoleucine, glutamic acid, phenylalanine, and arginine compared with other treatments. The results of ROC analysis between C and T groups revealed that the combination of arginine, alanine, methylhistidine, and citrulline had sufficient specificity and sensitivity (area under the curve = 0.986) to be excellent potential biomarkers of aflatoxin ingestion in dairy cows fed no sequestering agents. This study confirmed the protective effects of sequestering agents in dairy cows challenged with aflatoxin B_1.

Keywords: aflatoxin; biomarker; dairy cows

Key Contribution: The combination of plasma arginine, alanine, methylhistidine, and citrulline had sufficient specificity and sensitivity to be excellent biomarkers of aflatoxin ingestion in dairy cows.

1. Introduction

Fungal spoilage of livestock feeds continues to be a major problem for feed security because of reduced palatability and loss of nutritive value [1,2]. Worse still, the affected commodity may be contaminated with toxic fungal secondary metabolites such as mycotoxins [3]. Aflatoxin B1 is the most studied among the fungal secondary metabolites because it is carcinogenic and poses a serious public health issue due to its transfer from diet to animal products such as milk, meat, and eggs [4,5]. Consequently, most studies have focused on the use of sequestering agents such as clay and Saccharomyces cerevisiae-based additives to counteract the negative effects of aflatoxin on performance and reduce its transfer to animal products [6]. Most of these studies have evaluated the effects of aflatoxins with or without sequestering agents on the metabolic status of ruminants using few biochemical parameters such as plasma liver enzymes and blood cell counts [6,7], which offer very little in terms of metabolic inferences [8]. A comprehensive analysis of the metabolic profile of animals to aflatoxin exposure is needed to reveal a robust metabolic inference and identify biomarkers of aflatoxin ingestion, which may allow early detection of aflatoxicosis, poisoning caused by ingesting aflatoxins, in livestock.

In recent years, metabolomics has been extensively used in basic and applied research to study metabolic processes and identify biomarkers responsible for metabolic characteristics [9]. Metabolomics can reveal the metabolic response of a biological system to several factors including stress, environmental alterations, and dietary change [10,11]. Previously, our group applied high-resolution proton nuclear magnetic resonance spectroscopy (1H NMR)-based metabolomics of plasma to identify plasma metabolites such as acetic acid, arginine, ethanol, alanine, methylhistidine, and proline as biomarkers of aflatoxin ingestion in dairy cows fed no sequestering agents [12]. However, liquid chromatography coupled to tandem mass spectrometry (LC–MS/MS) offers several advantages including high sensitivity and specificity and the potential to analyze disease-associated metabolic changes and quantify hundreds of metabolites in one run [13,14]. Thus, the objective of this study was to evaluate the effects of supplementing clay with or without *Saccharomyces cerevisiae* fermentation product (SCFP) on the plasma metabolomics profile of dairy cows challenged with aflatoxin B_1 using a combination of direct injection and tandem mass spectrometry (DI–MS/MS) with a reverse-phase LC–MS/MS.

2. Results and Discussions

A total number of 127 metabolites belonging to groups such as biogenic amines, acylcarnitines, amino acids, glycerophospholipids, monosaccharides, organic acids, and hexoses were identified and quantified (Table S1). The partial least squares discriminant analysis modelling (Figure 1) revealed slight separations between the control and each of T (toxin), CL (clay), and YEA (CL with SCFP) groups, indicating that the dietary treatment altered the plasma metabolome of the dairy cows.

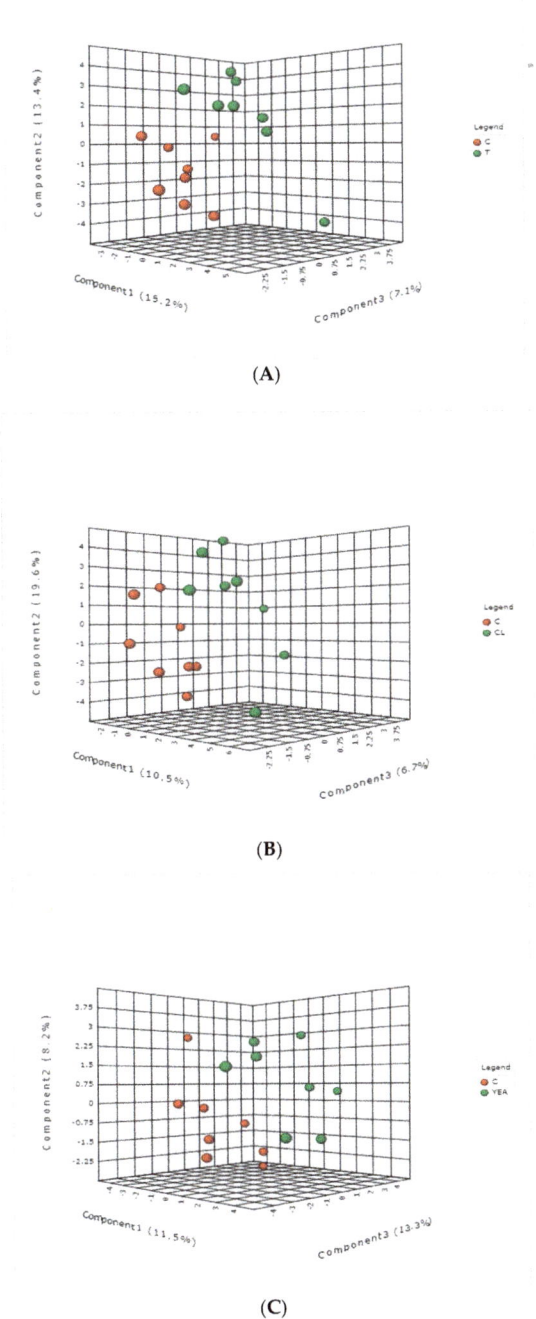

Figure 1. Partial least squares discriminant analysis score plots of (**A**) control vs. toxin groups, (**B**) control vs. clay groups, and (**C**) control vs. clay + *S. cerevisiae* fermentation product (YEA) groups.

The ranking of the metabolites by variable importance in projection (VIP) >1 showed that 40, 33, and 33 metabolites contributed to respective separations between control and each of T, CL, and YEA groups, respectively (Figure 2).

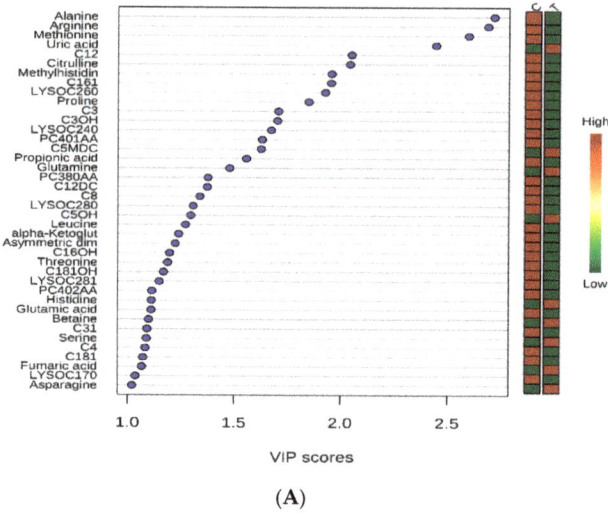

(A)

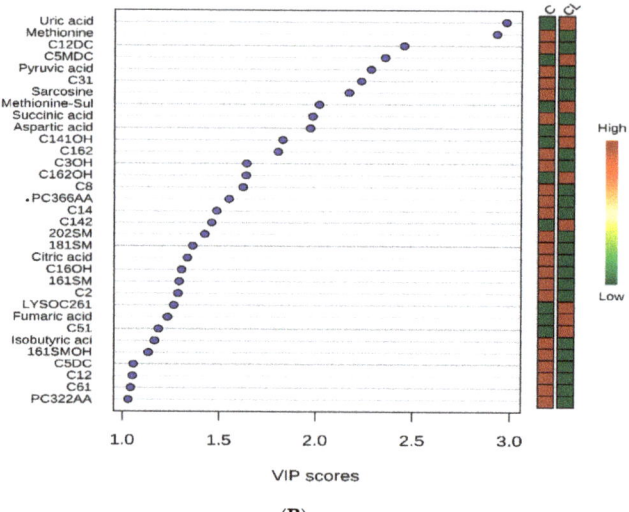

(B)

Figure 2. *Cont.*

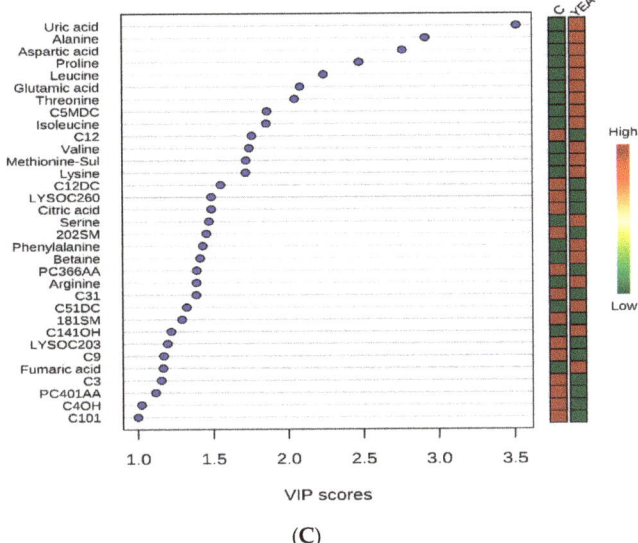

(C)

Figure 2. Variables ranked by variable importance in projection (VIP) between control and toxin groups (**A**), control and clay groups (**B**), and control and clay + *S. cerevisiae* fermentation product groups (**C**). Acylcarnitines: C12, C161, C3, C3OH, C12DC, C8, C5OH, C16OH, C18IOH, C31, C4, C181, C12DC, C5MDC, C31, C14IOH, C162, C3OH, C162OH, C8, C14, C142, C16OH, C2, C51, C5DC, C12, C61, C101, C4OH, C3, C9, C31, C12DC, C5MDC. Glycerophospholipids: LYSOC260, LYSOC240, PC401AA, LYSOC280, LYSOC281, PC402AA, LYSOC170, 202SM, 181SM, 161SM, LYSOC261, 161SMOH, PC322AA, PC401AA, LYSOC203.

When the metabolites with VIP >1 were statistically analyzed based on the design of this experiment, the concentrations of 13 metabolites were affected by dietary treatment. Relative to the control, T diet decreased ($p < 0.05$) the plasma concentrations of alanine, leucine, and arginine and tended to decrease ($p = 0.07$) that of citrulline (Table 1). These results agree with our earlier study that showed a similar trend using 1H-NMR [12]. This study also agrees with a recent study that reported reduced concentrations of some amino acids such as leucine, isoleucine, valine, and phenylalanine in dairy cows exposed to 40 µg/kg aflatoxin B_1 (AFB1) for 7 days [8].

Aflatoxins are known to impair protein formation by interfering with enzymes and substrates required for processes such as initiation, transcription, and translation that are involved in protein synthesis [15]. Pate et al. [16] reported reduced expression of mechanistic target of rapamycin (mTOR), a major regulator of protein synthesis in the tissues of mammals [17], in the liver of dairy cows fed 100 µg of AFB1/kg of dietary DMI for 3 days. This is probably a consequence of reduced plasma concentrations of leucine, which is known to activate the mTOR signaling pathway [18]. Mechanistic target of rapamycin plays a major role in regulating innate and adaptive immune responses in animals and humans because antibodies, interferons, and other immune cells are made up of proteins [18]. Arginine and its precursor, citrulline, play a vital role in regulating immune response during inflammatory stress because arginine serves as a sole precursor for synthesis of immune modulators such as polyamines, proline, and agmatine [19]. Taken together, this explains observed immunosuppression in animals exposed to AFB_1 in several studies [20,21]. Alanine is the major glucogenic amino acid vital for glucose metabolism in ruminants [22]. However, reduced concentration of alanine observed in this study is not an evidence that carbohydrate metabolism was affected by AFB_1 because plasma pyruvate and glucose concentrations were not affected. It is important to note that the concentration of AFB1 dosed (75 µg/kg) in this study exceeded that of the FDA action level in the feeds of dairy cattle (20 µg/kg).

However, it represents a typical natural level of AFB1 in corn samples [23] and is within the range (20–100 µg/kg) used in previous studies [7,24].

Table 1. The concentrations (µM) of plasma metabolites that were affected in dairy cows fed aflatoxin B_1 with or without clay and SCFP [1]-based sequestering agents.

Item	Treatment [2]				SEM	*p*-Value
	Control	T	CL	YEA		
Alanine	337 [b]	284 [c]	334 [b]	462 [a]	18.1	0.01
Valine	331 [y]	312 [y]	325 [y]	387 [x]	14.5	0.06
Proline	143 [b]	127 [b]	137 [b]	194 [a]	7.47	0.01
Threonine	152 [b]	136 [b]	140 [b]	172 [a]	7.82	0.01
Leucine	281 [b]	227 [b]	284 [b]	362 [a]	14.2	0.01
Isoleucine	129 [b]	131 [b]	128 [b]	148 [a]	6.30	0.03
Aspartic acid	23.5 [y]	26.9 [xy]	29.5 [xy]	43.5 [x]	5.62	0.09
Glutamic acid	236 [b]	219 [b]	206 [b]	305 [a]	9.95	0.01
Arginine	128 [b]	96 [c]	131 [b]	159 [a]	10.4	0.02
Phenylalanine	68.4 [b]	71.1 [b]	69.4 [b]	83.1 [a]	4.37	0.05
Citrulline	73.6 [xy]	62.6 [y]	81.0 [x]	71.6 [xy]	4.81	0.07
Sarcosine	1.83 [xy]	1.74 [xy]	1.50 [y]	1.95 [x]	0.12	0.06
Lysine	159 [b]	173 [ab]	170 [ab]	194 [a]	9.05	0.05

[1] *Saccharomyces cerevisiae* fermentation product–based sequestering agent (Diamond V, Cedar Rapids, IA), [2] T = control diet + aflatoxin B_1 (AFB1, 1725 µg/d); CL = T + 200 g/d of sodium bentonite clay; YEA = CL + 35 g/d of *Saccharomyces cerevisiae* fermentation product (SCFP). [a,b,c] Within a row, treatment means with different superscripts differ ($p \leq 0.05$). [x,y] Within a row, treatment means with different superscripts tend to differ, $0.05 < p \leq 0.10$.

The results of receiver–operator characteristic (ROC) analysis between C and T groups revealed five metabolites (arginine, alanine, methylhistidine, citrulline, and proline) with respective areas under the curve (AUC) of 0.88, 0.86, 0.86, 0.81, and 0.80. The utility of a biomarker is considered excellent at AUC = 0.9–1.0 and good at AUC = 0.8–0.9 [25]. Our previous study that applied 1H-NMR-based analysis revealed plasma acetic acid, arginine, ethanol, alanine, methylhistidine, and proline with AUC > 0.80 [12]; these results are similar except for ethanol and acetic acid, which were not quantified using DI/LC–MS/MS, and citrulline, which was not quantified in our previous study. This is an evidence that these metabolites, including ethanol and acetic acid reported in our companion paper, are good biomarkers of aflatoxin ingestion in dairy cows fed no sequestering agents. The combination of plasma concentrations of arginine and alanine gave a better ROC ability (AUC = 0.914; Figure 3a) compared with individual metabolites, whereas the combination of four metabolites (arginine, alanine, methylhistidine, and citrulline) with AUC = 0.986 was an excellent biomarker of aflatoxin ingestion in dairy cows fed no sequestering agents (Figure 3b). It is interesting to know that the use of multiple metabolites (arginine, alanine, methylhistidine, and citrulline) gave a better sensitivity and specificity to serve as potential biomarkers of aflatoxin ingestion in dairy cows fed no sequestering agents because it is likely that no single biomarker, as reported in our previous study using ^{1}H-NMR, will accurately predict a disease condition. However, the optimum range of plasma concentrations of these metabolites in healthy lactating dairy cows has to be established across different feeding regimens for them to be useful as biomarkers of aflatoxin ingestion.

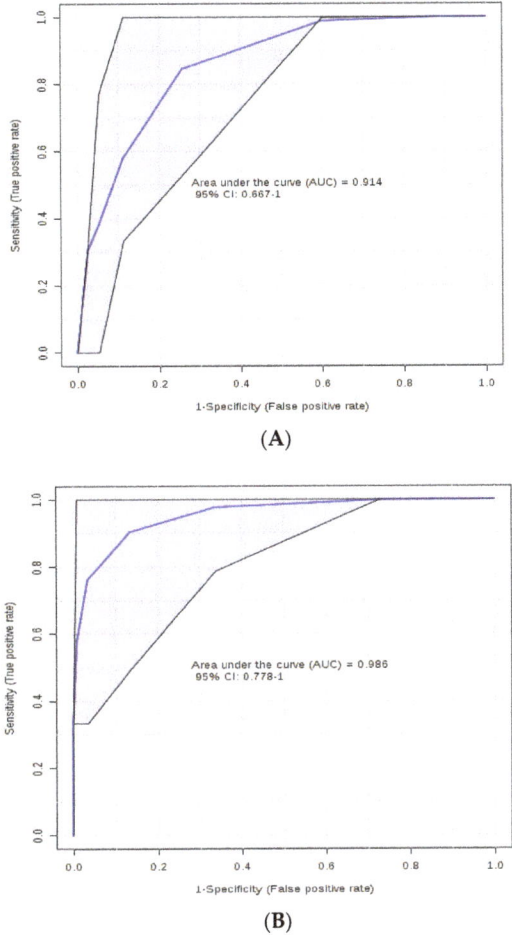

Figure 3. Receiver–operator characteristic curves of control vs. aflatoxin groups for (**A**) arginine and alanine and (**B**) arginine, alanine, methylhistidine, and citrulline.

Dietary treatment with CL had no effects on any of the metabolites relative to the control, but increased ($p < 0.05$) concentrations of alanine, leucine, and arginine, and tended to increase ($p = 0.07$) that of citrulline relative to T. This indicates that dietary supplementation of clay prevented the negative effects of AFB1. The gastrointestinal tract (GIT) is the major route for entry of aflatoxins into the bloodstream, where they are distributed to various tissues and liver. Clay is effective at ameliorating the negative effects of aflatoxins on the health and performance of animals by binding with aflatoxin in the GIT, thereby, preventing it from being absorbed and getting to the liver, where it causes increased stress of the liver cells due to toxic load [26]. Several studies have reported that clay supplementation reduced transfer of aflatoxins into animal products, improving liver health and immune response in animals exposed to aflatoxin [6,16].

Dietary treatment with YEA resulted in higher concentrations of aspartic acid (0.09) and lysine ($p = 0.05$) relative to the control, and the highest plasma concentrations of alanine, valine, proline, threonine, leucine, isoleucine, glutamic acid, phenylalanine, and arginine compared with other treatments. This confirms that feeding SCFP with clay is better than clay alone at improving the health and metabolic status of dairy cows exposed to aflatoxins. This explains the results of our companion paper [6] that reported that dietary supplementation of clay and SCFP was more effective than clay alone at maintaining the milk yield of dairy cows during aflatoxin challenge. Several studies have shown that dietary supplementation with SCFP has the potential to optimize the health and performance of cattle, especially during inflammatory stress. However, the effectiveness of SCFP at augmenting inflammatory stress response to aflatoxin exposure has been inconsistent [4]. It is possible that observed effects of YEA in this study are due to the synergistic effects of clay and SCFP. Clay supplementation plays the role of adsorbing aflatoxins in the gut, thereby allowing maximal effects of SCFP at improving the nutritional status of the cows. This explains the increased milk production by cows fed YEA relative to T in our companion study [6]. Supplementation of SCFP has been shown to improve gut health by stabilizing rumen pH and increasing microbial N yield; resulting in increased flow and quality of amino acids to the duodenum for intestinal absorption [27,28]. In addition, the SCFP used in this study is fortified with nutritional metabolites such as amino acids, B vitamins, nucleotides, lipids, and organic acids that may have contributed to improved metabolic status of dairy cows in this study [29].

In summary, this study gives a comprehensive insight into plasma metabolomics profile in response to aflatoxin challenge with or without sequestering agents. Aflatoxin challenge reduced plasma concentrations of some amino acids. Clay supplementation prevented the effects of AFB1, while supplementation of both clay and SCFP improved the metabolic status of the cows during aflatoxin exposure. The combination of arginine, alanine, citrulline, and leucine had sufficient sensitivity and specificity to serve as candidate biomarkers of aflatoxin ingestion in dairy cows fed no sequestering agents.

3. Materials and Methods

This study was part of a larger project designed to evaluate the effects of supplementing clay with or without SCFP on health and performance of dairy cows challenged with AFB1 [6]. The University of Florida Institutional Animal Care and Use Committee approved all experimental procedures used in this study. Details about cows and feeding have been reported previously [6,12]. Briefly, eight lactating multiparous Holstein cows (64 ± 11 days in milk) were randomly assigned to one of four treatment sequences in a balanced 4 × 4 Latin square design with two replicate squares, four 33 day periods, and a 5 day washout interval between periods. Treatments were (1) control (diet with no additives), (2) toxin (T; basal diet + 1725 µg of AFB1/head per day), (3) toxin with bentonite clay (CL; 200 g/head per day; Astra-Ben-20, Prince Agri Products Inc., Quincy, IL, USA), and (4) CL plus SCFP (YEA; 35 g of SCFP/head per day; Diamond V, Cedar Rapids, IA, USA). The basal diet was formulated and fed as a total mixed ration (TMR), to meet the nutrient requirements of dairy cows producing 30 kg/d or more of milk [30]. The basal diet contained 55.6% concentrate mix, 36.1% corn silage, and 8.3% alfalfa hay on a dry matter basis. Oral dose of 1725 µg of AFB1 was administered to each cow in treatments T, CL, and YEA from days 26 to 30 before the morning feeding to give a dietary concentration of 75 µg/kg based on estimated daily DMI of 23 kg/d. The sequestering agents were top-dressed on the respective TMR from days 1 to 33 of each period. Blood samples (15 mL) were obtained from the coccygeal vessels into vacutainer tubes containing sodium heparin anticoagulant before the morning feeding on day 30 of each experimental period. Plasma samples were prepared from the blood by centrifugation at 2500× g for 20 min at 4 °C, initially stored at −20 °C and then at −80 °C until LC-MS/MS analysis was done.

Plasma samples (20 µL) were analyzed using a commercial kit that uses direct injection and tandem mass spectrometry (DI–MS/MS) coupled with a reverse-phase liquid chromatography and tandem mass spectrometry (LC–MS/MS). The kit assay (AbsoluteIDQ p180; Biocrates Life Sci., Innsbruck, Austria), used with an ABI 4000 Q-Trap mass spectrometer (Applied Biosystems/MDS Sciex, Foster City, CA, USA), enables the quantification of 145 metabolites in as little of 10 µL of biofluid. Detailed information and description of the method has been reported elsewhere [14,31]. Mass spectrometric analysis was performed using an API4000 Qtrap® tandem mass spectrometry instrument (Applied Biosystems/MDS Analytical Technologies, Foster City, CA, USA) that is equipped with a solvent delivery system. Delivery of the samples to the mass spectrometer was done using an LC method, followed by a DI method.

4. Data and Statistical Analysis

Metabolite data were subjected to multivariate analysis using Metaboanalyst 4.0 software (www.metaboanalyst.ca) [24]. Prior to multivariate analysis, data were log-transformed and pareto-scaled. Partial least squares discriminant analysis (PLS-DA) was used to visualize differences between the control group and each of T, CL, and YEA groups. Based on the PLS-DA model, the metabolites that were important in discriminating cows in T, CL, and YEA from control group were ranked using variable importance in projection (VIP). Metabolites with VIP values ≥1 were considered powerful group discriminators [32]. Metabolites with VIP values ≥1 were analyzed using the GLIMMIX procedure of SAS version 9.4 (SAS Institute Inc., Cary, NC, USA, 2013). The model used for the analysis included the fixed effects of treatment, period, and random effects of cow and square, and their interactions. Significance was declared at $p \leq 0.05$, and tendency was declared at $0.10 \geq p > 0.05$. Biomarker profiles for aflatoxin ingestion in dairy cows fed no sequestering agents were determined using receiver–operator characteristic (ROC) curves, as calculated by the ROCCET web server [25]. Area under the curve (AUC), a value that combines sensitivity and specificity for a diagnostic test, was used to evaluate the utility of the biomarkers [25].

Supplementary Materials: The following are available online at http://www.mdpi.com/2072-6651/11/12/693/s1, Table S1: Average concentrations (μm) of the identified metabolites.

Author Contributions: Conceptualization, I.O.; investigation, Y.J., I.O. and A.P.C.; writing—original draft preparation, I.O..; writing—review and editing, I.O.

Funding: We gratefully acknowledge Diamond V Inc. (Cedar Rapids, IA) for funding the animal experiment. Cost of plasma metabolomics analysis was supported by funds from the US Department of Agriculture's National Institute of Food and Agriculture Evans-Allen project.

Conflicts of Interest: The authors declare no conflict of interest.

References

1. Gallo, A.; Giuberti, G.; Frisvad, J.C.; Bertuzzi, T.; Nielsen, K.F. Review on mycotoxin issues in ruminants: Occurrence in forages, effects of mycotoxin ingestion on health status and animal performance and ractical strategies to counteract their negative effects. *Toxins* **2015**, *7*, 3057–3111. [CrossRef] [PubMed]
2. Abdallah, M.F.; Girgin, G.; Baydar, T.; Krska, R.; Sulyok, M. Occurrence of multiple mycotoxins and other fungal metabolites in animal feed and maize samples from Egypt using LC-MS/MS. *J. Sci. Food Agric.* **2017**, *97*, 4419–4428. [CrossRef] [PubMed]
3. Richard, E.; Heutte, N.; Bouchart, V.; Garon, D. Evaluation of fungal contamination and mycotoxin production in maize silage. *Anim. Feed Sci. Technol.* **2009**, *148*, 309–320. [CrossRef]
4. Ogunade, I.M.; Arriola, K.G.; Jiang, Y.; Driver, J.P.; Staples, C.R.; Adesogan, A.T. Effects of 3 sequestering agents on milk aflatoxin M_1 concentration and the performance and immune status of dairy cows fed diets artificially contaminated with aflatoxin B_1. *J. Dairy Sci.* **2016**, *99*, 6263–6273. [CrossRef] [PubMed]
5. Herzallah, S.M. Determination of aflatoxins in eggs, milk, meat and meat products using HPLC fluorescent and UV detectors. *Food Chem.* **2009**, *114*, 1141–1146. [CrossRef]
6. Jiang, Y.; Ogunade, I.M.; Kim, D.H.; Li, X.; Pech-Cervantes, A.A.; Arriola, K.G.; Oliveira, A.S.; Driver, J.P.; Ferraretto, L.F.; Staples, C.R.; et al. Effect of sequestering agents based on a *Saccharomyces cerevisiae* fermentation product and clay on the health and performance of lactating dairy cows challenged with dietary aflatoxin B1. *J. Dairy Sci.* **2018**, *101*, 3008–3020. [CrossRef]
7. Xiong, J.L.; Wang, Y.M.; Nennich, Y.M.; Li, Y.; Liu, J.X. Transfer of dietary aflatoxin B1 to milk aflatoxin M1 and effect of inclusion of adsorbent in the diet of dairy cows. *J. Dairy Sci.* **2015**, *98*, 2545–2554. [CrossRef]
8. Wang, Q.; Zhang, Y.; Zheng, N.; Guo, L.; Song, X.; Zhao, S.; Wang, J. Biological system responses of dairy cows to aflatoxin B1 exposure revealed with metabolomic changes in multiple biofluids. *Toxins* **2019**, *11*, 77. [CrossRef]

9. Peng, B.; Li, H.; Peng, X.X. Functional metabolomics: from biomarker discovery to metabolome reprogramming. *Protein Cell* **2015**, *6*, 628–637. [CrossRef]
10. Patel, S.; Ahmed, S. Emerging field of metabolomics: big promise for cancer biomarker identification and drug discovery. *J. Pharm. Biomed. Anal.* **2015**, *107*, 63–74. [CrossRef]
11. Gibbons, H.; O'Gorman, A.; Brennan, L. Metabolomics as a tool in nutritional research. *Curr. Opin. Lipidol.* **2015**, *26*, 30–34. [CrossRef] [PubMed]
12. Ogunade, I.; Jiang, M.; Adeyemi, J.A.; Oliveira, A.; Vyas, D.; Adesogan, A.T. Biomarker of Aflatoxin Ingestion: 1H NMR-Based Plasma Metabolomics of Dairy Cows Fed Aflatoxin B1 with or without Sequestering Agents. *Toxins* **2018**, *10*, 545. [CrossRef] [PubMed]
13. Veenstra, T.D. Metabolomics: the final frontier? *Genome Med.* **2012**, *4*, 40. [CrossRef] [PubMed]
14. Zhang, G.; Dervishi, E.; Dunn, S.M.; Mandal, R.; Liu, P.; Han, B.; Wishart, D.S.; Ametaj, B.N. Metabotyping reveals distinct metabolic alterations in ketotic cows and identifies early predictive serum biomarkers for the risk of disease. *Metabolomics* **2017**, *13*, 43. [CrossRef]
15. Garvican, L.; Cajone, F.; Rees, K.R. The mechanism of action of aflatoxin B1 on protein synthesis; Observations on malignant, viral transformed and untransformed cells in culture. *Chem. Biol. Interact.* **1973**, *7*, 39–50. [CrossRef]
16. Pate, R.T.; Paulus Compart, D.M.; Cardoso, F.C. Aluminosilicate clay improves production responses and reduces inflammation during an aflatoxin challenge in lactating Holstein cows. *J. Dairy Sci.* **2018**, *101*, 11421–11434. [CrossRef]
17. Doelman, J.; Kim, J.J.M.; Carson, M.; Metcalf, J.A.; Cant, J.P. Branched chain amino acid and lysine deficiencies exert different effects on mammary translational regulation. *J. Dairy Sci.* **2015**, *98*, 7846–7855. [CrossRef]
18. Powell, J.D.; Pollizzi, K.N.; Heikamp, E.B.; Horton, M.R. Regulation of immune responses by mTOR. *Ann. Rev. Immunol.* **2012**, *30*, 39. [CrossRef]
19. Zhao, F.; Wu, T.; Zhang, H.; Loor, J.J.; Wang, M.; Peng, A.; Wang, H. Jugular infusion of arginine has a positive effect on antioxidant mechanisms in lactating dairy cows challenged intravenously with lipopolysaccharide. *J. Anim. Sci.* **2018**, *96*, 3850–3855. [CrossRef]
20. Queiroz, O.C.M.; Han, J.H.; Staples, C.R.; Adesogan, A.T. Effect of adding a mycotoxin-sequestering agent on milk aflatoxin M1 concentration and the performance and immune response of dairy cattle fed an aflatoxin B1-contaminated diet. *J. Dairy Sci.* **2012**, *95*, 5901–5908. [CrossRef]
21. Chaytor, A.C.; See, M.T.; Hansen, J.A.; de Souza, A.L.; Middleton, T.F.; Kim, S.W. Effects of chronic exposure of diets with reduced concentrations of aflatoxin and deoxynivalenol on growth and immune status of pigs. *J. Anim. Sci.* **2011**, *89*, 124–135. [CrossRef] [PubMed]
22. Reynolds, C.K. Glucose balance in cattle. Florida Ruminant Nutrition Symposium. Available online: http://dairy.ifas.ufl.edu/rns/2005/ReynoldAccessedonline:s.pdf (accessed on 14 November 2005).
23. Pietri, A.; Bertuzzi, T.; Pallaroni, L.; Piva, G. Occurrence of mycotoxins and ergosterol in maize harvested over 5 years in Northern Italy. *Food Addit. Contam.* **2004**, *21*, 479–487. [CrossRef] [PubMed]
24. Pantaya, D.; Morgavi, D.P.; Silberberg, M.; Chaucheyras-Durand, F.; Martin, C.; Wiryawan, K.G.; Boudra, H. Bioavailability of aflatoxin B1 and ochratoxin A, but not fumonisin B1 or deoxynivalenol, is increased in starch-induced low ruminal pH in nonlactating dairy cows. *J. Dairy Sci.* **2016**, *99*, 9759–9767. [PubMed]
25. Xia, J.; Wishart, D.S. Using metaboAnalyst 3.0 for comprehensive metabolomics data analysis. *Curr. Prot. Bioinform.* **2016**, *55*, 10–14. [CrossRef] [PubMed]
26. Guo, J.; Chang, G.; Zhang, K.; Xu, L.; Jin, D.; Bilal, M.S.; Shen, X. Rumen-derived lipopolysaccharide provoked inflammatory injury in the liver of dairy cows fed a high-concentrate diet. *Oncotarget* **2017**, *8*, 46769–46780. [CrossRef]
27. Erasmus, L.J.; Botha, P.M.; Kistner, A. Effect of yeast culture supplement on production, rumen fermentation, and duodenal nitrogen flow in dairy cows. *J. Dairy Sci.* **1992**, *75*, 3056–3065. [CrossRef]
28. Bach, A.; Iglesias, C.; Devant, M. Daily rumen pH pattern of loose-housed dairy cattle as affected by feeding pattern and live yeast supplementation. *Anim. Feed Sci. Technol.* **2007**, *136*, 146–153. [CrossRef]
29. Callaway, E.S.; Martin, S.A. Effects of a Saccharomyces cerevisiae culture on ruminal bacteria that utilize lactate and digest cellulose. *J. Dairy Sci.* **1997**, *80*, 2035–2044. [CrossRef]
30. NRC. *Nutrient Requirements of Dairy Cattle*, 7th ed.; National Academies Press: Washington, DC, USA, 2001.

31. Walsh, B.H.; Broadhurst, D.I.; Mandal, R.; Wishart, D.S.; Boylan, G.B.; Kenny, L.C.; Murray, D.M. The metabolomic Profile of umbilical cord blood in neonatal hypoxic ischaemic encephalopathy. *PLoS ONE* **2012**, *7*, e50520. [CrossRef]
32. Hailemariam, D.; Zhang, G.; Mandal, R.; Wishart, D.S.; Ametaj, B.N. Identification of serum metabolites associated with the risk of metritis in transition dairy cows. *Can. J. Anim. Sci.* **2018**, *98*, 525–537. [CrossRef]

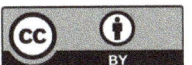

© 2019 by the authors. Licensee MDPI, Basel, Switzerland. This article is an open access article distributed under the terms and conditions of the Creative Commons Attribution (CC BY) license (http://creativecommons.org/licenses/by/4.0/).

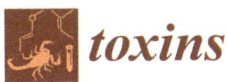 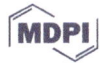

Article

Comparative In Vitro Assessment of a Range of Commercial Feed Additives with Multiple Mycotoxin Binding Claims

Oluwatobi Kolawole [1], Julie Meneely [1], Brett Greer [1], Olivier Chevallier [1], David S. Jones [2], Lisa Connolly [1] and Christopher Elliott [1,*]

[1] Institute for Global Food Security, Queens University Belfast, Belfast BT9 5DL, UK; okolawole01@qub.ac.uk (O.K.); j.p.meneely@qub.ac.uk (J.M.); brett.greer@qub.ac.uk (B.G.); o.chevallier@qub.ac.uk (O.C.); l.connolly@qub.ac.uk (L.C.)
[2] School of Pharmacy, Queens University Belfast, Belfast BT9 7BL, UK; D.Jones@qub.ac.uk
* Correspondence: chris.elliott@qub.ac.uk

Received: 20 October 2019; Accepted: 7 November 2019; Published: 12 November 2019

Abstract: Contamination of animal feed with multiple mycotoxins is an ongoing and growing issue, as over 60% of cereal crops worldwide have been shown to be contaminated with mycotoxins. The present study was carried out to assess the efficacy of commercial feed additives sold with multi-mycotoxin binding claims. Ten feed additives were obtained and categorised into three groups based on their main composition. Their capacity to simultaneously adsorb deoxynivalenol (DON), zearalenone (ZEN), fumonisin B1 (FB1), ochratoxin A (OTA), aflatoxin B1 (AFB1) and T-2 toxin was assessed and compared using an in vitro model designed to simulate the gastrointestinal tract of a monogastric animal. Results showed that only one product (a modified yeast cell wall) effectively adsorbed more than 50% of DON, ZEN, FB1, OTA, T-2 and AFB1, in the following order: AFB1 > ZEN > T-2 > DON > OTA > FB1. The remaining products were able to moderately bind AFB1 (44–58%) but had less, or in some cases, no effect on ZEN, FB1, OTA and T-2 binding (<35%). It is important for companies producing mycotoxin binders that their products undergo rigorous trials under the conditions which best mimic the environment that they must be active in. Claims on the binding efficiency should only be made when such data has been generated.

Keywords: mycotoxins; animal feed; mycotoxin binders; feed safety

Key Contribution: Only one out of ten commercial mycotoxin binders simultaneously adsorbed more than 50% of Aflatoxin B1, Deoxynivalenol, Zearalenone, Fumonisins B1, Ochratoxin A and T-2 in an in vitro model designed to mimic the gastrointestinal tract of a monogastric animal.

---

1. Introduction

Mycotoxins are toxic, low-molecular weight compounds produced as secondary metabolites by several fungi species belonging mainly to *Aspergillus, Fusarium, Penicillum, Alternaria* and *Clavicep* genera [1]. Under favourable environmental conditions such as moisture and temperature, these fungi can invade crops and proliferate (during growth, transportation and storage) to produce mycotoxins [2]. Other factors including climate change, poor harvesting practices, improper drying, handling and packaging may also predispose crops to fungal invasion and subsequent mycotoxin production [3]. Mycotoxins appear in the food and feed chain because forages and cereals, which are most susceptible crops to these fungi, are utilised as the main components of animal feed. Among the more than 400 mycotoxins currently identified, aflatoxin B1 (AFB1), deoxynivalenol (DON), zearalenone (ZEN), ochratoxin A (OTA), fumonisins B1 (FB1) and trichothecenes T-2/HT-2 toxin are considered the most economically significant mycotoxins in terms of their prevalence and their negative effects on human and animal health and performance [4,5]. In addition to the well characterised fungal mycotoxins, biological metabolism or modification of mycotoxins mainly by plants can lead to conjugated forms of mycotoxins widely known as masked mycotoxins. These mycotoxin derivatives are often not detected by analytical techniques, and several studies have shown them to be a potential threat to consumers, as they can be converted to their parent forms in the gastrointestinal tract (GIT) after ingestion [1].

DON, T-2, ZEN and FB1 are produced by *Fusarium* species including *Fusarium graminearum*, *Fusarium sporotrichioides*, *Fusarium verticilloides* and *Fusarium poae* [4]. DON and T-2 are potent DNA protein synthesis inhibitors and cause digestive disorders, oral lesions, immunologic effects and hematological disorder [6,7]. ZEN is estrogenic and impair reproductive performance [8]. FB1 is associated with liver necrosis, diarrhoea, intestinal disorder, nephritis and oedema [9]. OTA is produced by species of *Aspergillus* and *Penicillium* (mainly *Aspergillus ochraceus* and *Penicillium verrucosum*). OTA exerts several toxic effects including nephrotoxicity, hepatogenicity and genotoxicity; it can also affect carbohydrate metabolism and blood coagulation [10]. AFB1 is produced by *Aspergillus* species (*Aspergillus flavus* and *Aspergillus parasiticus*). AFB1 health effects include teratogenicity, mutagenicity and carcinogenicity, with the liver being the primarily affected organ [11]. In farm animals, ingestion of a diet contaminated with more than one mycotoxin may cause more complex additive, antagonistic or synergistic effect on health and performance [12]. The severity of symptoms depends on a number of factors including the type of mycotoxin and level present, animal species, gender, diet, age and duration of exposure. In addition, diagnosis is difficult as mycotoxicosis produces a very wide variety of clinical signs [13].

Mycotoxin occurrence in cereal crops sits at 25% in terms of breaches of European Union (EU) Codex limits and occurrence above the detectable levels ranges from to 60–80% depending on the crop type [4]. To minimise the negative effects of these mycotoxins in farm animals, several methods have been developed to reduce the occurrence of mycotoxins in animal feeds, these include physical (thermal and irradiation) [14,15]; chemical (ozonation and ammoniation) [16,17] and biological (microorganisms and enzymes) [18,19]. However, inclusion of binders or adsorbents to feed as a form of additive, appears to be the most prevalent strategy widely practiced by farmers and the feed industry, due to its economic feasibility [20]. The additives are added to the diet of animals to reduce the absorption of mycotoxins from the GIT and their distribution to blood and target organs [21]. The additives used for this purpose have been divided into two groups: binders and modifiers. Mycotoxin binders aim to prevent the absorption of the mycotoxins from the intestinal tract of the animal by adsorbing the toxins to their surface to form a mycotoxin-binder complexes, which are then excreted in animal faeces. Mycotoxin binders are mainly classified as: organic (yeast cell wall and glucommanan) and inorganic (clay minerals such as aluminosilicate, bentonite and zeolite) [22]. Mycotoxin modifiers are of biological origin (bacteria, fungi, enzymes and plants); they alter the chemical structure of mycotoxins (biotransformation) to produce metabolites that are less toxic than the parent mycotoxins or non-toxic [23]. Throughout this paper, terms including adsorption, binding and sequestering, will be used to describe the reduction or removal of mycotoxins by feed additives.

In the EU, there is a provision under European Commission (EC) regulation (EC 1831/2003), for the inclusion of a technical additive—"a substance that can suppress or reduce the absorption, promote the excretion of mycotoxins or modify their mode of action"- to animal feed. To register a feed additive in the EU, an application must be submitted to the EC, a technical dossier to European Food Safety Authority (EFSA) and three reference samples of the feed additive must be sent to European Union Reference Laboratory, who evaluates the safety and efficacy of the samples before they can be authorized for use in the EU. However, in many other parts of the world, there are no regulations regarding the use of feed additives or substances that can counteract the toxic effects of mycotoxins in farm animals [20].

Several of these products are registered as digestibility enhancers, antioxidants and generic or catalogue names such as montmorillonite, bentonite and hydrated sodium calcium aluminosilicate

(HSCAS), with mycotoxin binding claims [24,25]. Many researchers have investigated mycotoxin sequestering potentials of some of these products, which are commercially available worldwide. However, most of the studies are focused on only one or two mycotoxins, particularly AFB1 [26–28]. As mycotoxins are often co-occurring in animal feed [29,30], the current study aims to evaluate and compare the efficacy of ten commercial feed additives with multi-mycotoxin binding claims on DON, T-2, ZEN, OTA, FB1 and AFB1 using an in vitro model simulated to mimic the gastro-intestinal tract (GIT) of a monogastric animal. Results showed that only one of the products (a modified yeast cell wall) effectively adsorbed more than 50% of DON, ZEN, FB1, OTA, T-2 and AFB1, in the following order: AFB1 > ZEN > T-2 > DON > OTA > FB1. The remaining products were able to moderately bind AFB1 (44–58%) but had less, or in some cases, no effect on ZEN, FB1, OTA and T-2 binding (<35%).

2. Results and Discussion

Contamination of different agricultural commodities with multi-mycotoxins, as well as adverse health effects and reduction in animal performance, due to mycotoxicosis are still prevalent, despite the prevention strategies currently employed [31–33]. Additives are added to the diets of livestock animals to bind mycotoxins and reduce their bioavailability in GIT and distribution to blood and target organs. The most prevalent adsorbing agents are polymers, yeast cell wall, cholestyramine and clay minerals [21,22]. In vitro analysis of mycotoxin adsorption is a very useful tool for rapid screening and identification of agents that may have mycotoxin sequestering potentials [22]. Several researchers have investigated different mycotoxin binders, however, most of the studies have focused on a single mycotoxin and carried out using buffer solutions mostly at pH 3 and 7, to simulate physiological pH in stomach and intestine, respectively. This does not truly reflect the conditions in a farm animal GIT as other factors including temperature, digestive enzymes, feed, bile salts and nutrients may interfere with the adsorption (ion-exchange) process [21].

In the current study, ten commercial feed additives with adsorption, inactivation or detoxification claims on DON, ZEN, FB1, OTA, T-2 and AFB1 were obtained and categorised into three groups based on their composition. Their capacity to simultaneously bind or adsorb DON, ZEN, FB1, OTA, T-2 and AFB1, which often co-occur in complete feed or feed ingredients such as maize, wheat and barley was assessed and compared. The ratio of additive:binder used in this study is based on the maximum permitted/guidance levels for mycotoxins in European pig feed [34] and the conventional binder inclusion level of 2 g/kg feed [35]. In order to assess the mycotoxin binding capacity of the adsorbents, an in vitro system with buffer solutions at pH 3 and 7—to simulate stomach and intestine respectively, was used to study mycotoxin adsorption/desorption. Furthermore, a robust in vitro model relative to the GIT of a monogastric animal in terms of compartment, enzymes, feed, gastric fluids, temperature, pH and transit time was designed, to investigate the adsorption efficacy of the feed additives. The percentage adsorption of DON, ZEN, FB1, OTA, T-2 and AFB1 by various feed additives in buffer solutions as well as in vitro GIT model are presented in Tables 1 and 2, respectively.

Table 1. Percentage adsorption of deoxynivalenol (DON), zearalenone (ZEN), fumonisin B1 (FB1), ochratoxin A (OTA), T-2 toxin and aflatoxin B1 (AFB1) by ten commercial feed additives in pH 3 and pH 7 buffer solutions *.

Category	Product	Adsorbed Mycotoxin (%) (mean ± SD) **											
		DON		ZEN		FB1		OTA		T-2		AFB1	
		pH 3	pH 7	pH 3	pH 7	pH 3	pH 7	pH 3	pH 7	pH 3	pH 7	pH 3	pH 7
Inorganic Additives	1	58 ± 0.5 b	50 ± 2.9 b	52 ± 0.9 b	49 ± 1.1 a,b	38 ± 1.2 b,c	47 ± 0.9 a	40 ± 1.6 b,c	37 ± 1.1 b	38 ± 0.7 b	29 ± 1.1 c	68 ± 0.8 a	68 ± 1.6 a
	2	33 ± 2.5 d	31 ± 0.7 c	32 ± 0.4 d	31 ± 1.4 c	33 ± 2.5 d	30 ± 0.8 c	12 ± 2.1 d	12 ± 1.4 d	08 ± 1.2 d	06 ± 1.1 d	49 ± 1.9 b	41 ± 3.2 d
	3	53 ± 1.3 c	53 ± 1.8 b	44 ± 1.2 c	39 ± 2.3 c	32 ± 3.1 d	28 ± 0.6 c	41 ± 1.4 b,c	28 ± 1.6 c	22 ± 1.5 c	10 ± 1.2 d	61 ± 3.4 a	52 ± 2.7 c
	4	29 ± 1.2 d	22 ± 1.2 d	27 ± 2.3 d	20 ± 0.7 d	29 ± 1.4 d	22 ± 1.4 d	05 ± 0.3 e	02 ± 0.7 e	09 ± 0.9 d	09 ± 1.6 d	51 ± 3.1 b	47 ± 1.9 c,d
Organic Additives	5	56 ± 1.9 c	54 ± 1.5 b	36 ± 1.4 d	29 ± 0.9 c	45 ± 0.9 b	40 ± 1.9 b	38 ± 0.8 b	25 ± 2.3 c	40 ± 2.2 b	31 ± 1.1 c	53 ± 4.2 b	53 ± 2.1 c
	6	55 ± 4.7 c	55 ± 0.5 b	56 ± 2.2 a	56 ± 1.5 a	51 ± 2.9 a	50 ± 1.6 a	60 ± 1.4 a	56 ± 0.8 a	55 ± 0.7 a	56 ± 1.3 a	65 ± 2.2 a	65 ± 1.9 a
	7	36 ± 3.2 c	38 ± 1.1 c	28 ± 0.3 d	19 ± 1.2 d	19 ± 1.7 e	18 ± 2.2 d	35 ± 2.5 c	28 ± 1.2 c	10 ± 1.3 d	09 ± 1.3 d	50 ± 1.9 b	55 ± 1.6 c
Mixed Additives	8	52 ± 1.2 c	50 ± 0.6 b	46 ± 1.9 c	40 ± 1.6 b,c	39 ± 2.3 b	31 ± 0.7 c	20 ± 2.2 d	20 ± 1.3 c,d	43 ± 1.6 b	40 ± 2.1 b	61 ± 2.3 a	56 ± 1.9 c
	9	72 ± 2.4 a	71 ± 1.5 a	55 ± 1.8 b	52 ± 1.4 a,b	42 ± 1.3 b	25 ± 1.7 c	49 ± 1.6 b	37 ± 1.6 b	55 ± 1.4 a	53 ± 1.3 a	63 ± 3.1 a	60 ± 2.2 a,b
	10	32 ± 1.6 d	32 ± 1.4 c	22 ± 1.2 e	20 ± 1.1 d	19 ± 1.9 e	10 ± 1.7 e	15 ± 1.4 d	12 ± 0.9 d	14 ± 1.6 d	06 ± 1.9 d	52 ± 2.5 b	30 ± 1.6 e

* Calculated in comparison to the control treatment with no feed additives. ** Values are means of three replicates. a–f Values labelled with the same superscript in a column are not significantly different ($p > 0.05$).

Table 2. Percentage adsorption of deoxynivalenol (DON), zearalenone (ZEN), fumonisin B1 (FB1), ochratoxin A (OTA), T-2 toxin and aflatoxin B1 (AFB1) by 10 commercially available feed additives in an in vitro model designed to mimic the gastrointestinal tract of a monogastric animal *.

Category		Adsorbed Mycotoxin (%) (mean ± SD) **					
	Product	DON	ZEN	FB1	OTA	T-2	AFB1
Inorganic Additives	1	55 ± 3.1 [b]	40 ± 2.2 [b]	33 ± 3.6 [c]	25 ± 2.5 [c]	26 ± 1.3 [c]	51 ± 2.9 [b]
	2	39 ± 1.3 [d]	29 ± 2.6 [d]	20 ± 1.9 [d]	18 ± 3.2 [d]	04 ± 1.4 [d]	53 ± 2.1 [b]
	3	41 ± 1.6 [d]	12 ± 1.2 [f]	21 ± 2.3 [d]	00	00	38 ± 1.5 [c]
	4	31 ± 1.7 [e]	18 ± 2.2 [e]	20 ± 3.1 [d]	00	02 ± 0.4 [d]	42 ± 1.2 [c]
Organic Additives	5	47 ± 1.9 [c]	40 ± 2.4 [b]	45 ± 2.1 [b]	29 ± 1.5 [b]	28 ± 1.3 [c]	54 ± 2.2 [b]
	6	55 ± 1.6 [b]	53 ± 1.1 [a]	51 ± 1.5 [a]	52 ± 2.3 [a]	56 ± 1.4 [a]	62 ± 0.9 [a]
	7	36 ± 2.2 [e]	41 ± 2.5 [b]	19 ± 0.6 [d]	26 ± 0.9 [c]	00	39 ± 1.4 [c]
Mixed Additives	8	41 ± 3.3 [d]	36 ± 1.7 [c]	23 ± 1.4 [d]	10 ± 2.1 [e]	28 ± 1.6 [c]	48 ± 1.9 [b,c]
	9	61 ± 2.4 [a]	53 ± 1.4 [a]	35 ± 2.6 [c]	32 ± 1.2 [b]	35 ± 0.7 [b]	58 ± 3.2 [a]
	10	22 ± 1.8 [f]	08 ± 1.9 [f]	00	00	00	29 ± 0.8 [d]

* Calculated in comparison to the control treatment with no feed additives. ** Values are means of three replicates.
[a–f] Values labelled with the same superscript in a column are not significantly different ($p > 0.05$).

2.1. Inorganic Additives

Aluminosilicate constitute the most abundant group of rock-forming minerals [36]. The basic structural unit of silicate clay minerals consists of the combination of aluminium octahedral and silica tetrahedral sheets, both with hydroxyl and oxygen groups [37]. Most studies (both in vivo and in vitro) on mycotoxin binders using clay minerals have focused on aluminosilicates such as bentonite, montmorillonite, zeolite and hydrated sodium calcium aluminosilicates (HSCAS). They possess high cation exchange capacity, pore volume and large surface area, which enable them to adsorb low-molecular weight compounds such as mycotoxins to their surfaces, edges and interlayer spaces [27]. Four commercial clay-based products (1, 2, 3 and 4) were investigated for their multi-mycotoxin binding potentials. Results obtained for in vitro buffer solutions showed that all the 4 products bound DON, ZEN, FB1, OTA, T-2 and AFB1 at adsorption rates of 29–58%, 27–42%, 29–47%, 5–40%, 9–38%, 51–68% respectively (Table 1). Product 1 and 3 had a significant adsorption on AFB1 (68% and 61%), DON (53% and 49%) and ZEN (42% and 46%) respectively, compared to product 2 and 4 ($p < 0.05$). There was no significant difference ($p > 0.05$) in the adsorption of DON, ZEN, FB1, OTA, T-2 and AFB1 by product 2 and 4, as they sequestered <34% of DON, ZEN and FB1; <13% of OTA and T-2, and approximately 50% of AFB1. Within this category, AFB1 was the most adsorbed mycotoxin followed by DON, ZEN, FB1, OTA and T-2 at pH 3 and 7. Several studies on adsorption of mycotoxins using buffer solutions at different pH (mostly 3, 5 and 7) have shown that AFB1 is highly adsorbed by clay minerals at acidic and alkaline pH with little to no adsorption of other mycotoxins [26,38,39]. A recent study on the efficacy of commercial clay minerals to sequester 0.1 μg/mL of AFB1, DON and ZEN showed that 1% of a commercial smectite and an aluminosilicate clays significantly adsorbed AFB1 (95–100%) and ZEN (56–82%) in acidic pH, with no significant effect on DON (<10%) [40]. Similarly, 50 mg of a commercial bentonite adsorbed 99% of 10 ng/mL AFB1 and 1% of 250 ng/mL DON in buffer solution (pH 5) [41]. The difference in the ability of clay minerals to sequester mycotoxin has been attributed to their origin and physiochemical properties such as cation exchange capacity, pore volume and expandability [21,22].

For the in vitro GIT experiment, 22–100% reduction in the efficacy of all the four clay-based products to adsorb multi-mycotoxins was observed (Table 2). Adsorption capacities of product 2 and 4 on DON, ZEN and FB1 were the most severely affected. Their adsorption rates were reduced to less than 23%, 18% and 16% for DON, ZEN and FB1, respectively, with no observed adsorption of OTA and T-2. However, both products (2 and 4) were still able to significantly bind >42% of AFB1 ($p < 0.05$) (Table 2). Product 1 performed better than other products within this group, with a simultaneous adsorption rate of 46%, 33%, 29%, 25%, 26% and 51% for DON, ZEN, FB1, OTA, T-2 and AFB1 respectively, followed by product 3: DON (37%), ZEN (29%), FB1 (22%), OTA (18%), T-2 (15%) and AFB1 (53%). A similar study carried out by Vekiru et al. [42], showed that the sequestering potential of HSCAS, activated charcoal and bentonites against AFB1 strongly decreased in the presence of swine gastric juice. The percentage adsorption dropped from 98% to 72% for HSCAS, 88% to 35% for activated charcoal and by more than 15% for bentonites [42]. Also, the capacity of 1 mg of smectite to reduce 8 µg/mL aflatoxin was reduced from 0.5 mol/kg in distilled water to 0.2 mol/kg in simulated gastric fluid [43].

Although, the adsorption capacity of product 1 and 3 were reduced in the GIT model, they still significantly adsorbed DON, ZEN, FB1, OTA, T-2 and AFB1 ($p < 0.05$) when compared with product 2 and 4. These products (1 and 3) are chemically modified clay minerals. Modified clay minerals have been shown to possess high mycotoxin-sequestering ability compare to natural clay minerals (product 2 and 4). Modified adsorbents are prepared by alteration of surface properties such as cation exchange capacity using acids, alkalis, organic compounds and heat, that consequently increase their contaminant removal capacity and efficacy [44]. Nevertheless, their safety and interaction with nutrients and veterinary substances remain a concern [45].

2.2. Organic Additives

The three products (5, 6 and 7) within this category of feed additives, were able to bind DON, ZEN, FB1, OTA, T-2 and AFB1 in the range of 36–56%, 28–69%, 19–55%, 35–60%, 10–56% and 55–65%, respectively, mostly at pH 3 ($p < 0.05$) (Table 1). Only product 6 was able to adsorb more than 50% of each toxin simultaneously: DON (55%), ZEN (56%), FB1 (55%), OTA (60%), T-2 (56%) and AFB1 (65%). Product 5 adsorbed DON (56%) and AFB1 (51%), with moderate binding on ZEN, FB1, OTA and T-2 (<45%). Product 7 also adsorbed AFB1 (55%), but its multi-mycotoxin adsorption capacity on DON (36%), ZEN (28%), FB1 (19%), OTA (35%), T-2 (10%) was significantly lower when compared to product 5 and 6 ($p < 0.05$). In terms of percentage adsorption under in vitro GIT model, again, all the products binding capacities were reduced, but to a much lesser extent compared with products under inorganic additives (Table 2). Only product 6 had a significant binding ($p < 0.05$) on ZEN (56%), FB1 (55%), OTA (60%), T-2 (56%) and AFB1 (63%). However, no significant difference was observed in the adsorption of DON, FB1 and AFB1 by products 5 and 6 ($p > 0.05$). Interestingly, the percentage adsorption of ZEN by product 6 in buffer solutions (56%) was similar to that which was found in the in vitro GIT model, which indicates a good additive with high mycotoxin specificity. Similar results were obtained by Joannis-Casssan et al. [46]. This group tested the binding efficacy of a commercial yeast cell wall obtained from baker's yeast on OTA, AFB1 and ZEN and found it to effectively adsorb up to 62%, 29% and 68%, respectively, in a dose-dependent manner [46]. Also, a commercial inactivated yeast-based product sandwiched with glutathione bound 45% of AFB1 and more than 50% of OTA and ZEN [47].

Organic additives such as yeast cell wall and glucommanan have been shown to have a high binding activity across a wide spectrum of mycotoxins compare to inorganic minerals [48]. The cell wall of the yeast *Saccharomyces cerevisiae* is composed of lipids, protein and polysaccharide fraction, with glucans and mannans being the two main constituents of the latter fraction [47]. Glucomannan is a water-soluble polysaccharide composed of hemicellulose, it is present in the cell wall of some plant species. Several authors have suggested that the cell wall components of these substances could be responsible for the adsorption of mycotoxins through non-covalent, hydrogen bonds, ionic or hydrophobic interactions [49–51]. Rignot et al. [50] showed that β-D-glucans are the yeast component largely responsible for the complexation of mycotoxins, and that the reticular organization of β-D-glucans and the distribution between β-(1,6)-D-glucans and β-(1,3)-D-glucans plays a vital role in mycotoxin adsorption [50]. Furthermore, Van der Waals forces and weak hydrogen bonding maybe involved in the adsorption of mycotoxins by β-D-glucans [49]. The efficacy and type of mycotoxins a yeast cell wall product can adsorb is dependent on the origin of yeast, strain, pH, binding sites or accessible surface area, growth condition and percentage of cell wall components (mannoproteins, chitins, lipids and β-glucan) [51]. Glucomannan is commonly used as a dietary fibre, however, there are very limited studies published regarding the types of mycotoxins adsorbed and mechanisms of adsorption.

2.3. Mixture of Additives

Due to the affinity of most technical additives towards a single mycotoxin, a mixture of additives has been developed and used recently, to counteract adverse health effects of multiple mycotoxins in farm animals, the most prevalent one being mixture of clay minerals and yeast cell wall [26]. Three commercial products with mixed additives (product 8—mixed silicates and yeast cell wall; product 9—yeast cell wall and enzyme; product 10—natural clay minerals and algae) were assessed for their multi-mycotoxin binding capacity in the present study. Results of in vitro buffer solution testing showed that the three products adsorbed DON (32–72%), ZEN (22–55%), FB1 (19–56%) OTA (15–49%), T-2 (38–55%) and AFB1 (32–63%), mostly at pH 3 ($p < 0.05$) (Table 1). Product 9 significantly sequestered DON (72%), ZEN (55%) and T-2 (55%), however, compared to product 8, no significant adsorption was observed ($p > 0.05$) for FB1 (42%) and AFB1 (63%). Product 10 had a poor binding capacity on DON, ZEN, FB1, OTA and T-2 with an adsorption rate of 32%, 22%, 19%, 15% and 38%, respectively. Under in vitro GIT conditions, product 10 lost its binding potential as mycotoxins adsorption rates were reduced to 22%, 8%, 0%, 0% and 24% for DON, ZEN, FB1, OTA and T-2, respectively. Similar results were obtained for product 8, with a reduction from 52–41%, 46–35%, 39–23%, 20–9%, 43–28% and 61–48% for DON, ZEN, FB1, OTA, T-2 and AFB1, respectively. Product 9 significantly adsorbed DON (61%), ZEN (55%), OTA (33%), T-2 (36%) and AFB1 (58%) compared to product 8 and 10 ($p < 0.05$) (Table 2). Results obtained for products within this category suggest that mere mixing of additives does not guarantee multi-mycotoxin binding as the mixture may either lead to synergistic or antagonistic effect. When mixing additives, it is important to investigate the efficacy of individual agent and their mixtures to identify the mycotoxins they can adsorb effectively.

Generally, all the commercial binder or feed additive products assessed for their capacity to bind multi-mycotoxin in the current study adsorbed DON, ZEN, FB1, OTA, T-2 and AFB1 simultaneously at different rates under both acidic and alkaline pH. However, percentage adsorption at pH 3 was more significant when compare with adsorption at pH 7 ($p < 0.05$), this indicates that products investigated can form a stable mycotoxin-binder complex at pH 3 and to some extent at pH 7. Under in vitro GIT model, adsorption efficacies of all the products were reduced (except product 6, for ZEN) possibly due to interaction of binder products with other components of GIT such as pepsin, HCl and feed [43,52,53]. For instance, Barrientos et al. [43] showed that the adsorption of a globular protein (pepsin) by a smectite clay significantly reduced the adsorption rate of AFB1 in simulated acidic gastrointestinal fluid [43]. Also, a corn protein interfered with AFB1 adsorption to a smectite clay in corn fermentation solution [53].

Regarding the performances of investigated feed additives under the in vitro GIT model, product 1—a modified aluminosilicate had a good multi-mycotoxin binding capacity on DON (46%), ZEN (33%), T-2 (29%), FB1 (25%), OTA (25%) and AFB1 (51%) when compared with other products in this category ($p < 0.05$). Within category of organic additives, a modified yeast extract (product 6) had a broad significant mycotoxin adsorption spectrum, with adsorption rate of 55%, 56%, 51%, 53%, 56% and 65% for DON, ZEN, FB1, OTA, T-2 and AFB1, respectively. Within category of mixture of additives, product 9 (a mixed yeast cell wall and enzymes) adsorbed 61%, 55%, 28%, 33%, 36% and 58% of DON, ZEN, FB1, OTA, T-2 and AFB1, respectively ($p < 0.05$). Overall, in terms of multi-mycotoxin binding efficiency, only product 6 performed well, as it was able to simultaneously sequester more than 50% of mycotoxins in the following order: AFB1 > ZEN > T-2 > DON > OTA > FB1; followed by product 9 (yeast cell wall and enzyme) and product 5 (glucomannan).

Mycotoxin binders adsorb mycotoxin at the surface, to form a mycotoxin-binder complex, the bound mycotoxins are then excreted along with the binder in animal faeces. The adsorption capacity and stability of the complex through the GIT is influenced by physiochemical properties of the binder including polarity, size of the pores and accessible surface area as well as physicochemical properties of mycotoxins including polarity, solubility, size and charge [38]. AFB1 is relatively hydrophilic with aromatic planar molecules, therefore it is easily bound by most binders, particularly clay minerals, under both acidic and alkaline conditions, by formation of a coordination bonds with the beta-carbonyl system [26]. However, other mycotoxins—ZEN, OTA, FB1, T-2 and DON range from being moderately hydrophilic to high hydrophobic compounds, therefore being very difficult to adsorb [26]. However, emerging nanocomposites [54], modified organic and inorganic adsorbents [55] are being used to sequester these mycotoxins.

3. Conclusions

In light of the high co-occurrence of fungi and mycotoxins in agricultural commodities, exacerbated by climate change, products with wide spectrum mycotoxin adsorption or detoxification are in great demand from farmers and animal feed producers, to minimise the economic losses caused by mycotoxicosis. In the current study, an in vitro GIT model was designed to assess and compare the efficacy of ten commercially available binder products with multiple mycotoxin claims on DON, ZEN, FB1, OTA, T-2 and AFB1. Results showed that most of the products were able to significantly bind DON, ZEN, FB1, OTA, T-2 and AFB1 in both alkaline and acidic buffer solutions. However, under the in vitro model simulating the conditions in the GIT of monogastric animals such as chicken and pig, the efficacy of all the products were significantly reduced and only one of the products tested (6—a modified yeast cell wall) was still able to simultaneously adsorb more than 50% of DON, ZEN, FB1, OTA, T-2 and AFB1, in the following order AFB1 > ZEN > T-2 > DON > OTA > FB1. The remaining products were able to moderately bind AFB1 (44–58%) but had less than 35% or in some cases no binding effect on ZEN, FB1, OTA and T-2 binding. A robust method that mimics the GIT condition of a farm animal must be used to study the efficiency of a potential mycotoxin binder, not the conventional use of buffers at different pH. Furthermore, producers of feed additives with mycotoxin binding claims should ensure appropriate and detailed labelling of their products such as the composition, physicochemical properties, mode of action, dosage and importantly the specific mycotoxin(s) their product can bind, adsorb or detoxify, to ensure farmers and animal nutrition companies are not misled.

4. Materials and Methods

4.1. Chemicals and Reagents

Hydrochloric acid (HCl), citric acid, monobasic sodium phosphate (NaH_2PO_4), pancreatin, pepsin, polytetrafluoroethylene (PTFE) filter, formic acid, bile salt, sodium chloride (NaCl), sodium bicarbonate ($NaHCO_3$), LC-MS grade methanol and acetonitrile were supplied by Sigma-Aldrich (Gillingham, UK). Mycotoxins—AFB1, ZEN, FB1, OTA, T-2 and DON—crystalline solids were obtained from Romer Labs GmBH (Tulln, Austria). Ultra-pure water was obtained from a Milli-Q Gradient A10 water purification device (Millipore, Molsheim, France). All chemicals used were of analytical grade unless otherwise stated.

4.2. Feed Additives

Ten commercially available products claiming multiple mycotoxin adsorption or binding on DON, T-2, ZEN, AFB1 and FB1 were obtained and categorised into three groups (inorganic, organic and mixture of additives) based on their main functional composition. The products were coded with numbers to preserve the confidentiality of the source. Products 1, 3 and 4 were purchased online, while products 2, 5, 6, 7, 8, 9 and 10 were obtained directly from the companies. Product details including mode of action and main composition (as stated on the product labels and manufacturers' websites) are listed in Table 3.

Table 3. Composition and mode of actions (as stated on the product labels and manufacturers' websites) of commercial feed additives claiming multiple-mycotoxin binding.

Category	Product	Main Composition	Mode of Action
Inorganic adsorbent	1	Modified aluminosilicates	Adsorption
	2	Bentonite	***
	3	Activated clay	Adsorption and Inactivation
	4	Montmorillonite	Adsorption
Organic adsorbent	5	Glucomannan	Adsorption and complexation
	6	Modified yeast cell wall	Adsorption
	7	Esterified glucomannan	***
Mixed adsorbent	8	Mixed silicates and yeast cell wall	***
	9	Aluminosilicate and enzyme	Adsorption and biotransformation
	10	Natural minerals and algae	Adsorption and degradation

*** no information provided.

4.3. Multi-Mycotoxins Adsorption Experiment

4.3.1. Buffer Solution

Mycotoxin stock solutions (1 mg/mL) of AFB1, DON, ZEN, T-2 and OTA were prepared by dissolving pure solid standards in methanol and FB1 in acetonitrile/water (50:50, v/v). A mixed-mycotoxin working solution was prepared in 10 mL acetonitrile and stored at −20 °C until use. To evaluate adsorption efficacy of the binding products and stability (adsorption/desorption) of mycotoxin-binders complex in both acidic and alkaline conditions, adsorption capacity of each product was studied at pH 3 and 7 to simulate physiologic pH in the stomach and intestine of monogastric animal respectively. The buffer solutions (pH 3 and 7) were prepared by using 0.1 M citrate and 0.2 M phosphate buffers. Each product (20 mg) was weighed into a 30 mL flask containing 10 mL of buffer solution; 20 µL of multi-mycotoxin working standard solution was added to reach a final concentration of 20 ng/mL, 50 ng/mL, 900 ng/mL, 5000 ng/mL, 100 ng/mL and 250 ng/mL for AFB1, OTA, DON, FB1, ZEN and T-2 respectively, this was performed for each pH in triplicate. A blank control was prepared using only multi-mycotoxin working solution in buffers without any mycotoxin binder. The flasks were shaken and incubated for 3 h at 37 °C in an incubator shaker. Thereafter, samples were centrifuged (30 min, 1000× g, 25 °C), and 1 mL of supernatant was mixed with an equal volume of acetonitrile and evaporated to dryness under gentle nitrogen stream (40 °C). The residue was reconstituted in 1 mL of methanol, filtered through 0.2 µm PTFE filter and transferred to a glass vial for LC-MS/MS analyses.

4.3.2. In Vitro Gastrointestinal Model

An artificially contaminated feed was made by spiking 1 g of finely ground feed material with 200 µL of multi-mycotoxin stock solution to reach approximately the following mycotoxin concentrations, based on EU permitted/regulated limit for mycotoxins in pig feed: AFB1 (21.2 µg/kg), OTA (48.9 µg/kg), DON (997.2 µg/kg), FB1 (5582.3 µg/kg), T-2 (243.1 µg/kg) and ZEN (152.8 µg/kg). The spiked material was incubated overnight in the dark at 40 °C to evaporate to dryness. To check the homogeneity of the batch, three samples taken randomly were extracted and analysed for multi-mycotoxins using a previously validated QuEChERS-based LC-MS/MS method [56]. To assess the efficacy of commercial feed additives to adsorb multiple mycotoxins, an in vitro model was designed to simulate the GIT conditions of monogastric animal using an automated dissolution USP Apparatus 2 (Vankel VK 7010, Erweka, Germany) with an auto-controlled multi-channel peristaltic pump (Vankel VK 810, England). Temperature of 40 °C and rotation speed of 100 rpm were used throughout the experiment. The first GIT compartment simulated was the crop/oesophagus, 1.0 g of multi-mycotoxin contaminated feed and 20 mg of each feed additive were mixed with 40 mM of acetic acid, 0.2 M $Na_2 HPO_4$ and 5 M NaCl buffer. Each tube was mixed to reach a pH value of 4.5–5.3 and incubated for 60 min. Subsequent stomach/proventriculus simulation was performed by addition of 0.23 M HCl, 0.034 M NaCl and 5000 U of purified pepsin derived from pig stomach mucosa, to reach a pH between 1.9 and 3.7, tubes were further incubated for 90 min. The final GIT compartment simulated was the intestine; here, 0.05 M $NaHCO_3$, pancreatin (0.5 mg/mL) and 0.4% bile salt were added to the tubes, the pH was increased and ranged between 5.3 and 7.5. All samples were incubated further for 120 min. The total incubation time for the in vitro digestion was 4 h and 30 min. Blank controls were prepared without the addition of any feed additive, and all experiments were performed in quintuplicate. After incubation, 1 mL of sample was withdrawn and mixed with 1 mL of 0.01% formic acid in acetonitrile, followed by a rigorous vortex and centrifugation at $10,000\times g$ for 30 min. Subsequently, 1 mL of supernatant was dried under gentle nitrogen stream (35 °C) and residue was re-dissolved in 0.5 mL of methanol, filtered through 0.2 µm PTFE filter and transferred to a glass vial for LC-MS/MS analysis.

4.4. LC-MS/MS Analysis of Mycotoxins

AFB1, DON, ZEN, T-2, FB1 and OTA were analysed using an Acquity UPLC I-Class system coupled to a Xevo TQ-S triple quadrupole mass spectrometer (MS) (both from Waters, Milford, USA), which allowed the simultaneous determination of the toxins. Data acquisition and instrument control were performed by Masslynx software (Waters, Milford, MA). For the UPLC, the column used was a Cortecs C18 100 mm × 2.1 mm i.d., 1.6 µm (Waters, Milford, USA) and mobile phases consisted of A —water and B—methanol: acetonitrile (1:1, v/v). Both contained 0.1% formic acid and 1mM ammonium formate. Chromatographic separation was achieved through a gradient elution program as follows: 0–2 min, 99% A/1% B; 2–3 min 30% A/70% B, 3–5.5 min, 1% A/99% B; 5.5–6.5 min, 99%A/1% B; 6.5–7 min, 99% A/1% B. Column temperature was maintained at 40 °C, and the flow rate and injection volume were set at 0.4 mL/min and 1 µL respectively. ESI-MS/MS was performed in a multiple reaction monitoring mode (MRM) at positive polarity. The m/z transitions for quantification were 313.2 > 241.2, 297.3 > 249.5, 319.3 > 282.9, 466.5 > 245.1, 721.83 > 335.1, 403.8 > 238.8 for AFB1, DON, ZEN, T-2, FB1 and OTA respectively. The ion source parameters were as follows: capillary voltage, 1 kV; desolvation temperature, 600 °C; source temperature, 150 °C; cone gas flow, 50 L/h; desolvation gas flow, 1000 L/h. Collision energy and cone voltage were optimised by an infusion of each compound using the IntelliStart function.

4.5. Method Performance

For quantification, a seven-point calibration curve was prepared for each mycotoxin in the following concentration range: 0.5–50 ng/mL for AFB1, 10–5000 ng/mL for FB1, 5–500 ng/mL for ZEN, T-2 and OTA, and 10–2000 ng/mL for DON. To evaluate the effects of the matrix on MS quantification, matrix-induced suppression/enhancement (SSE) was determined by comparing the response of matrix spiked with seven different concentrations of each mycotoxin to a neat solvent standard at the same concentrations. The experiment was performed for buffer solutions (pH 3, pH 7) and gastrointestinal fluid (GF) in triplicate at three different times. SSE was calculated as the ratio of calibration curve slope for matrix-matched standards and neat solvent standards multiplied by 100. Limits of detection and limits of quantification (LOQ) of each mycotoxin were calculated at a signal-to-noise ratio of 3:1 and 10:1, respectively, based on a matrix-matched calibration in buffer solutions and GF. The coefficients of determination (R^2) for selected mycotoxins in the three matrices (pH 3, pH 7 and GF) ranged from 0.9901 to 0.9995. The retention times of the analyte in the sample extract were checked to correspond to that of the calibration standards and was within a tolerance of ± 0.1 min. Also, the ion ratios were within 25% of that obtained from the calibration standard for all analytes. SSE and LOQs values obtained for mycotoxins in the three matrices are reported in Table 4. Figure 1 shows chromatograms obtained for the six mycotoxins in a spiked feed sample.

Table 4. Signal suppression-enhancement/relative standard deviation (SSE/RSD) and limit of quantification (LOQ) obtained for deoxynivalenol (DON), zearalenone (ZEN), fumonisins B1 (FB1), ochratoxin A (OTA), T-2 and aflatoxin B1 (AFB1) and validated matrices—pH 3, pH 7 and gastrointestinal fluid (GF).

Matrix		DON	ZEN	FB1	OTA	T-2	AFB1
pH 3	SSE/RSD (%)	95/2.1	98/2.4	113/3.2	97/3.9	78/2.7	96/0.9
	LOQ (ng/mL)	2.5	2.5	5	0.4	2.5	0.13
pH 7	SSE/RSD (%)	78/2.6	97/2.7	83/3.1	102/4.1	88/3.4	100/1.2
	LOQ (ng/mL)	2.5	2.5	5	0.4	2.5	0.13
GF	SSE/RSD (%)	89/3.2	92/6.8	123/5.7	103/4.9	79/7.4	87/4.6
	LOQ (ng/mL)	2.5	5	5	0.8	5	0.25

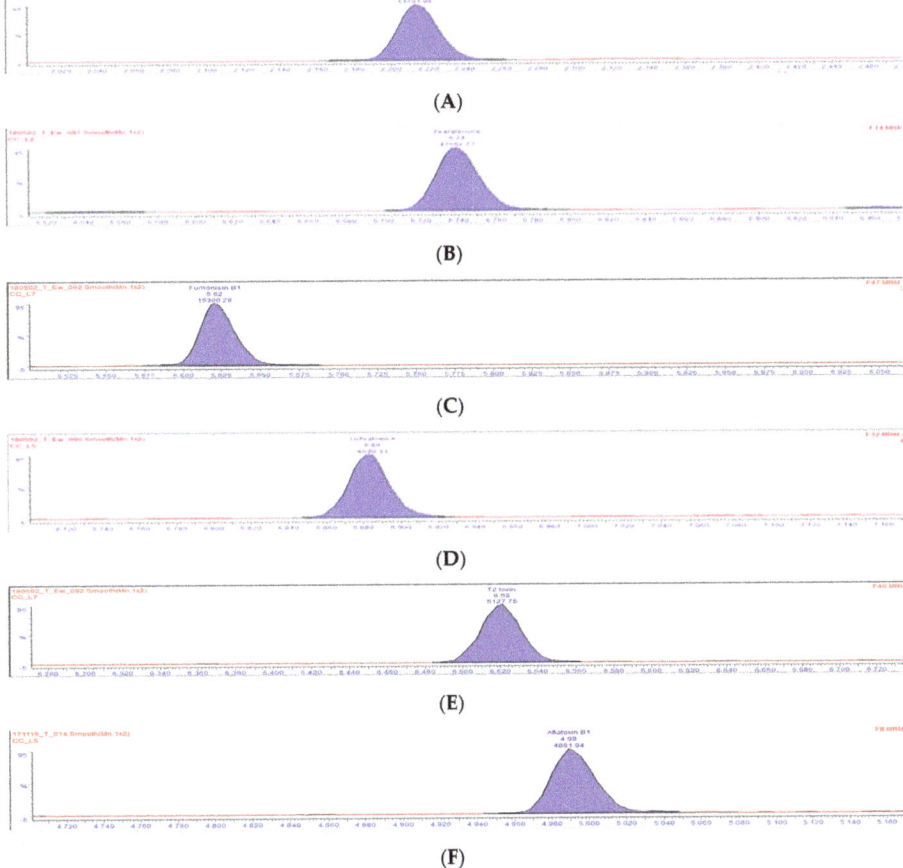

Figure 1. UPLC-MS/MS chromatograms of spiked feed sample (**A**) at 10 µg/kg for deoxynivalenol (DON), (**B**) 5 µg/kg for zearalenone (ZEN), (**C**) 10 µg/kg for fumonisin (FB1), (**D**) 2 µg/kg for ochratoxin A (OTA), (**E**) 5 µg/kg for T-2 toxin, (**F**) 0.5 µg/kg for aflatoxin B1 (AFB1).

4.6. Quantification of Mycotoxins and Statistical Analysis

The percentage adsorption of mycotoxins by each product was calculated as follows:

$$\text{Adsorption (\%)} = (C_b - C_t)/C_t \times 100.$$

where C_b is the mycotoxin concentration in blank spiked buffer solutions (ng/mL); and C_t, the amount of mycotoxin in the supernatant of sample (ng/mL). The data obtained were analysed using TargetLynx processing software (Waters, Wilmslow, UK) and Prism® version 8 (San Diego, CA, USA). The means of treatments showing significant differences in two and three-way ANOVA were compared using Tukey's honestly significance difference multiple-comparisons post-test. All statements of significance are based on the 0.05 level of probability.

Author Contributions: Conceptualization, C.E., D.S.J. and O.K.; Methodology, O.K. and C.E.; Formal analysis, D.S.J. and O.K.; Data curation, O.K. and D.S.J.; Writing—original draft preparation, O.K and C.T.; Writing—review and editing, C.T., D.S.J., L.C. and O.C.; Supervision, C.E., D.S.J., J.M. and O.C.; Funding acquisition, L.C. and C.E.; Project administration, B.G. and J.M.; Resources, B.G., J.M. and O.K.

Funding: This project has received funding from the European Union's Horizon 2020 research and innovation programme under the Marie Skłodowska-Curie grant agreement No. 722634.

Conflicts of Interest: The authors declare no conflict of interest.

References

1. Kovač, M.; Šubarić, D.; Bulaić, M.; Kovač, T.; Šarkanj, B. Yesterday masked, today modified; what do mycotoxins bring next? *Arch. Ind. Hyg. Toxicol.* **2018**, *69*, 196–214. [CrossRef] [PubMed]
2. Mannaa, M.; Kim, K. Influence of temperature and water activity on deleterious fungi and mycotoxin production during grain storage. *Mycobiology* **2017**, *45*, 240–254. [CrossRef] [PubMed]
3. Milani, J. Ecological conditions affecting mycotoxin production in cereals: A review. *Veterinární Med.* **2013**, *58*, 405–411. [CrossRef]
4. Eskola, M.; Gregor, K.; Christopher, E.; Hájslová, J.; Mayar, S.; Krska, R. Worldwide contamination of food-crops with mycotoxins: Validity of the widely cited 'FAO estimate' of 25%. *Crit. Rev. Food Sci. Nutr.* **2019**, 1–17. [CrossRef] [PubMed]
5. Pitt, J. Toxigenic fungi: Which are important? *Med. Mycol.* **2000**, *38*, 17–22. [CrossRef] [PubMed]
6. Sobrova, P.; Adam, V.; Vasatkova, A.; Beklova, M.; Zeman, L.; Kizek, R. Deoxynivalenol and its toxicity. *Interdiscip. Toxicol.* **2010**, *3*, 94–99. [CrossRef] [PubMed]
7. Li, Y.; Wang, Z.; Beier, R.; Shen, J.; Smet, D.; De Saeger, S. T-2 toxin, a trichothecene mycotoxin: Review of toxicity, metabolism, and analytical methods. *J. Agric. Food Chem.* **2011**, *59*, 3441–3453. [CrossRef] [PubMed]
8. Frizzell, C.; Ndossi, D.; Verhaegen, S.; Dahl, E.; Eriksen, G.; Sørlie, M.; Ropstand, E.; Muller, M.; Elliott, C.; Connolly, L. Endocrine disrupting effects of zearalenone, alpha-and beta-zearalenol at the level of nuclear receptor binding and steroidogenesis. *Toxicol. Lett.* **2011**, *206*, 210–217. [CrossRef] [PubMed]
9. Henry, M.; Wyatt, R. The toxicity of fumonisin B1, B2, and B3, individually and in combination, in chicken embryos. *Poult. Sci.* **2001**, *80*, 401–407. [CrossRef] [PubMed]
10. Bui-Klimke, T.; Wu, F. Ochratoxin A and human health risk: A review of the evidence. *Crit. Rev. Food Sci. Nutr.* **2014**, *55*, 1860–1869. [CrossRef] [PubMed]
11. Rushing, B.; Selim, M. Aflatoxin B1: A review on metabolism, toxicity, occurrence in food, occupational exposure, and detoxification methods. *Food Chem. Toxicol.* **2019**, *124*, 81–100. [CrossRef] [PubMed]
12. Sobral, M.; Faria, M.; Cunha, S.; Ferreira, I. Toxicological interactions between mycotoxins from ubiquitous fungi: Impact on hepatic and intestinal human epithelial cells. *Chemosphere* **2018**, *202*, 538–548. [CrossRef] [PubMed]
13. Schiefer, H. Mycotoxicoses of domestic animals and their diagnosis. *Can. J. Physiol. Pharmacol.* **1990**, *68*, 987–990. [CrossRef] [PubMed]
14. Raters, M.; Matissek, R. Thermal stability of aflatoxin B1 and ochratoxin A. *Mycotoxin Res.* **2008**, *24*, 130–134. [CrossRef] [PubMed]

15. Calado, T.; Venâncio, A.; Abrunhosa, L. Irradiation for mold and mycotoxin control: A review. *Compr. Rev. Food Sci. Food Saf.* **2014**, *13*, 1049–1061. [CrossRef]
16. Trombete, F.; Porto, Y.; Freitas-Silva, O.; Pereira, R.; Direito, G.; Saldanha, T.; Fraga, E. Efficacy of ozone treatment on mycotoxins and fungal reduction in artificially contaminated soft wheat grains. *J. Food Process. Preserv.* **2016**, *41*, e12927. [CrossRef]
17. Gomaa, M.; Ayesh, A.; Abdel-Galil, M.; Naguib, K. Effect of high pressure ammoniation procedure on the detoxification of aflatoxins. *Mycotoxin Res.* **1997**, *13*, 23–34. [CrossRef] [PubMed]
18. Ben Taheur, F.; Kouidhi, B.; Al Qurashi, Y.; Ben Salah-Abbès, J.; Chaieb, K. Review: Biotechnology of mycotoxins detoxification using microorganisms and enzymes. *Toxicon* **2019**, *160*, 12–22. [CrossRef] [PubMed]
19. Lyagin, I.; Efremenko, E. Enzymes for detoxification of various mycotoxins: Origins and mechanisms of catalytic action. *Molecules* **2019**, *24*, 2362. [CrossRef] [PubMed]
20. De Mil, T.; Devreese, M.; De Baere, S.; Van Ranst, E.; Eeckhout, M.; De Backer, P.; Croubels, S. Characterization of 27 mycotoxin binders and the relation with in vitro zearalenone adsorption at a single concentration. *Toxins* **2015**, *7*, 21–33. [CrossRef] [PubMed]
21. Di Gregorio, M.; Neeff, D.; Jager, A.; Corassin, C.; Carão, Á.; Albuquerque, R. Mineral adsorbents for prevention of mycotoxins in animal feeds. *Toxin Rev.* **2014**, *33*, 125–135. [CrossRef]
22. Vila-Donat, P.; Marín, S.; Sanchis, V.; Ramos, A. A review of the mycotoxin adsorbing agents, with an emphasis on their multi-binding capacity, for animal feed decontamination. *Food Chem. Toxicol.* **2018**, *114*, 246–259. [CrossRef] [PubMed]
23. Loi, M.; Fanelli, F.; Liuzzi, V.; Logrieco, A.; Mulè, G. Mycotoxin biotransformation by native and commercial enzymes: Present and Future Perspectives. *Toxins* **2017**, *9*, 111. [CrossRef] [PubMed]
24. Kolosova, A.; Stroka, J. Evaluation of the effect of mycotoxin binders in animal feed on the analytical performance of standardised methods for the determination of mycotoxins in feed. *Food Addit. Contam. Part A* **2012**, *29*, 1959–1971. [CrossRef] [PubMed]
25. Mutua, F.; Lindahl, J.; Grace, D. Availability and use of mycotoxin binders in selected urban and peri-urban areas of Kenya. *Food Secur.* **2019**, *11*, 359–369. [CrossRef]
26. Boudergue, C.; Burel, C.; Dragacci, C.; Favrot, M.; Fremy, J.; Massimi, C.; Prigent, P.; Debongnie, P.; Pussemier, L.; Boudra, H.; et al. Review of mycotoxin-detoxifying agents used as feed additives: Mode of action, efficacy and feed/food safety. *EFSA Support. Publ.* **2009**, *6*, 192. [CrossRef]
27. Jaynes, W.; Zartman, R.; Hudnall, W. Aflatoxin B1 adsorption by clays from water and corn meal. *Appl. Clay Sci.* **2007**, *36*, 197–205. [CrossRef]
28. Tengjaroenkul, U.; Pimpukdee, K.; Tengjaroenkul, B. Adsorption study for the detoxification of aflatoxin B1 by using the different clay minerals in Thailand. *Mycotoxins* **2006**, *2006*, 240–244. [CrossRef]
29. Binder, E.; Tan, L.; Chin, L.; Handl, J.; Richard, J. Worldwide occurrence of mycotoxins in commodities, feeds and feed ingredients. *Anim. Feed Sci. Technol.* **2007**, *137*, 265–282. [CrossRef]
30. Streit, E.; Schatzmayr, G.; Tassis, P.; Tzika, E.; Marin, D.; Taranu, I.; Tabu, C.; Nicolau, A.; Aprodu, I.; Puel, O.; et al. Current situation of mycotoxin contamination and co-occurrence in animal feed—Focus on Europe. *Toxins* **2012**, *4*, 788–809. [CrossRef] [PubMed]
31. Hassan, Z.; Al Thani, R.; Balmas, V.; Migheli, Q.; Jaoua, S. Prevalence of fusarium fungi and their toxins in marketed feed. *Food Control* **2019**, *104*, 224–230. [CrossRef]
32. Gruber-Dorninger, C.; Jenkins, T.; Schatzmayr, G. Global mycotoxin occurrence in feed: A ten-year survey. *Toxins* **2019**, *11*, 375. [CrossRef] [PubMed]
33. Khatoon, A.; Khan, M.; Abidin, Z.; Bhatti, S. Effects of feeding bentonite clay upon ochratoxin A–induced immunosuppression in broiler chicks. *Food Addit. Contam. Part A* **2017**, *35*, 538–545. [CrossRef] [PubMed]
34. Pinotti, L.; Ottoboni, M.; Giromini, C.; Dell'Orto, V.; Cheli, F. Mycotoxin contamination in the EU feed supply chain: A focus on cereal by-products. *Toxins* **2016**, *8*, 45. [CrossRef] [PubMed]
35. Scientific opinion on the safety and efficacy of a preparation of bentonite-and sepiolite (Toxfin®Dry) as feed additive for all species. *EFSA J.* **2013**, *11*, 3179. [CrossRef]
36. Alaniz, C.; Regil, E.; Cruz, G.; Torres, J.; Monroy, J. Composition and properties of tectosilicate-uranium layers of soil. *Eur. J. Chem.* **2012**, *3*, 32–36. [CrossRef]
37. Kerr, G. Chemistry of crystalline aluminosilicates. I. Factors affecting the formation of zeolite A. *J. Phys. Chem.* **1966**, *70*, 1047–1050. [CrossRef]

38. Deng, Y.; Velázquez, A.; Billes, F.; Dixon, J. Bonding mechanisms between aflatoxin B1 and smectite. *Appl. Clay Sci.* **2010**, *50*, 92–98. [CrossRef]
39. Ayo, E.; Matemu, A.; Laswai, G.; Kimanya, M. An in vitro evaluation of the capacity of local tanzanian crude clay and ash-based materials in binding aflatoxins in solution. *Toxins* **2018**, *10*, 510. [CrossRef] [PubMed]
40. Prapapanpong, J.; Udomkusonsri, P.; Mahavorasirikul, W.; Choochuay, S.; Tansakul, N. In vitro studies on gastrointestinal monogastric and avian models to evaluate the binding efficacy of mycotoxin adsorbents by liquid chromatography-tandem mass spectrometry. *J. Adv. Vet. Anim. Res.* **2019**, *6*, 125–132. [CrossRef] [PubMed]
41. Kong, C.; Shin, S.; Kim, B. Evaluation of mycotoxin sequestering agents for aflatoxin and deoxynivalenol: An in vitro approach. *SpringerPlus* **2014**, *3*, 346. [CrossRef] [PubMed]
42. Vekiru, E.; Fruhauf, S.; Sahin, M.; Ottner, F.; Schatzmayr, G.; Krska, R. Investigation of various adsorbents for their ability to bind aflatoxin B1. *Mycotoxin Res.* **2007**, *23*, 27–33. [CrossRef] [PubMed]
43. Barrientos-Velázquez, A.; Arteaga, S.; Dixon, J.; Deng, Y. The effects of pH, pepsin, exchange cation, and vitamins on aflatoxin adsorption on smectite in simulated gastric fluids. *Appl. Clay Sci.* **2016**, *120*, 17–23. [CrossRef]
44. De Paiva, L.; Morales, A.; Valenzuela Díaz, F. Organoclays: Properties, preparation and applications. *Appl. Clay Sci.* **2008**, *42*, 8–24. [CrossRef]
45. Elliott, C.; Connolly, L.; Kolawole, O. Potential adverse effects on animal health and performance caused by the addition of mineral adsorbents to feeds to reduce mycotoxin exposure. *Mycotoxin Res.* **2019**. [CrossRef] [PubMed]
46. Joannis-Cassan, C.; Tozlovanu, M.; Hadjeba-Medjdoub, K.; Ballet, N.; Pfohl-Leszkowicz, A. Binding of zearalenone, aflatoxin B1, and ochratoxin A by yeast-based products: A method for quantification of adsorption performance. *J. Food Prot.* **2011**, *74*, 1175–1185. [CrossRef] [PubMed]
47. Faucet-Marquis, V.; Joannis-Cassan, C.; Hadjeba-Medjdoub, K.; Ballet, N.; Pfohl-Leszkowicz, A. Development of an in vitro method for the prediction of mycotoxin binding on yeast-based products: Case of aflatoxin B1, zearalenone and ochratoxin A. *Appl. Microbiol. Biotechnol.* **2014**, *98*, 7583–7596. [CrossRef] [PubMed]
48. Firmin, S.; Morgavi, D.; Yiannikouris, A.; Boudra, H. Effectiveness of modified yeast cell wall extracts to reduce aflatoxin B1 absorption in dairy ewes. *J. Dairy Sci.* **2011**, *94*, 5611–5619. [CrossRef] [PubMed]
49. Jouany, J. Methods for preventing, decontaminating and minimizing the toxicity of mycotoxins in feeds. *Anim. Feed Sci. Technol.* **2007**, *137*, 342–362. [CrossRef]
50. Ringot, D.; Lerzy, B.; Chaplain, K.; Bonhoure, J.; Auclair, E.; Larondelle, Y. In vitro biosorption of ochratoxin A on the yeast industry by-products: Comparison of isotherm models. *Bioresour. Technol.* **2007**, *98*, 1812–1821. [CrossRef] [PubMed]
51. Yiannikouris, A.; André, G.; Poughon, L.; François, J.; Dussap, C.; Jeminet, G. Chemical and conformational study of the interactions involved in mycotoxin complexation with β-d-Glucans. *Biomacromolecules* **2006**, *7*, 1147–1155. [CrossRef] [PubMed]
52. Ralla, K.; Sohling, U.; Riechers, D.; Kasper, C.; Ruf, F.; Scheper, T. Adsorption and separation of proteins by a smectitic clay mineral. *Bioprocess Biosyst. Eng.* **2010**, *33*, 847–861. [CrossRef] [PubMed]
53. Alam, S.; Deng, Y. Protein interference on aflatoxin B1 adsorption by smectites in corn fermentation solution. *Appl. Clay Sci.* **2017**, *144*, 36–44. [CrossRef]
54. González-Jartín, J.; de Castro Alves, L.; Alfonso, A.; Piñeiro, Y.; Vilar, S.; Gomez, M.; Vargas, Z.; María, O.; Mercedes, J.; Vieytesd, R.; et al. Detoxification agents based on magnetic nanostructured particles as a novel strategy for mycotoxin mitigation in food. *Food Chem.* **2019**, *294*, 60–66. [CrossRef] [PubMed]
55. Hailu, S.; Nair, B.; Redi-Abshiro, M.; Diaz, I.; Tessema, M. Preparation and characterization of cationic surfactant modified zeolite adsorbent material for adsorption of organic and inorganic industrial pollutants. *J. Environ. Chem. Eng.* **2017**, *5*, 3319–3329. [CrossRef]
56. Oplatowska-Stachowiak, M.; Haughey, S.; Chevallier, O.; Galvin-King, P.; Campbell, K.; Magowan, E. Determination of the mycotoxin content in distiller's dried grain with soluble using a multianalyte UHPLC–MS/MS method. *J. Agric. Food Chem.* **2015**, *63*, 9441–9451. [CrossRef] [PubMed]

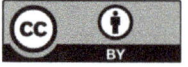

© 2019 by the authors. Licensee MDPI, Basel, Switzerland. This article is an open access article distributed under the terms and conditions of the Creative Commons Attribution (CC BY) license (http://creativecommons.org/licenses/by/4.0/).

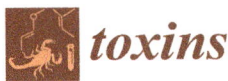

Article

Efficacy of a Yeast Cell Wall Extract to Mitigate the Effect of Naturally Co-Occurring Mycotoxins Contaminating Feed Ingredients Fed to Young Pigs: Impact on Gut Health, Microbiome, and Growth

Sung Woo Kim [1],*, Débora Muratori Holanda [1], Xin Gao [1], Inkyung Park [1] and Alexandros Yiannikouris [2]

[1] Department of Animal Science, North Carolina State University, Raleigh, NC 27695, USA; dmurato@ncsu.edu (D.M.H.); xgao@ncsu.edu (X.G.); ipark2@ncsu.edu (I.P.)
[2] Alltech Inc, Center for Animal Nutrigenomics and Applied Animal Nutrition, 3031 Catnip Hill Road, Nicholasville, KY 40356, USA; ayiannikouris@alltech.com
* Correspondence: sungwoo_kim@ncsu.edu

Received: 28 September 2019; Accepted: 28 October 2019; Published: 31 October 2019

Abstract: Mycotoxins are produced by fungi and are potentially toxic to pigs. Yeast cell wall extract (YCWE) is known to adsorb mycotoxins and improve gut health in pigs. One hundred and twenty growing (56 kg; experiment 1) and 48 nursery piglets (6 kg; experiment 2) were assigned to four dietary treatments in a 2 × 2 factorial design for 35 and 48 days, respectively. Factors were mycotoxins (no addition versus experiment 1: 180 µg/kg aflatoxins and 14 mg/kg fumonisins; or experiment 2: 180 µg/kg aflatoxins and 9 mg/kg fumonisins, and 1 mg/kg deoxynivalenol) and YCWE (0% versus 0.2%). Growth performance, blood, gut health and microbiome, and apparent ileal digestibility (AID) data were evaluated. In experiment 1, mycotoxins reduced ADG and G:F, and duodenal IgG, whereas in jejunum, YCWE increased IgG and reduced villus width. In experiment 2, mycotoxins reduced BW, ADG, and ADFI. Mycotoxins reduced ADG, which was recovered by YCWE. Mycotoxins reduced the AID of nutrients evaluated and increased protein carbonyl, whereas mycotoxins and YCWE increased the AID of the nutrients and reduced protein carbonyl. Mycotoxins reduced villus height, proportion of Ki-67-positive cells, and increased IgA and the proportion of bacteria with mycotoxin-degrading ability, whereas YCWE tended to increase villus height and reduced IgA and the proportion of pathogenic bacteria in jejunum. The YCWE effects were more evident in promoting gut health and growth in nursery pigs, which showed higher susceptibility to mycotoxin effects.

Keywords: mycotoxin; prevention; reduction strategies

Key Contribution: The current study suggests that susceptibility of pigs to mycotoxins depends on their ages and health status of gastrointestinal and immune systems. The YCWE showed a protective role against mycotoxins, improving pig growth and health mainly in nursery pigs in comparison to growing pigs.

1. Introduction

Mycotoxins are toxic secondary metabolites produced by certain species of fungi growing on cereal grains and feedstuffs [1]. Cereal grains such as corn, sorghum, and wheat have been used in the United States as the main feedstuffs in swine production. However, these feedstuffs are frequently contaminated with several types of co-occurring mycotoxins and contribute significantly to the overall contamination in compound feeds and potential impact on animal performance and health. Amongst hundreds of mycotoxins potentially contaminating feedstuffs, the response in pigs to the presence of aflatoxin B1 (AFB1), deoxynivalenol (DON), and fumonisin B1 (FB1) has been well documented [1]. Mycotoxicosis can impact gut health, alter immune function, and susceptibility of the animal to other contaminants or pathogens causing organ damage in pigs. The harmful effects of mycotoxin eventually lead to reduced growth performance of pigs [1–4].

Although feeding pigs without mycotoxins is the ultimate approach to counteract their impact, mycotoxin contamination in feeds is unavoidable [5]. In the United States, the Food and Drug Administration (FDA) limits aflatoxins (AF) concentration for immature pigs at 20 µg/kg of feed. For DON and fumonisins (FUM), there is no upper limit, but the FDA has advisory levels of 1 mg/kg of feed and 2 mg/kg of feed for DON and FUM, respectively. Therefore, various strategies to reduce mycotoxicosis have been investigated in pig production. Adsorbents have been used to mitigate mycotoxicosis by directly decreasing the mycotoxin bioavailability, and consequently, by indirectly reducing the inflammatory response, improving intestinal health, and by preventing oxidative stress [1–4]. Organic adsorbents, such as yeast cell wall and algae-based carbohydrates have shown that their ß-D-glucans composition and tridimensional network were able to chemically adsorb mycotoxins in vitro [6–9], reduce the absorption of mycotoxins in the small intestine [10], decrease the accumulation of mycotoxins in specific organs, and increase their clearance [11], thus protecting the vital organs against mycotoxin exposure. Thus, it is hypothesized that yeast cell wall extract (YCWE) supplementation might mitigate the adverse effects of pig diets naturally contaminated with mycotoxins.

The objective of this study was to determine the effects of YCWE (Mycosorb™ A+, Alltech, KY, USA) derived from the cell wall of *Saccharomyces cerevisiae* and a heterotrophically grown microalgae on the growth performances and gut health variables, such as gut integrity and permeability, oxidative stress, immune response, and microbiome in pigs fed diets with naturally contaminated mycotoxins (AFB1, DON, and FB1).

2. Results

2.1. Experiment 1

2.1.1. Growth Performance

There were no effects of mycotoxins, YCWE, or interaction in body weights of pigs during the first 7 days (Table 1). From day 7 to 14, feeding diets with mycotoxins tended to reduce ($p = 0.099$) body weight, but this trend did not continue during the later periods. From day 21 to 35, there were no effects of mycotoxins, YCWE, or interaction in body weights of pigs.

During the first 7 days, feeding diets with mycotoxins reduced ($p < 0.05$) average daily gain (ADG) and feeding diets with YCWE tended to reduce ($p = 0.088$) ADG. However, there were no effects of mycotoxins, YCWE, or interaction in ADG of pigs after the first 7 days. There were no effects of mycotoxins, YCWE, or interaction in average daily feed intake (ADFI) of pigs until day 28, whereas feeding diets with YCWE tended to further reduce ($p = 0.073$) the ADFI of pigs during days 28 to 35. Feeding diets with mycotoxins reduced ($p < 0.05$) the gain to feed ratio (G:F) of pigs during the first 7 days, whereas it tended to increase ($p = 0.098$) G:F during days 14 to 21. During the entire 35-day period, there were no effects of mycotoxins, YCWE, or interaction in ADG, ADFI, and G:F of pigs.

Table 1. Growth performance of pigs fed diets with mycotoxins (MT) and yeast cell wall extract (YCWE[1]) (YC) in experiment 1.

Mycotoxins (MT)	-		+			p Value		
YCWE (YC)	0%	0.2%	0%	0.2%	SEM	MT	YC	MT × YC
Body Weight, kg								
Initial	55.7	55.6	55.7	55.8	3.1	0.687	0.929	0.608
Day 7	59.7	58.8	58.8	58.6	3.6	0.151	0.176	0.405
Day 14	68.9	68.0	67.8	67.2	3.8	0.099	0.178	0.758
Day 21	75.8	74.7	74.7	74.8	4.1	0.444	0.409	0.335
Day 28	82.5	80.8	81.2	82.1	4.3	0.547	0.262	0.197
Day 35	90.5	88.3	88.5	88.4	4.5	0.255	0.205	0.228
ADG[2], kg								
Day 0 to 7	1.342	1.078	1.047	0.937	0.211	0.048	0.088	0.470
Day 7 to 14	1.311	1.303	1.282	1.229	0.054	0.271	0.506	0.626
Day 14 to 21	0.985	0.956	0.987	1.083	0.118	0.221	0.520	0.231
Day 21 to 28	0.963	0.880	0.928	0.933	0.067	0.879	0.492	0.442
Day 28 to 35	1.142	1.074	1.037	1.012	0.105	0.220	0.484	0.745
Overall	1.124	1.055	1.057	1.052	0.071	0.201	0.178	0.249
ADFI[3], kg								
Day 0 to 7	2.733	2.502	2.597	2.579	0.142	0.788	0.256	0.330
Day 7 to 14	3.075	2.825	2.828	2.847	0.170	0.174	0.166	0.107
Day 14 to 21	2.889	2.774	2.813	2.785	0.232	0.741	0.472	0.659
Day 21 to 28	2.588	2.606	2.430	2.683	0.233	0.781	0.358	0.421
Day 28 to 35	3.093	2.828	2.872	2.672	0.252	0.145	0.073	0.796
Overall	2.894	2.733	2.713	2.721	0.183	0.165	0.272	0.225
G:F[4]								
Day 0 to 7	0.472	0.423	0.396	0.364	0.064	0.044	0.216	0.798
Day 7 to 14	0.434	0.461	0.457	0.435	0.024	0.925	0.896	0.151
Day 14 to 21	0.340	0.346	0.353	0.390	0.022	0.098	0.209	0.372
Day 21 to 28	0.381	0.344	0.390	0.355	0.026	0.683	0.137	0.960
Day 28 to 35	0.369	0.382	0.358	0.379	0.019	0.697	0.339	0.788
Overall	0.389	0.388	0.390	0.387	0.007	0.937	0.627	0.865

[1] YCWE: yeast cell wall extract; [2] ADG: average daily gain; [3] ADFI: average daily feed intake; [4] G:F: gain to feed ratio. MT-: diet without aflatoxin B1 and fumonisin B1; MT+: inclusion of 180 µg/kg aflatoxin B1 and 14 mg/kg fumonisin B1 by replacing the clean corn with naturally mycotoxin-contaminated corn; YC 0%: no addition of YCWE (Mycosorb A+, Alltech, Nicholasville, KY, USA); YC 0.2%: YCWE added at 2 g/kg of feed.

2.1.2. Hematological Measurements

Feeding diets with mycotoxins reduced ($p < 0.05$) neutrophils blood levels on day 28 (Table 2). Feeding diets with YCWE did not influence cell counts in blood on day 28. There was a tendency ($p = 0.099$) for an interaction between feeding diets with mycotoxins and with YCWE in the lymphocyte count in blood, indicating that YCWE tended to increase ($p < 0.10$) lymphocyte count in pigs fed diets without mycotoxins, whereas this tendency disappeared when mycotoxins were introduced. There were no effects of mycotoxins, YCWE, or interaction in red or white blood cells, hemoglobin, hematocrit, mean corpuscular volume, mean corpuscular hemoglobin, mean corpuscular hemoglobin concentration, platelet, monocytes, eosinophils, or basophils of pigs.

Table 2. Cell counts in blood of pigs fed diets with mycotoxins (MT) and YCWE[1] (YC) on day 28 in experiment 1.

Mycotoxins (MT)	-	-	+	+		p Value		
YCWE (YC)	0%	0.2%	0%	0.2%	SEM	MT	YC	MT × YC
RBC[2], 10⁶/µL	6.84	6.90	7.05	6.80	0.23	0.687	0.601	0.387
Hemoglobin, g/dL	12.43	12.48	12.64	11.95	0.45	0.709	0.317	0.254
Hematocrit, %	40.91	40.63	41.05	38.79	1.38	0.495	0.189	0.317
MCV[3], fL	59.70	58.70	58.39	57.22	1.19	0.124	0.286	0.988
MCH[4], pg	18.22	18.12	17.96	17.62	0.36	0.217	0.527	0.755
MCHC[5], g/dL	30.47	30.81	30.79	30.79	0.21	0.492	0.420	0.412
Platelet count, mL	185.9	144.0	133.7	152.4	27.1	0.394	0.618	0.237
WBC[6], 10³/µL	20.52	21.43	19.91	18.83	1.36	0.236	0.950	0.470
Neutrophils, cell/mL	7.89	6.66	5.89	5.77	0.72	0.003	0.139	0.225
Lymphocytes, cell/mL	10.97^A	13.05^B	12.47^{AB}	11.30^{AB}	0.97	0.868	0.614	0.099
Monocytes, cell/mL	1.04	1.13	0.96	1.13	0.15	0.777	0.397	0.781
Eosinophils, cell/µL	543	499	518	484	84	0.812	0.636	0.949
Basophils, cell/µL	109	128	130	66	45	0.585	0.545	0.271

[1] YCWE: yeast cell wall extract; [2] RBC: red blood cells; [3] MCV: mean corpuscular volume; [4] MCH: mean corpuscular hemoglobin; [5] MCHC: mean corpuscular hemoglobin concentration; [6] WBC: white blood cells. MT-: diet without aflatoxin B1 and fumonisin B1; MT+: inclusion of 180 µg/kg aflatoxin B1 and 14 mg/kg fumonisin B1 by replacing the clean corn with naturally mycotoxin-contaminated corn; YC 0%: no addition of YCWE (Mycosorb A+, Alltech, Nicholasville, KY, USA); YC 0.2%: YCWE added at 2 g/kg of feed. ^{AB} Means within a row lacking a common superscript tend to differ ($0.05 \leq p < 0.1$).

2.1.3. Serum Biochemical Measurements

Feeding diets with mycotoxins increased ($p < 0.05$) serum albumin concentration of pigs, and there was a tendency ($p = 0.074$) for an interaction between feeding diets with mycotoxins and with YCWE for albumin on day 28 (Table 3). Feeding diets with YCWE reduced serum albumin in pigs fed diets without mycotoxins, whereas feeding diets with YCWE increased serum albumin in pigs fed diets with mycotoxins. There were no effects of mycotoxins, YCWE, or interaction in globulin, albumin-to-globulin ratio, total protein, or most hepatic enzymes evaluated (aspartate aminotransferase, alanine aminotransferase, and creatine phosphokinase) in serum of pigs. Feeding diets with mycotoxins tended to increase ($p = 0.098$) alkaline phosphatase, tended to reduce ($p = 0.088$) blood urea nitrogen (BUN), and tended to increase ($p = 0.051$) glucose in serum of pigs. Feeding diets with mycotoxins decreased ($p < 0.05$) cholesterol level in serum of pigs. There were no effects of mycotoxins, YCWE, or interaction in creatinine or BUN-to-creatinine ratio in serum of pigs. Feeding diets with YCWE tended to increase chloride ($p = 0.081$) and sodium ($p = 0.064$) in serum. Feeding diets with mycotoxins tended to decrease ($p = 0.064$) potassium and tended to increase ($p = 0.053$) sodium-to-potassium ratio in serum. There were no effects of mycotoxins, YCWE, or interaction in calcium levels of pigs.

Table 3. Hematological measurements in serum of pigs fed diets with mycotoxins (MT) and YCWE[1] (YC) on day 28 in experiment 1.

Mycotoxins (MT)	-	-	+	+		p Value		
YCWE (YC)	0%	0.2%	0%	0.2%	SEM	MT	YC	MT × YC
Total protein, g/dL	6.44	6.18	6.49	6.36	0.12	0.309	0.090	0.573
Albumin, g/dL	3.60	3.48	3.62	3.73	0.08	0.042	0.950	0.074
Globulin, g/dL	2.84	2.70	2.87	2.66	0.11	0.948	0.106	0.731
A to G ratio[2]	1.28	1.29	1.27	1.40	0.06	0.389	0.231	0.319
AST[3], U/L	23.25	27.88	22.72	20.36	2.71	0.111	0.712	0.144
ALT[4], U/L	19.38	20.63	20.03	17.83	1.76	0.507	0.769	0.291
ALP[5], U/L	132	143	149	157	10	0.098	0.301	0.947
CPK[6], U/L	1,230	1,749	1,119	1,358	254	0.287	0.113	0.552
BUN[7], mg/dL	14.75	13.75	13.08	12.33	1.84	0.088	0.336	0.868
Creatinine, mg/dL	1.30	1.40	1.30	1.25	0.08	0.197	0.629	0.189
BUN-to-creatinine ratio	11.50	10.25	10.07	10.34	1.85	0.385	0.526	0.330
Cholesterol, mg/dL	86.13	85.25	79.89	74.29	3.65	0.019	0.354	0.497
Glucose, mg/dL	72.50	77.13	82.90	79.27	4.14	0.051	0.873	0.189
Ca, mg/dL	10.59	10.54	10.66	10.76	0.13	0.232	0.821	0.519
Cl, mEq/L	100.6	101.5	100.0	101.1	0.86	0.384	0.081	0.807
Na, mEq/L	145.4	147.5	145.8	146.0	0.65	0.374	0.064	0.129
K, mEq/L	5.28	5.35	5.06	4.95	0.22	0.064	0.914	0.566
Na to K ratio	27.63	27.75	28.96	29.90	1.06	0.053	0.553	0.652
P, mg/dL	9.16	9.03	8.82	8.86	0.16	0.100	0.721	0.577

[1] YCWE: yeast cell wall extract; [2] A to G ratio: albumin to globulin ratio; [3] AST: aspartate aminotransferase; [4] ALT: alanine aminotransferase; [5] ALP: alkaline phosphatase; [6] CPK: creatine phosphokinase; and [7] BUN: blood urea N. MT-: diet without aflatoxin B1 and fumonisin B1; MT+: inclusion of 180 µg/kg aflatoxin B1 and 14 mg/kg fumonisin B1 by replacing the clean corn with naturally mycotoxin-contaminated corn; YC 0%: no addition of YCWE (Mycosorb A+, Alltech, Nicholasville, KY, USA); YC 0.2%: YCWE added at 2 g/kg of feed.

2.1.4. Immunological and Oxidative Stress Measurements

No effects of mycotoxins, YCWE, or interaction were found in the concentrations of tumor necrosis factor-alpha (TNF-α) in duodenal and jejunal mucosa as well as in serum of pigs (Table 4). Feeding diets with mycotoxins increased ($p < 0.05$) duodenal immunoglobulin G (IgG). Feeding diets with YCWE reduced ($p < 0.05$) serum 8-hydroxy-2′-deoxyguanosine (8-OHdG) of pigs. For instance, in pigs fed diets with mycotoxins, there was a reduction of the levels of serum 8-OHdG down to 0.26 ng/mL when YCWE was included, whereas when no YCWE was added, there was increased oxidation with up to 1.66 ng/mL of 8-OHdG. There was an interaction ($p < 0.05$) between mycotoxins and YCWE, where a reduced ($p < 0.05$) jejunal IgG concentration was observed in pigs fed diets with mycotoxins with the addition of YCWE, whereas feeding with YCWE increased ($p < 0.05$) jejunal IgG levels in animals not challenged with mycotoxins. A tendency ($p = 0.096$) for an interaction was observed for serum IgG, indicating that YCWE increased ($p < 0.05$) serum IgG concentration in pigs, whereas this effect disappeared when mycotoxins were introduced. No effects of mycotoxins, YCWE, or interaction were observed on oxidative stress, concentrations of malondialdehydes (MDA) in duodenal and jejunal mucosa or in serum of pigs.

Table 4. Immunological and oxidative stress parameters in duodenal and jejunal mucosa and serum of pigs fed diets with mycotoxins (MT) and YCWE[1] (YC) in experiment 1.

Mycotoxins (MT)	-	-	+	+		p Value		
YCWE (YC)	0%	0.2%	0%	0.2%	SEM	MT	YC	MT × YC
Immunological Parameters								
Duodenal TNF-α[2], pg/mg protein	8.79	6.96	8.69	8.91	0.81	0.261	0.331	0.217
Jejunal TNF-α, pg/mg protein	6.56	5.53	5.36	5.80	0.75	0.490	0.659	0.281
Serumal TNF-α, pg/mL	183	187	169	173	11	0.206	0.726	0.959
Duodenal IgG[3], μg/mg protein	2.77	4.26	5.36	4.61	0.71	0.049	0.605	0.128
Jejunal IgG, μg/mg protein	1.75 [a]	2.95 [b]	2.96 [b]	2.40 [ab]	0.37	0.255	0.274	0.005
Serumal IgG, mg/mL	7.92	8.04	9.49	7.75	0.85	0.240	0.143	0.096
Oxidative Stress Parameters								
Duodenal MDA[4], nmol/mg protein	0.82	0.73	0.68	0.96	0.12	0.701	0.415	0.123
Jejunal MDA, nmol/mg protein	1.14	1.20	0.99	1.08	0.38	0.561	0.747	0.959
Serumal MDA, μM	15.94	14.74	15.80	15.22	5.39	0.915	0.575	0.845
Serumal 8-OHdG[5], ng/mL	1.29	0.93	1.66	0.26	0.49	0.737	0.049	0.235

[1] YCWE: yeast cell wall extract; [2] TNF-α: tumor necrosis factor-alpha; [3] IgG: immunoglobulin G; [4] MDA: malondialdehydes; [5] 8-OHdG: 8-hydroxy-2'-deoxyguanosine. MT-: diet without aflatoxin B1 and fumonisin B1; MT+: inclusion of 180 μg/kg aflatoxin B1 and 14 mg/kg fumonisin B1 by replacing the clean corn with naturally mycotoxin-contaminated corn; YC 0%: no addition of YCWE (Mycosorb A+, Alltech, Nicholasville, KY, USA); YC 0.2%: YCWE added at 2 g/kg of feed. [ab] Means within a row lacking a common superscript differ ($p < 0.05$).

2.1.5. Histomorphometry of Duodenum and Jejunum

There were no effects of mycotoxins, YCWE, or interaction on villus height or villus width in duodenum of pigs (Table 5). Feeding diets with YCWE showed a tendency ($p = 0.051$) for reducing crypt depth in duodenum histomorphometry. No effects of mycotoxins, YCWE, or interaction were observed on villus height-to-crypt depth ratio in duodenum of pigs. Feeding diets with YCWE reduced ($p < 0.05$) villus width in jejunum. There were no effects of mycotoxins, YCWE, or interaction on villus height, crypt depth, and villus height-to-crypt depth ratio in jejunum of pigs.

Table 5. Intestinal morphology of pigs fed diets with mycotoxins (MT) and YCWE[1] (YC) in experiment 1.

Mycotoxins (MT)	-	-	+	+		p Value		
YCWE (YC)	0%	0.2%	0%	0.2%	SEM	MT	YC	MT × YC
Duodenum								
Villus height (VH), μm	516	484	498	491	19	0.770	0.306	0.509
Villus width, μm	115	112	111	108	5.8	0.323	0.442	1.000
Crypt depth (CD), μm	295	253	275	268	13	0.840	0.051	0.141
VH to CD ratio	1.77	1.93	1.83	1.83	0.08	0.761	0.192	0.233
Jejunum								
Villus height, μm	482	495	495	495	36	0.845	0.845	0.842
Villus width, μm	119	101	116	108	5.3	0.685	0.018	0.324
Crypt depth, μm	238	235	243	245	8.9	0.368	0.950	0.798
VH-to-CD ratio	2.04	2.11	2.05	2.01	0.16	0.758	0.899	0.646

[1] YCWE: yeast cell wall extract. MT-: diet without aflatoxin B1 and fumonisin B1; MT+: inclusion of 180 μg/kg aflatoxin B1 and 14 mg/kg fumonisin B1 by replacing the clean corn with naturally mycotoxin-contaminated corn; YC 0%: no addition of YCWE (Mycosorb A+, Alltech, Nicholasville, KY, USA); YC 0.2%: YCWE added at 2 g/kg of feed.

2.2. Experiment 2

2.2.1. Growth Performance

There were no effects of mycotoxins, YCWE, or interaction on body weight of pigs during the first 5 days among pigs in treatment groups (Table 6). Feeding diets with mycotoxins tended to reduce ($p = 0.079$) pig body weight at day 15 and significantly reduced ($p < 0.05$) pig body weight in all periods between days 20 and 48. Feeding diets with YCWE showed a tendency ($p = 0.057$) for reducing body weight of pig on days 10 and 20, and significantly decreased ($p < 0.05$) pig body weight on day 15. Feeding diets with mycotoxins tended to decrease ($p = 0.020$) ADG of pigs from day 10 to 15 and significantly reduced ($p < 0.05$) ADG from day 15 to 20, as well as for all periods between days 20 and 48. Feeding diets with YCWE decreased ($p < 0.05$) ADG from day 0 to 5, from day 5 to 10, and for the phase 1 period. There were no effects of mycotoxins, YCWE, or interaction on ADG of pigs from 20 to 27 days. There was a tendency ($p = 0.096$) for an interaction on ADG of pigs from 27 to 34 days, indicating that mycotoxins tended to reduce ADG but the tendency disappeared with YCWE addition. There was an interaction ($p < 0.05$) on pig ADG from day 34 to 41, indicating that mycotoxins reduced ADG but YCWE successfully recovered ADG reduction. Feeding diets with mycotoxins reduced ($p < 0.05$) ADG of pigs for all periods from day 27 until the end of the experimental period, phase 2, and the overall period. Feeding diets with YCWE reduced ($p < 0.05$) ADFI of pigs for the periods evaluated during the first 15 days of the study and tended to decrease ($p = 0.065$) ADFI during phase 1. Feeding diets with mycotoxins reduced ($p < 0.05$) ADFI of pigs for all periods from day 5 to the end of the study, for phase 1, phase 2, and the overall periods. Feeding diets with YCWE tended to lower ($p = 0.054$) G:F for the first 5 days of the study. There was a tendency ($p = 0.054$) for an interaction from day 5 to 10, where feeding diets with mycotoxins alone tended to increase G:F, whereas feeding diets with mycotoxins and YCWE tended to reduce G:F of pigs. There were no effects of mycotoxins, YCWE, or interaction for G:F from day 10 to 34 or for phase 1 of pigs. Feeding diets with mycotoxins tended to increase ($p = 0.078$) G:F of pigs from day 41 to 48, and significantly increased ($p < 0.05$) G:F during phase 2 and the overall periods. Feeding diets with YCWE increased ($p < 0.05$) G:F of pigs from day 35 to 48, as well as for phase 2, and tended to increase ($p = 0.079$) G:F in the overall period.

Table 6. Growth performance of weanling pigs fed diets with mycotoxins (MT) and YCWE[1] (YC) in experiment 2.

Mycotoxins (MT)	-		+			p Value		
YCWE (YC)	0%	0.2%	0%	0.2%	SEM	MT	YC	MT × YC
Body Weight, kg								
Initial	6.0	6.0	6.0	6.0	0.2	1.000	0.632	0.905
Day 5	6.1	5.9	5.9	5.9	0.3	0.364	0.258	0.569
Day 10	6.9	6.7	6.8	6.4	0.3	0.293	0.057	0.473
Day 15	8.5	8.1	8.2	7.6	0.4	0.079	0.037	0.779
Day 20	10.8	10.3	10.2	9.3	0.4	0.030	0.066	0.638
Day 27	14.5	14.3	13.7	14.4	0.6	0.017	0.156	0.327
Day 34	19.6	18.6	17.4	16.4	0.7	0.001	0.129	0.940
Day 41	25.4	24.3	22.2	22.0	0.8	<0.001	0.370	0.514
Day 48	31.7	30.4	27.6	27.9	1.0	<0.001	0.589	0.348
ADG[2], kg								
Day 0 to 5	0.017	−0.017	−0.008	−0.024	0.014	0.205	0.048	0.489
Day 5 to 10	0.165	0.155	0.180	0.104	0.021	0.390	0.047	0.122
Day 10 to 15	0.321	0.278	0.265	0.243	0.029	0.082	0.210	0.673
Day 15 to 20	0.462	0.445	0.403	0.343	0.033	0.020	0.249	0.527
Day 20 to 27	0.529	0.567	0.506	0.444	0.044	0.103	0.783	0.259
Day 27 to 34	0.728 [A]	0.614 [AB]	0.521 [B]	0.569 [AB]	0.047	0.011	0.488	0.096
Day 34 to 41	0.831 [a]	0.819 [a]	0.686 [b]	0.795 [a]	0.034	0.006	0.110	0.045
Day 41 to 48	0.895	0.876	0.778	0.852	0.036	0.046	0.420	0.180
Phase 1 (day 0 to 20)	0.241	0.215	0.210	0.166	0.017	0.025	0.048	0.612
Phase 2 (day 20 to 48)	0.746	0.719	0.623	0.665	0.024	0.001	0.750	0.151
Overall	0.494	0.467	0.416	0.416	0.017	<0.001	0.420	0.440
ADFI[3], kg								
Day 0 to 5	0.083 [c]	0.053 [d]	0.066	0.049	0.008	0.212	0.005	0.403
Day 5 to 10	0.234	0.201	0.201	0.145	0.019	0.027	0.027	0.564
Day 10 to 15	0.433	0.402	0.372	0.303	0.024	0.002	0.039	0.428
Day 15 to 20	0.642	0.625	0.523	0.488	0.039	0.001	0.475	0.805
Day 20 to 27	0.786	0.805	0.643	0.630	0.043	<0.001	0.944	0.722
Day 27 to 34	1.060	0.944	0.783	0.789	0.056	<0.001	0.328	0.281
Day 34 to 41	1.245	1.136	1.036	1.046	0.064	0.010	0.327	0.284
Day 41 to 48	1.529	1.406	1.275	1.262	0.055	<0.001	0.156	0.245

Table 6. Cont.

Mycotoxins (MT)	-		+			p Value		
YCWE (YC)	0%	0.2%	0%	0.2%	SEM	MT	YC	MT × YC
Phase 1 (day 0 to 20)	0.348	0.320	0.291	0.247	0.019	0.001	0.065	0.679
Phase 2 (day 20 to 48)	1.155	1.073	0.934	0.932	0.042	<0.001	0.301	0.324
Overall	0.752	0.700	0.613	0.589	0.028	<0.001	0.149	0.554
G:F[4]								
Day 0 to 5	−0.043	−1.346	−0.299	−1.109	0.542	0.986	0.054	0.646
Day 5 to 10	0.718	0.769	0.873 [A]	0.632 [B]	0.074	0.904	0.210	0.055
Day 10 to 15	0.732	0.693	0.721	0.806	0.061	0.352	0.678	0.256
Day 15 to 20	0.731	0.705	0.771	0.709	0.036	0.547	0.226	0.632
Day 20 to 27	0.666	0.695	0.791	0.703	0.045	0.140	0.501	0.190
Day 27 to 34	0.689	0.640	0.663	0.716	0.034	0.447	0.949	0.117
Day 34 to 41	0.675	0.731	0.663	0.769	0.022	0.547	<0.001	0.263
Day 41 to 48	0.587	0.626	0.604	0.678	0.019	0.078	0.006	0.366
Phase 1 (day 0 to 20)	0.693	0.666	0.716	0.673	0.032	0.579	0.186	0.766
Phase 2 (day 20 to 48)	0.649	0.673	0.666	0.717	0.012	0.016	0.003	0.287
Overall	0.660	0.673	0.679	0.708	0.012	0.023	0.079	0.495

[1] YCWE: yeast cell wall extract; [2] ADG: average daily gain; [3] ADFI: average daily feed intake; [4] G:F: gain to feed ration. MT-: diet without aflatoxin B1 and fumonisin B1; MT+: inclusion of 180 μg/kg aflatoxin B1, 1 mg/kg deoxynivalenol, and 9 mg/kg fumonisin B1 by replacing the clean corn and clean wheat with naturally mycotoxin-contaminated corn and wheat; YC 0%: no addition of YCWE (Mycosorb A+, Alltech, Nicholasville, KY, USA); YC 0.2%: YCWE added at 2 g/kg of feed. [ab] Means within a row lacking a common superscript differ ($p < 0.05$). [AB] Means within a row lacking a common superscript tend to differ ($0.05 \leq p < 0.1$).

2.2.2. Apparent Ileal Digestibility

There were no effects of mycotoxins, YCWE, or interaction for dry matter apparent ileal digestibility of pigs (Table 7). There was a tendency ($p = 0.091$) for an interaction, where feeding diets with mycotoxins alone reduced ($p < 0.05$) apparent ileal digestibility of crude protein, whereas feeding diets with mycotoxins and YCWE increased ($p < 0.05$) apparent ileal digestibility of crude protein of pigs. Similarly, there was a tendency ($p = 0.096$) for an interaction, where feeding diets with mycotoxins alone reduced ($p < 0.05$) apparent ileal digestibility of gross energy, whereas feeding diets with mycotoxins and YCWE increased ($p < 0.05$) apparent ileal digestibility of gross energy of pigs. There was an interaction ($p < 0.05$), where feeding diets with mycotoxins alone reduced ($p < 0.05$) apparent ileal digestibility of ether extract, whereas feeding diets with mycotoxins and YCWE increased ($p < 0.05$) apparent ileal digestibility of ether extract of pigs.

Table 7. Apparent ileal digestibility (AID) in weanling pigs fed diets with mycotoxins (MT) and YCWE[1] (YC) in experiment 2.

Mycotoxins (MT)	-		+			p Value		
YCWE (YC)	0%	0.2%	0%	0.2%	SEM	MT	YC	MT × YC
AID, %								
Dry matter	69.7	70.0	64.0	70.7	2.39	0.243	0.106	0.144
Crude protein	78.5	78.9	75.5 [b]	80.1 [a]	1.25	0.479	0.049	0.091
Gross energy	70.9 [AB]	70.9 [AB]	65.1 [B]	72.6 [A]	2.35	0.354	0.097	0.096
Ether extract	81.8 [ab]	80.8 [ab]	76.6 [b]	83.5 [a]	1.88	0.483	0.113	0.032

[1] YCWE: yeast cell wall extract. MT-: diet without aflatoxin B1 and fumonisin B1; MT+: inclusion of 180 μg/kg aflatoxin B1, 1 mg/kg deoxynivalenol, and 9 mg/kg fumonisin B1 by replacing the clean corn and clean wheat with naturally mycotoxin-contaminated corn and wheat; YC 0%: no addition of YCWE (Mycosorb A+, Alltech, Nicholasville, KY, USA); YC 0.2%: YCWE added at 2 g/kg of feed. [ab] Means within a row lacking a common superscript differs ($p < 0.05$). [AB] Means within a row lacking a common superscript tend to differ ($0.05 \leq p < 0.1$).

2.2.3. Hematological Measurements

There were no effects of mycotoxins, YCWE, or interaction for hematological measurements on day 14 of pigs, except for neutrophils, where feeding diets with mycotoxins decreased ($p < 0.05$) the concentration in blood (Table 8). Feeding diets with YCWE increased ($p < 0.05$) red blood cell count, whereas it tended to increase ($p = 0.071$) white blood cell count at 45 days. Feeding diets with mycotoxins tended to increase ($p = 0.052$) hemoglobin concentration, whereas feeding diets with YCWE tended to reduce ($p = 0.086$) hemoglobin concentration on day 45. Feeding diets with YCWE reduced ($p < 0.05$) the percentage of hematocrit on day 45. There were no effects of mycotoxins, YCWE, or interaction for mean corpuscular volume, mean corpuscular hemoglobin, or mean corpuscular hemoglobin concentration of pigs on day 45. Feeding diets with YCWE tended to lower ($p = 0.058$) platelet count on day 45. Feeding diets with YCWE decreased ($p < 0.05$) lymphocyte count on day 45. There were no effects of mycotoxins, YCWE, or interaction for monocyte or eosinophil concentrations of pigs on day 45.

Table 8. Hematology of weanling pigs fed diets containing mycotoxins (MT) and YCWE[1] (YC) on days 14 and 45 in experiment 2.

Mycotoxins (MT)	−	−	+	+		p Value		
YCWE (YC)	0%	0.2%	0%	0.2%	SEM	MT	YC	MT × YC
RBC[2], 10^6/μL								
Day 14	6.84	6.90	7.05	6.80	0.23	0.687	0.601	0.387
Day 45	6.86	6.30	6.91	6.68	0.17	0.194	0.023	0.313
Hemoglobin, g/dL								
Day 14	12.43	12.48	12.64	11.95	0.45	0.709	0.317	0.254
Day 45	12.11	11.51	12.53	12.18	0.27	0.052	0.086	0.659
Hematocrit, %								
Day 14	40.91	40.63	41.05	38.79	1.38	0.495	0.189	0.317
Day 45	41.58	38.92	42.33	40.17	1.15	0.392	0.043	0.830
MCV[3], fL								
Day 14	59.70	58.70	58.39	57.22	1.19	0.124	0.286	0.988
Day 45	60.50	61.75	61.25	60.25	0.85	0.660	0.883	0.192
MCH[4], pg								
Day 14	18.22	18.12	17.96	17.62	0.36	0.217	0.527	0.755
Day 45	17.67	18.31	18.14	18.32	0.25	0.330	0.104	0.347
MCHC[5], g/dL								
Day 14	30.47	30.81	30.79	30.79	0.21	0.492	0.420	0.412
Day 45	29.21	29.70	29.66	30.40	0.41	0.170	0.147	0.757
Platelet count, cell/mL								
Day 14	185.9	144.0	133.7	152.4	27.1	0.394	0.618	0.237
Day 45	230.4	174.0	220.3	154.1	31.4	0.635	0.058	0.876
WBC[6], 10^3/μL								
Day 14	20.52	21.43	19.91	18.83	1.36	0.236	0.950	0.470
Day 45	18.62	16.30	18.68	16.25	1.28	0.997	0.071	0.966
Neutrophils, cell/mL								
Day 14	7.89	6.66	5.89	5.77	0.72	0.003	0.139	0.225
Day 45	3.64	4.21	3.89	3.45	0.44	0.545	0.882	0.233
Lymphocytes, cell/mL								
Day 14	10.97	13.05	12.47	11.30	0.97	0.868	0.614	0.100
Day 45	13.33	9.96	12.96	11.37	1.19	0.662	0.042	0.452
Monocytes, cell/mL								
Day 14	1.04	1.13	0.96	1.13	0.15	0.777	0.397	0.781
Day 45	1.07	1.04	1.32	0.98	0.18	0.580	0.285	0.377
Eosinophils, cell/μL								
Day 14	543	499	518	484	84	0.812	0.636	0.949
Day 45	502	451	478	434	78	0.786	0.529	0.954

[1] YCWE: yeast cell wall extract; [2] RBC: red blood cells; [3] MCV: mean corpuscular volume; [4] MCH: mean corpuscular hemoglobin; [5] MCHC: mean corpuscular hemoglobin concentration; [6] WBC: white blood cells. MT−: diet without aflatoxin B1 and fumonisin B1; MT+: inclusion of 180 μg/kg aflatoxin B1, 1 mg/kg deoxynivalenol, and 9 mg/kg fumonisin B1 by replacing the clean corn and clean wheat with naturally mycotoxin-contaminated corn and wheat; YC 0%: no addition of YCWE (Mycosorb A+, Alltech, Nicholasville, KY, USA); YC 0.2%: YCWE added at 2 g/kg of feed.

2.2.4. Serum Biochemical Measurements

Feeding diets with mycotoxins tended to decrease ($p = 0.077$) total protein concentration in serum on day 45 (Table 9). Likewise, feeding diets with YCWE tended to reduce ($p = 0.077$) total protein concentration in serum at 45 days. Feeding diets with mycotoxins tended to increase ($p = 0.078$) albumin concentration on day 45 and to decrease ($p = 0.071$) globulin concentration on day 14. Feeding diets with mycotoxins increased ($p < 0.05$) the albumin-to-globulin ratio on day 14. There was an interaction ($p < 0.05$) for the albumin-to-globulin ratio on day 45, indicating that there was a reduction of the albumin-to-globulin ratio when YCWE was added for pigs fed diets with no mycotoxins. There was an interaction for cholesterol on day 45, indicating that there was a decrease in cholesterol level when pigs were fed diets with mycotoxins and YCWE, in comparison to when pigs were fed diets without mycotoxins but with YCWE. There was a tendency ($p = 0.067$) for an interaction for serum AST on day 14, indicating that YCWE tended to reduce serum AST in pigs fed diets with mycotoxins but the tendency disappeared in pigs fed diets without mycotoxins. Feeding diets with YCWE tended to decrease ($p = 0.091$) serum alkaline phosphatase on day 14. Feeding diets with mycotoxins increased ($p < 0.05$) creatinine concentration in serum on day 14. Feeding diets with mycotoxins reduced ($p < 0.05$) cholesterol in serum on day 14. Feeding diets with YCWE decreased ($p < 0.05$) calcium levels, tended to decrease ($p = 0.083$) sodium levels, and tended to increase ($p = 0.081$) chloride levels in serum on day 14. Feeding diets with mycotoxins tended to decrease ($p = 0.064$) potassium concentration and tended to increase ($p = 0.053$) sodium-to-potassium in serum on day 14. There were no effects of mycotoxins, YCWE, or interaction for alkaline phosphatase, BUN, BUN-to-creatinine ratio, phosphorus, glucose, and creatine phosphokinase in serum of pigs neither on day 14 nor 45.

Table 9. Biochemical blood assay of weanling pigs fed diets containing mycotoxins (MT) or and YCWE[1] (YC) on days 14 and 45 in experiment 2.

Mycotoxins (MT)	-	-	+	+		p Value		
YCWE (YC)	0%	0.2%	0%	0.2%	SEM	MT	YC	MT × YC
Total protein, g/dL								
Day 14	4.65	4.64	4.67	4.57	0.09	0.742	0.542	0.606
Day 45	5.18	5.14	5.14	4.87	0.110	0.077	0.077	0.163
Albumin, g/dL								
Day 14	2.65	2.58	2.70	2.69	0.06	0.164	0.506	0.605
Day 45	3.33	2.98	7.64	5.27	1.96	0.078	0.457	0.583
Globulin, g/dL								
Day 14	2.00	2.06	1.97	1.82	0.08	0.071	0.539	0.167
Day 45	1.84	3.50	3.88	1.78	1.16	0.895	0.850	0.114
Albumin to globulin ratio								
Day 14	1.34	1.27	1.42	1.51	0.06	0.012	0.891	0.175
Day 45	1.84 [a]	1.47 [b]	1.62 [ab]	1.76 [ab]	0.09	0.723	0.218	0.009
AST[2], U/L								
Day 14	33.92 [AB]	38.83 [AB]	41.42 [A]	32.42 [B]	3.69	0.884	0.583	0.067
Day 45	21.33	23.42	31.08	23.50	4.60	0.193	0.463	0.201
ALT[3], U/L								
Day 14	22.17	25.50	22.42	24.33	1.85	0.806	0.165	0.704
Day 45	22.08	21.50	22.17	28.75	2.30	0.120	0.201	0.128
ALP[4], U/L								
Day 14	381	352	375	332	21	0.535	0.091	0.718
Day 45	311	256	271	278	22	0.693	0.278	0.165
CPK[5], U/L								
Day 14	1230	1749	1119	1358	254	0.287	0.113	0.552
Day 45	1224	1161	1931	1454	403	0.223	0.508	0.610
BUN[6], mg/dL								
Day 14	15.42	17.75	16.50	17.67	1.61	0.751	0.270	0.711
Day 45	10.83	11.50	10.33	11.00	0.52	0.345	0.210	1.000

Table 9. Cont.

Mycotoxins (MT)	-		+			p Value		
YCWE (YC)	0%	0.2%	0%	0.2%	SEM	MT	YC	MT × YC
Creatinine, mg/dL								
Day 14	0.75	0.75	0.78	0.88	0.04	0.035	0.154	0.154
Day 45	0.88	0.89	0.89	0.82	0.04	0.351	0.351	0.245
BUN-to-creatinine ratio								
Day 14	20.42	24.08	21.33	20.42	2.09	0.455	0.455	0.216
Day 45	12.67	13.25	11.75	13.58	0.791	0.715	0.135	0.435
Cholesterol, mg/dL								
Day 14	86.13	85.25	79.89	74.29	3.65	0.019	0.354	0.497
Day 45	82.83 [ab]	86.25 [a]	83.92 [ab]	77.08 [b]	2.19	0.072	0.439	0.024
Glucose, mg/dL								
Day 14	101.3	104.3	99.1	99.4	4.0	0.377	0.680	0.741
Day 45	110.8	113.1	112.9	113.0	3.9	0.757	0.719	0.738
Ca, mg/dL								
Day 14	11.64	11.12	11.30	10.79	0.25	0.153	0.030	0.971
Day 45	11.31	10.96	11.02	11.13	0.14	0.683	0.416	0.108
Cl, mEq/L								
Day 14	100.6	101.5	100.0	101.1	0.86	0.384	0.081	0.807
Day 45	101.6	102.8	101.3	102.1	0.615	0.442	0.112	0.726
Na, mEq/L								
Day 14	144.4	143.3	145.3	143.5	0.86	0.534	0.083	0.678
Day 45	141.9	142.8	140.5	142.3	0.790	0.217	0.099	0.552
K, mEq/L								
Day 14	5.28	5.35	5.06	4.95	0.22	0.064	0.914	0.566
Day 45	5.57	6.08	5.68	5.53	0.25	0.381	0.479	0.181
Na-to-K ratio								
Day 14	27.63	27.75	28.96	29.90	1.06	0.053	0.553	0.652
Day 45	26.00	24.00	25.42	26.42	1.06	0.363	0.618	0.140
P, mg/dL								
Day 14	9.20	9.06	9.03	8.52	0.27	0.184	0.227	0.493
Day 45	10.76	10.91	10.55	10.54	0.24	0.246	0.773	0.748

[1] YCWE: yeast cell wall extract; [2] AST: aspartate aminotransferase; [3] ALT: alanine aminotransferase; [4] ALP: alkaline phosphatase; [5] BUN: blood urea N; and [6] CPK: creatine phosphokinase. MT-: diet without aflatoxin B1 and fumonisin B1; MT+: inclusion of 180 µg/kg aflatoxin B1, 1 mg/kg deoxynivalenol, and 9 mg/kg fumonisin B1 by replacing the clean corn and clean wheat with naturally mycotoxin-contaminated corn and wheat; YC 0%: no addition of YCWE (Mycosorb A+, Alltech, Nicholasville, KY, USA); YC 0.2%: YCWE added at 2 g/kg of feed. [ab] Means within a row lacking a common superscript differ ($p < 0.05$). [AB] Means within a row lacking a common superscript tend to differ ($0.05 \leq p < 0.1$).

2.2.5. Jejunal Histomorphometry and Crypt Cell Proliferation

Feeding diets with mycotoxins reduced ($p < 0.05$) villus height in pig jejunum (Table 10). However, feeding diets with YCWE tended to increase ($p = 0.088$) villus height in pig jejunum. Feeding diets with mycotoxins tended to increase ($p = 0.096$) the width at the top of jejunal villus. There were no effects of mycotoxins, YCWE, or interaction for the width in the middle or bottom of the villus, nor for crypt depth and villus height/crypt depth ratio of pigs. Feeding diets with mycotoxins tended to reduce ($p = 0.091$) the percentage of Ki-67 staining-positive cells in jejunum. Whereas, feeding diets with YCWE tended to increase ($p = 0.052$) the percentage of cells positive to Ki-67 staining.

Table 10. Jejunal morphology and crypt cell proliferation of weanling pigs fed diets with mycotoxins (MT) or and YCWE[1] (YC) in experiment 2.

Mycotoxins (MT)	-		+			p Value		
YCWE (YC)	0%	0.2%	0%	0.2%	SEM	MT	YC	MT × YC
Villus height (VH), μm	521	525	509	520	4.4	0.047	0.088	0.448
Villus width (top), μm	91	89	91	100	3.1	0.096	0.246	0.130
Villus width (middle), μm	118	113	111	114	3.3	0.401	0.673	0.258
Villus width (bottom), μm	124	119	121	117	4.3	0.476	0.257	0.870
Crypt depth (CD), μm	239	239	232	234	4.3	0.101	0.764	0.820
VH-to-CD ratio[2]	2.19	2.20	2.20	2.23	0.04	0.759	0.632	0.788
Ki-67, %	26.0	28.7	22.0	26.5	2.01	0.091	0.052	0.646

[1] YCWE: yeast cell wall extract; [2] Ki-67: technique for staining proliferating cells in the crypt where results are showed as a percentage of proliferating cells in comparison to all cells in the crypt. MT-: diet without aflatoxin B1 and fumonisin B1; MT+: inclusion of 180 μg/kg aflatoxin B1, 1 mg/kg deoxynivalenol, and 9 mg/kg fumonisin B1 by replacing the clean corn and clean wheat with naturally mycotoxin-contaminated corn and wheat; YC 0%: no addition of YCWE (Mycosorb A+, Alltech, Nicholasville, KY, USA); YC 0.2%: YCWE added at 2 g/kg of feed.

2.2.6. Immunological and Oxidative Stress Measurements

Feeding diets with mycotoxins increased ($p < 0.05$) immunoglobulin A (IgA) concentration in jejunal mucosa of pigs. In the other hand, feeding diets with YCWE reduced ($p < 0.05$) IgA concentration in jejunal mucosa of pigs. Feeding diets with YCWE tended to reduce ($p = 0.055$) TNF-α concentration in jejunal mucosa of pigs. There was a tendency for an interaction ($p = 0.083$) for TNF-α concentration in pig serum on day 14, where feeding diets with mycotoxins alone increased ($p < 0.05$) TNF-α concentration in comparison to feeding diets with mycotoxins and YCWE (Table 11). There were no effects of mycotoxins, YCWE, or interaction for serum concentrations of TNF-α, IgA, protein carbonyl, or MDA on day 45 of pigs. On day 14, there were no effects of mycotoxins, YCWE, or interaction for serum concentrations of IgA, IgG, protein carbonyl, or MDA of pigs. There was a tendency ($p = 0.057$) for an interaction, where IgG concentration tended to be higher in pigs fed diets with only mycotoxins than in diets with mycotoxins and YCWE on day 45. There were no effects of mycotoxins, YCWE, or interaction for jejunal mucosa concentrations of IgG and MDA of pigs. There was an interaction ($p < 0.05$), where feeding mycotoxins alone increased protein carbonyl concentration in jejunal mucosa of pigs, whereas feeding mycotoxins and YCWE reduced the amount of protein carbonyl.

Table 11. Immune response and oxidative stress markers of serum and jejunum in weanling pigs fed diets with mycotoxins (MT) or and YCWE[1] (YC) in experiment 2.

Mycotoxins (MT)	-		+			p Value		
YCWE (YC)	0%	0.2%	0%	0.2%	SEM	MT	YC	MT × YC
Tumor necrosis factor-α								
Serum at day 14, pg/mL	124 [A]	124 [A]	151 [B]	127 [A]	6.8	0.031	0.084	0.083
Serum at day 45, pg/mL	61	61	68	61	2.5	0.180	0.115	0.147
Jejunal mucosa, ng/mg protein	708	668	730	562	58	0.429	0.055	0.233
Immunoglobulin A								
Serum at day 14, mg/mL	0.42	0.33	0.41	0.37	0.05	0.701	0.183	0.554
Serum at day 45, mg/mL	0.57	0.55	0.67	0.61	0.06	0.187	0.515	0.752
Jejunal mucosa, µg/mg protein	5.83	5.57	6.85	6.12	0.24	0.002	0.037	0.318
Immunoglobulin G								
Serum at day 14, mg/mL	3.19	3.59	3.33	3.05	0.30	0.469	0.831	0.226
Serum at day 45, mg/mL	2.62 [AB]	2.83 [AB]	3.04 [A]	2.51 [B]	0.21	0.787	0.418	0.057
Jejunal mucosa, µg/mg protein	1.04	1.42	1.11	1.02	0.19	0.379	0.441	0.208
Protein carbonyl								
Serum at day 14, nmol/mg protein	1.91	2.00	2.16	1.85	0.15	0.730	0.458	0.189
Serum at day 45, nmol/mg protein	1.76	2.01	2.02	1.87	0.12	0.605	0.668	0.108
Jejunal mucosa, nmol/mg protein	2.33	2.31	2.83 [a]	2.51 [b]	0.08	0.001	0.026	0.047
Malondialdehydes								
Serum at day 14, µM	8.90	9.49	11.17	9.91	1.23	0.255	0.774	0.429
Serum at day 45, µM	8.89	9.57	10.25	9.83	1.43	0.542	0.922	0.682
Jejunal mucosa, nmol/g protein	511	542	488	579	78	0.925	0.401	0.679

[1] YCWE: yeast cell wall extract. MT-: diet without aflatoxin B1 and fumonisin B1; MT+: inclusion of 180 µg/kg aflatoxin B1, 1 mg/kg deoxynivalenol, and 9 mg/kg fumonisin B1 by replacing the clean corn and clean wheat with naturally mycotoxin-contaminated corn and wheat; YC 0%: no addition of YCWE (Mycosorb A+, Alltech, Nicholasville, KY, USA); YC 0.2%: YCWE added at 2 g/kg of feed. [ab] Means within a row lacking a common superscript differ ($p < 0.05$). [AB] Means within a row lacking a common superscript tend to differ ($0.05 \leq p < 0.1$).

2.2.7. Microbiome Analysis in Jejunal Mucosa

There were no effects of mycotoxins, YCWE, or interaction on pigs for the following bacterial phylum sequences from jejunal mucosa: Actinobacteria, Firmicutes, Proteobacteria, Chlamydiae, Deinococcus-Thermus, Fusobacteria, Nitrospirae, Tenericutes, and Verrucomicrobia (Table 12 and Figure 1). There was an interaction ($p < 0.05$) for Bacteriodetes indicating that YCWE increased Bacteriodetes in pigs fed diets with mycotoxins. There was a tendency ($p = 0.062$) for an interaction for Spirochaetes, indicating that YCWE tended to increase Spirochaetes in pigs fed diets with mycotoxins.

Table 12. Bacterial phyla (expressed as a percentage of sequences) collected from jejunal mucosa of weanling pigs fed diets with mycotoxins (MT) or and YCWE[1] (YC), based on 16S rRNA gene sequencing in experiment 2.

Mycotoxins (MT)	-		+			p Value		
YCWE (YC)	0%	0.2%	0%	0.2%	SEM	MT	YC	MT × YC
Actinobacteria	5.65	7.69	7.71	6.01	1.90	0.915	0.922	0.288
Bacteroidetes	8.64 [ab]	7.66 [ab]	5.93 [b]	19.63 [a]	3.52	0.182	0.069	0.037
Firmicutes	57.49	59.40	62.92	46.44	6.68	0.514	0.210	0.116
Proteobacteria	20.06	25.01	21.88	26.57	4.90	0.733	0.331	0.979
Spirochaetes	0.74 [AB]	0.16 [AB]	0.10 [A]	1.07 [B]	0.45	0.737	0.632	0.062
Chlamydiae	7.37	0.08	1.34	0.25	2.80	0.302	0.142	0.275
Deinococcus-Thermus	0.00	0.00	0.11	0.00	0.06	0.324	0.324	0.324
Fusobacteria	0.02	0.00	0.00	0.00	0.01	0.324	0.324	0.324
Nitrospirae	0.01	0.00	0.00	0.03	0.01	0.467	0.467	0.231
Tenericutes	0.01	0.00	0.00	0.01	0.01	0.965	0.965	0.161
Verrucomicrobia	0.00	0.00	0.01	0.00	0.01	0.324	0.324	0.324

[1] YCWE: yeast cell wall extract. MT-: diet without aflatoxin B1 and fumonisin B1; MT+: inclusion of 180 µg/kg aflatoxin B1, 1 mg/kg deoxynivalenol, and 9 mg/kg fumonisin B1 by replacing the clean corn and clean wheat with naturally mycotoxin-contaminated corn and wheat; YC 0%: no addition of YCWE (Mycosorb A+, Alltech, Nicholasville, KY, USA); YC 0.2%: YCWE added at 2 g/kg of feed. [ab] Means within a row lacking a common superscript differ ($p < 0.05$). [AB] Means within a row lacking a common superscript tend to differ ($0.05 \leq p < 0.1$).

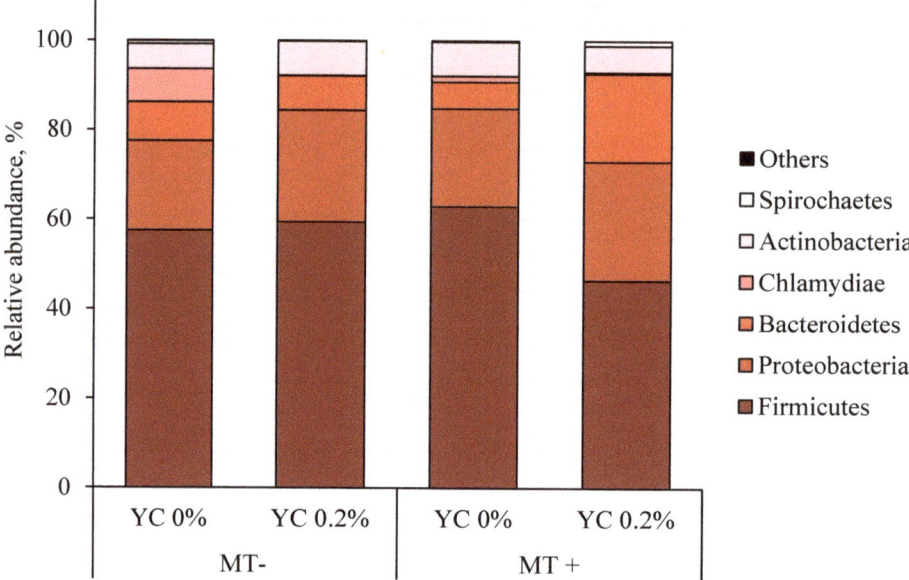

Figure 1. Bacterial phyla (expressed as a percentage of relative abundance of sequences) collected from jejunal mucosa of weanling pigs fed diets with mycotoxins (MT) or and yeast cell wall extract (YC), based on 16S rRNA gene sequencing in experiment 2. Each pattern represents a particular bacterial phylum. Phylum sequences that did not achieve 1% within each phylum were combined as "Others". MT-: diet without aflatoxin B1 and fumonisin B1; MT+: inclusion of 180 μg/kg aflatoxin B1, 1 mg/kg deoxynivalenol, and 9 mg/kg fumonisin B1 by replacing the clean corn and clean wheat with naturally mycotoxin-contaminated corn and wheat; YC 0%: no addition of yeast cell wall extract (YCWE; Mycosorb A+, Alltech, Nicholasville, KY, USA); YC 0.2%: YCWE added at 2 g/kg of feed.

There were no effects of mycotoxins, YCWE, or interaction on pigs for the percentage of bacterial sequences from jejunal mucosa in pigs for the following bacterial families: Clostridiaceae, Veillonellaceae, Ruminococcaceae, Propionibacteriaceae, Helicobacteraceae, Moraxellaceae, Oxalobacteraceae, Oxalobacteraceae, Chlamydiaceae, Staphylococcaceae, Pseudomonadaceae, Streptococcaceae, Paenibacillaceae, Succinivibrionaceae, Xanthomonadaceae, and for the total percent of all families lower than 1.0% in each family (Table 13). Feeding diets with mycotoxins increased ($p < 0.05$) the percentage of sequences from the family Lactobacillaceae. Feeding diets with YCWE reduced ($p < 0.05$) the proportion of sequences from the family Prevotellaceae. Feeding diets with YCWE tended to decrease ($p = 0.064$) the proportion of sequences from *Eubacterium*. Feeding diets with YCWE decreased ($p < 0.05$) the percentage of sequences from Erysipelotrichaceae and tended to decrease ($p = 0.064$) the proportion for *Eubacterium* in that family.

Table 13. Bacterial families and genera (expressed as a percentage of sequences) collected from jejunal mucosa of weanling pigs fed diets with mycotoxins (MT) or and YCWE[1] (YC), based on 16S rRNA gene sequencing in experiment 2.

Mycotoxins (MT)	-	-	+	+		p Value		
YCWE (YC)	0%	0.2%	0%	0.2%	SEM	MT	YC	MT × YC
Lactobacillaceae	13.95	20.02	32.20	35.86	6.68	0.011	0.451	0.851
Lactobacillus	13.95	20.02	32.20	35.86	6.68	0.011	0.451	0.851
Clostridiaceae	12.94	7.53	7.81	11.60	3.99	0.895	0.841	0.256
Clostridium	12.94	7.53	7.81	11.60	3.99	0.895	0.841	0.256
Prevotellaceae	14.84	7.77	11.38	3.73	3.78	0.295	0.044	0.935
Prevotella	14.84	7.77	11.38	3.73	3.78	0.295	0.044	0.935
Veillonellaceae	3.81	4.32	4.18	4.98	1.66	0.758	0.696	0.929
Dialister	0.10	0.31	0.22	0.13	0.10	0.762	0.576	0.129
Mitsuokella	0.52	1.56	1.75	2.75	0.91	0.192	0.271	0.981
Ruminococcaceae	2.37	3.54	2.65	4.57	2.03	0.707	0.379	0.831
Faecalibacterium	0.52	2.23	1.03	3.29	1.68	0.581	0.169	0.849
Ruminococcus	1.85	1.31	1.62	1.28	0.62	0.830	0.471	0.870
Propionibacteriaceae	2.46	5.03	2.59	2.86	0.93	0.249	0.110	0.194
Propionibacterium	0.02	0.00	0.01	0.00	0.01	0.542	0.215	0.542
Helicobacteraceae	2.50	5.10	0.80	3.92	2.90	0.623	0.329	0.930
Helicobacter	2.50	5.10	0.80	3.92	2.90	0.623	0.329	0.930
Bacillaceae	2.33	4.13	2.97	2.76	1.78	0.835	0.658	0.575
Anoxybacillus	0.50	1.63	1.32	0.12	0.69	0.615	0.957	0.097
Bacillus	1.65	2.35	1.55	2.46	1.66	0.999	0.631	0.949
Moraxellaceae	1.89	2.01	2.57	4.44	1.16	0.188	0.397	0.453
Acinetobacter	1.89	2.01	2.57	4.44	1.16	0.188	0.397	0.453
Lachnospiraceae	2.78	2.28	3.37	1.97	0.89	0.871	0.267	0.601
Roseburia	1.31	1.24	0.88	0.99	0.54	0.533	0.973	0.868
Oxalobacteraceae	1.06	0.25	0.16	0.34	0.34	0.244	0.365	0.160
Massilia	0.00	0.00	0.01	0.00	0.00	0.324	0.324	0.324
Enterobacteriaceae	3.65	0.83	1.42	2.90	1.29	0.919	0.632	0.097
Leclercia	0.12	0.00	0.00	0.00	0.06	0.324	0.324	0.324
Proteus	0.38	0.00	0.01	0.2	0.15	0.233	0.217	0.187
Trabulsiella	0.03	0.00	0.00	0.00	0.01	0.175	0.175	0.175
Turicibacter	0.34	0.19	1.35	0.38	0.52	0.125	0.144	0.241
Chlamydiaceae	0.04	8.24	0.70	0.05	2.79	0.185	0.184	0.121
Chlamydia	0.04	8.24	0.70	0.05	2.79	0.185	0.184	0.121
Staphylococcaceae	1.17	5.08	0.81	1.91	2.13	0.413	0.247	0.513
Staphylococcus	0.01	0.10	0.02	0.05	0.06	0.742	0.319	0.627
Pseudomonadaceae	0.68	3.19	1.61	1.63	1.04	0.752	0.212	0.216
Pseudomonas	0.58	2.96	1.52	1.43	1.03	0.760	0.247	0.212
Erysipelotrichaceae	2.72	0.45	2.93	0.98	0.92	0.665	0.017	0.853
Streptococcaceae	1.72	0.88	2.85	1.07	1.02	0.481	0.166	0.615
Streptococcus	1.72	0.88	2.85	1.07	1.02	0.481	0.166	0.615
Paenibacillaceae	6.17	0.75	0.17	0.15	2.08	0.121	0.198	0.201
Succinivibrionaceae	1.65	2.04	1.00	1.16	0.62	0.206	0.642	0.841
Succinivibrio	1.65	2.04	1.00	1.16	0.62	0.206	0.642	0.841
Xanthomonadaceae	3.88	0.20	0.35	0.53	1.79	0.369	0.326	0.279
Stenotrophomonas	0.04	0.00	0.00	0.03	0.02	0.673	0.673	0.121
Others[2]	17.44	16.36	17.60	12.62	3.74	0.634	0.423	0.604

[1] YCWE: yeast cell wall extract; [2] Total percent combined of all family lower than 1.0% in each family. MT-: diet without aflatoxin B1 and fumonisin B1; MT+: inclusion of 180 μg/kg aflatoxin B1, 1 mg/kg deoxynivalenol, and 9 mg/kg fumonisin B1 by replacing the clean corn and clean wheat with naturally mycotoxin-contaminated corn and wheat; YC 0%: no addition of YCWE (Mycosorb A+, Alltech, Nicholasville, KY, USA); YC 0.2%: YCWE added at 2 g/kg of feed.

There were no effects of mycotoxins, YCWE, or interaction on pigs for the percentage of bacterial sequences from jejunal mucosa for the following bacterial species: *Lactobacillus mucosae, Clostridium perfringens, Propionibacterium acnes, Lactobacillus delbrueckii, Chlamydia suis, Lactobacillus sp., Clostridium butyricum, Dialister succinatiphilus, Faecalibacterium prausnitzii, Succinivibrio dextrinosolvens, Massilia niabensis, Acinetobacter radioresistens, Streptococcus hyointestinalis, Mitsuokella jalaludinii, Ruminococcus gauvreauii, Helicobacter equorum, Staphylococcus sciuri, Stenotrophomonas rhizophila,*

Helicobacter mastomyrinus, Mitsuokella multacida, Prevotella sp., Helicobacter rappini, Bacillus coagulans, Eubacterium multiforme, Roseburia faecis, Clostridium hiranonis, Eubacterium biforme, and *Lactobacillus johnsonii* (Table 14). Feeding diets with mycotoxins reduced ($p < 0.05$) the percentage of sequences from *Lactobacillus kitasatonis* in jejunal mucosa of pigs. Feeding diets with YCWE increased ($p < 0.05$) the proportion of sequences from *Prevotella copri* and *Prevotella stercorea*, whereas it decreased ($p < 0.05$) the proportion from *Lactobacillus equicursoris*. Feeding diets with YCWE tended to increase the proportion of sequences from *Turicibacter sanguinis* ($p = 0.064$) and *Clostridium sp.* ($p = 0.075$). Feeding diets with mycotoxins tended to decrease the proportion of sequences from *Leclercia adecarboxylata* ($p = 0.064$) and *Trabulsiella odontotermitis* ($p = 0.067$).

Table 14. Bacterial species (expressed as a percentage of sequences) collected from jejunal mucosa of weanling pigs fed diets with mycotoxins (MT) or and YCWE[1] (YC), based on 16S rRNA gene sequencing in experiment 2[2].

Mycotoxins (MT)	-		+			p Value		
YCWE (YC)	0%	0.2%	0%	0.2%	SEM	MT	YC	MT × YC
Lactobacillus mucosae	8.18	16.63	7.17	9.19	3.83	0.259	0.164	0.389
Prevotella copri	2.49	8.85	5.62	11.62	3.02	0.306	0.036	0.951
Lactobacillus kitasatonis	17.58	5.50	3.01	1.06	4.51	0.031	0.107	0.241
Clostridium perfringens	7.07	3.18	5.34	8.56	3.82	0.636	0.930	0.358
Propionibacterium acnes	2.85	2.55	5.00	2.43	0.92	0.245	0.104	0.197
Lactobacillus delbrueckii	2.35	2.64	2.57	1.59	0.50	0.386	0.476	0.190
Chlamydia suis	0.05	0.70	8.22	0.04	2.78	0.184	0.184	0.120
Lactobacillus sp.	2.04	2.38	2.01	1.19	0.49	0.159	0.582	0.179
Lactobacillus equicursoris	2.99	0.37	3.90	0.13	1.49	0.820	0.039	0.701
Clostridium butyricum	2.15	2.77	1.00	1.05	0.93	0.133	0.725	0.759
Dialister succinatiphilus	2.75	1.75	1.56	0.52	0.91	0.192	0.271	0.981
Faecalibacterium prausnitzii	1.28	1.62	1.31	1.85	0.62	0.830	0.471	0.870
Succinivibrio dextrinosolvens	1.16	1.00	2.04	1.65	0.62	0.206	0.642	0.841
Massilia niabensis	1.51	1.60	1.49	1.23	0.56	0.679	0.858	0.715
Acinetobacter radioresistens	2.43	1.49	0.94	0.72	0.75	0.139	0.441	0.631
Prevotella stercorea	0.70	1.95	0.89	2.03	0.58	0.813	0.047	0.921
Streptococcus hyointestinalis	0.90	2.04	0.51	1.52	0.96	0.597	0.217	0.938
Mitsuokella jalaludinii	0.95	1.02	1.25	1.57	0.52	0.414	0.713	0.808
Ruminococcus gauvreauii	2.22	0.29	1.88	0.38	1.42	0.917	0.161	0.859
Helicobacter equorum	0.08	0.00	2.94	1.65	1.66	0.182	0.681	0.718
Staphylococcus sciuri	0.00	0.67	3.52	0.22	1.79	0.396	0.465	0.273
Turicibacter sanguinis	0.59	1.18	0.26	2.37	0.71	0.544	0.064	0.286
Stenotrophomonas rhizophila	0.24	0.24	0.10	3.73	1.77	0.349	0.311	0.312
Helicobacter mastomyrinus	2.22	0.41	1.25	0.41	1.04	0.642	0.207	0.643
Mitsuokella multacida	0.99	0.83	0.96	1.28	0.55	0.696	0.875	0.659
Leclercia adecarboxylata	1.65	0.73	0.48	0.64	0.40	0.064	0.257	0.106
Prevotella sp.	0.49	0.54	1.17	1.17	0.54	0.160	0.965	0.958
Helicobacter rappini	1.61	0.39	0.90	0.39	0.82	0.665	0.296	0.659
Bacillus coagulans	1.35	0.81	0.18	0.51	0.68	0.285	0.875	0.529
Clostridium sp.	0.21	0.41	0.19	1.74	0.48	0.182	0.075	0.164
Eubacterium multiforme	0.40	0.22	0.79	1.10	0.45	0.170	0.891	0.593
Roseburia faecis	0.46	0.70	0.65	0.68	0.34	0.806	0.684	0.749
Trabulsiella odontotermitis	1.11	0.53	0.33	0.40	0.28	0.067	0.292	0.190
Clostridium hiranonis	0.18	0.13	0.85	1.11	0.56	0.118	0.839	0.771
Eubacterium biforme	0.34	1.37	0.18	0.30	0.40	0.124	0.148	0.255
Anoxybacillus kestanbolensis	0.06	0.97	1.06	0.08	0.48	0.913	0.945	0.056
Lactobacillus johnsonii	0.52	0.96	0.38	0.17	0.32	0.324	0.324	0.324

[1] YCWE: yeast cell wall extract; [2] Species that are lower than 0.5% in each species had their values combined in the common genera. MT-: diet without aflatoxin B1 and fumonisin B1; MT+: inclusion of 180 µg/kg aflatoxin B1, 1 mg/kg deoxynivalenol, and 9 mg/kg fumonisin B1 by replacing the clean corn and clean wheat with naturally mycotoxin-contaminated corn and wheat; YC 0%: no addition of YCWE (Mycosorb A+, Alltech, Nicholasville, KY, USA); YC 0.2%: YCWE added at 2 g/kg of feed.

2.2.8. Tight Junction Proteins in Jejunum

There were no effects of mycotoxins, YCWE, or interaction for tight junction proteins in jejunal mucosa of pigs (Figure 2).

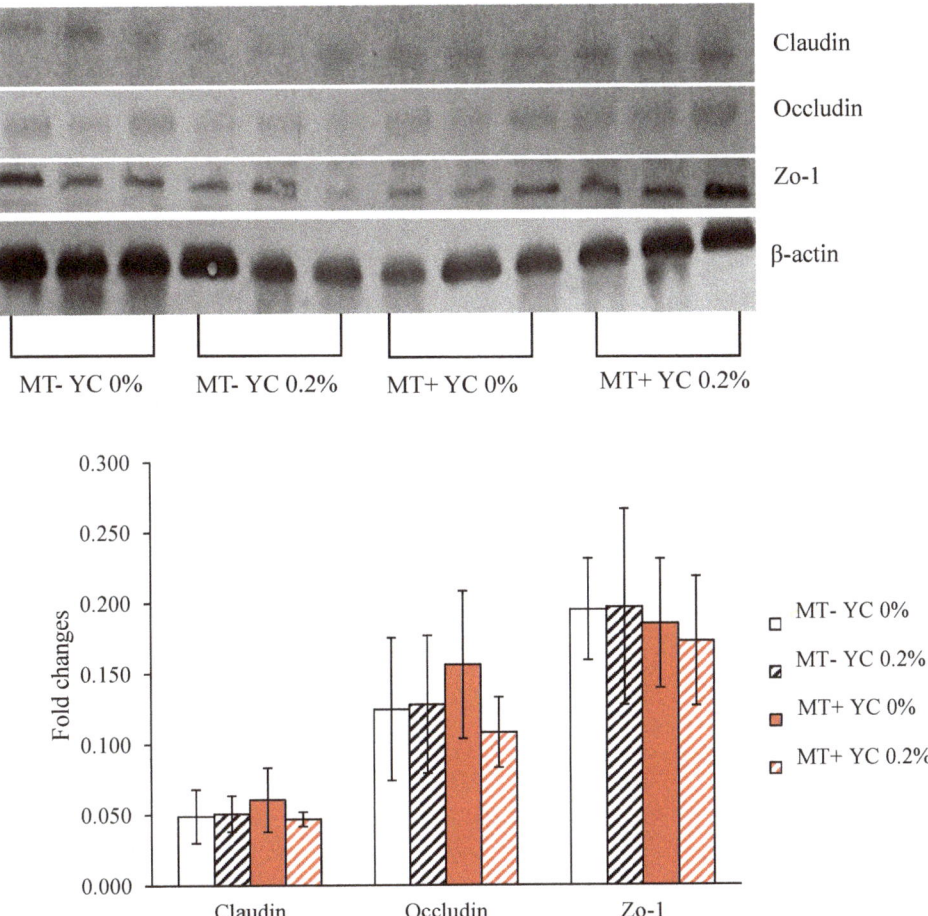

Figure 2. Tight junction proteins of jejunal mucosa in weanling pigs fed diets with mycotoxin or/and yeast cell wall extract. Zo-1: zona occludens-1 protein; MT-: diet without aflatoxin B1 and fumonisin B1; MT+: inclusion of 180 µg/kg aflatoxin B1, 1 mg/kg deoxynivalenol, and 9 mg/kg fumonisin B1 by replacing the clean corn and clean wheat with naturally mycotoxin-contaminated corn and wheat; YC 0%: no addition of yeast cell wall extract (YCWE; Mycosorb A+, Alltech, Nicholasville, KY, USA); YC 0.2%: YCWE added at 2 g/kg of feed.

3. Discussion

The present study was designed to test the efficacy of the YCWE (Mycosorb A+, Alltech Inc. Kentucky) derived from the cell wall of *Saccharomyces cerevisiae* and algal material in nursery and growing pigs challenged with AFB1, DON, and FB1 in naturally contaminated diets (Table 15).

Table 15. Experimental design and mycotoxin contamination in feedstuff and diets for experiments 1 and 2.

Experiment	1				2			
Treatments	MT- YC 0%	MT- YC 0.2%	MT+ YC 0%	MT+ YC 0.2%	MT- YC 0%	MT- YC 0.2%	MT+ YC 0%	MT+ YC 0.2%
Factor								
Mycotoxin (MT)	-	-	+	+	-	-	+	+
YCWE[1] (YC)	-	+	-	+	-	+	-	+
Pigs								
Per treatment	30	30	30	30	12	12	12	12
Per pen	3	3	3	3	1	1	1	1
Period, d	35	35	35	35	48	48	48	48
Feedstuff								
Ground yellow corn								
Aflatoxins, mg/kg	ND	ND	2.8	2.8	ND	ND	2.8	2.8
Fumonisins, mg/kg	ND	ND	170.2	170.2	ND	ND	170.2	170.2
Zearalenone, mg/kg	ND	ND	1.1	1.1	ND	ND	1.1	1.1
Wheat, soft red								
Deoxynivalenol, mg/kg	-	-	-	-	ND	ND	7.3	7.3
Zearalenone, mg/kg	-	-	-	-	ND	ND	1.8	1.8
Diet[2]								
YCWE, %	-	0.2	-	0.2	-	0.2	-	0.2
Aflatoxin B1, µg/kg	-	-	180	180	-	-	180	180
Fumonisin B1, mg/kg	-	-	14	14	-	-	9	9
Deoxynivalenol, mg/kg	-	-	-	-	-	-	1	1

[1] YCWE: yeast cell wall extract; [2] Contaminated corn and wheat were blended with corn and wheat without mycotoxins in order to reach desired levels of mycotoxins in diets. Mycotoxin levels in feedstuff were detected by UPLC-MS/MS using Alltech 37+ program at Alltech (Nicholasville, KY, USA). ND: Not detected.

In nursery pigs, aflatoxin concentration up to 20 µg/kg has shown no impact on the growth of pigs [3]. Nevertheless, the aflatoxin concentration at 180 µg/kg used in experiment 2 has shown impairment on growth performance of nursery pigs, where a stronger impairment on growth performance was noticed in comparison to growing pigs from experiment 1. In experiment 2, feeding diets with mycotoxins had an obvious and negative effect on growth performance in nursery pigs by reducing BW, ADG, and ADFI by 11%, 13%, and 17%, respectively. However, mycotoxins increased G:F by 4% during the entire period. The compensatory improvement of G:F is possibly due to the reduction in feed intake [12]. Mycotoxin impact was weaker in growing pigs, where mycotoxins decreased ADG by 18% and G:F by 15% during only the first seven days. These results along with the absence of change in ADFI during the first seven days are indicative that mycotoxins impaired animal growth by affecting nutrient absorption or utilization during acute challenge. As a result, mycotoxins tended to reduce pig BW on day 14. Challenges with aflatoxin and fumonisin in growing pigs have been shown to reduce BW, ADG, and ADFI when in higher concentrations (2.5 mg of aflatoxin and 100 mg of FB1/kg) than the concentrations used in experiment 1 (180 µg/kg AFB1 and 14 mg/kg FB1) [13]. A compensatory improvement of G:F of 8% was observed in growing pigs from day 14 to 21 in experiment 1 from the current study. Of interest, the interaction observed from day 27 to 34 and from day 34 to 41 showed that the reduction on ADG in nursery pigs fed diets with mycotoxins was ceased by the inclusion of YCWE in diets, suggesting a protective role of YCWE against mycotoxins with an impact on pig growth performance. The effects of YCWE on growth performance of nursery pigs fed diets with mycotoxins is supported by the results obtained for nutrient digestibility, where the apparent ileal digestibility of crude protein, gross energy, and ether extract was reduced in pigs fed diets with mycotoxins but increased when YCWE was included in the diets.

Comparing the results of both experiments, along with results previously reported in the scientific field, the severity and persistence of the effects of the mycotoxin challenge on growth performance of pigs seems to depend on age, being more severe in nursery pigs in comparison to growing pigs. In addition, nursery pigs can be more susceptible to the mycotoxin challenge due to weaning stress [14].

Besides age and weaning stress factors, the presence of deoxynivalenol in the experimental diets fed to nursery pigs in experiment 2 may have intensified mycotoxins impairment on growth performance. Piglets weaned with 24 days (older than in experiment 2) and challenged with 3 mg/kg of DON, have shown impaired growth performance during the 14 days of the challenge [15]. However, deoxynivalenol-challenged pigs presented impaired growth performance when fed values as low as 0.6 mg/kg [16]. Deoxynivalenol impairment on growth performance seems to be caused specially by its anorexigenic effect. The reduction on feed intake caused by deoxynivalenol is due to an increased release of proinflammatory cytokines [17,18] satiety hormones [19], and neuroendocrine regulation [20]. Satiety hormones such as peptide YY and cholecystokinin have increased levels in serum after deoxynivalenol challenge in mice, resulting in reduced feed intake [19]. Resistance to deoxynivalenol was developed by adult mice where no anorexigenic effect was observed for at least two days after ceasing the challenge with the mycotoxin [21]. The same study showed that animals developed a dose-dependent increase in feed intake after the challenge, reinforcing animal ability of acclimation to mycotoxins. The neuroendocrine regulation is mediated by serotonin receptor activation in rats, reducing digesta transit time, and thus, feed intake [20]. Feeding higher concentrations of deoxynivalenol can even cause emesis. High serum levels of peptide YY and serotonin were described as responsible for the deoxynivalenol emetic effect in mice [22].

The YCWE from *S. cerevisiae* is composed of an inner layer of insoluble β-D-glucans arranged in a network [23]. Insoluble property and structural conformation allow the β-D-glucans to survive digestion and to mitigate the impact of mycotoxins in the lower gastrointestinal tract. Directly related to mycotoxins, β-D-glucans [8,24] and a mixture of YCWE, clay, and organic acids [15] have previously shown binding efficacy on *Fusarium* toxins, resulting in reduced deoxynivalenol impact on growth performance of nursery pigs [15]. Even though previous studies have shown improved animal performance, minor effects were observed in pigs fed diets with YCWE considering growth performance for nursery and growing pigs. In growing pigs, YCWE tended to reduce animal ADG during the first seven days and ADFI during the last seven days, suggesting a mild detrimental effect of YCWE on growth performance. In experiment 2 with nursey pigs, YCWE reduced feed intake during phase 1, which may have caused the reduced ADG for the same phase. The lower G:F for nursery pigs fed diets with YCWE during the first seven days may have enhanced G:F during the last days of the study, after day 34, as a compensatory mechanism [12], as observed as a tendency of increased G:F for the overall period for pigs fed diets with YCWE. The results regarding YCWE and growth performance were unexpected, since a combination of fermented media by *S. cerevisiae* and hydrolyzed yeast cell wall from *S. cerevisiae* [25] or *S. cerevisiae* cell wall [26] demonstrated enhanced nutrient digestibility and utilization in weaned pigs. Likewise, pigs fed YCWE had greater digestibility than pigs fed a basal diet without *S. cerevisiae* cell wall [26]. The production of total volatile fatty acids in ileum and cecum was also reported to be increased in pigs fed β-D-glucans from *S. cerevisiae* [27].

Growing pigs consuming mycotoxins showed increased serum albumin and reduced serum cholesterol and BUN. The observed increase in serum albumin could be due to the ability of the serum protein to hydrolyze *Fusarium* toxins [28] and to its antioxidant role [29], properties that may help with handling the mycotoxin challenge. Cholesterol and urea are primarily synthesized by hepatocytes and their decrease is indicative of impaired liver function [1]. In experiment 2, the interaction observed on day 45, where mycotoxins a decreased cholesterol level among pigs fed YCWE, is indicative that the supplementation with YCWE was not able to recover cholesterol synthesis by hepatocytes. Although, YCWE showed a tendency to reduce serum AST in pigs fed diets with mycotoxins. The aspartate aminotransferase is more sensitive than alanine aminotransferase for hepatic damage in pigs [30]. Therefore, YCWE could improve liver function in pigs with moderate hepatic damage, as shown in experiment 2 of the current study. The reduction on glucose and K levels, with a consequent impact on the Na-to-K ratio, might indicate kidney damage, due to inefficient glucose and K reabsorption after glomerular filtration [31–33]. The YCWE was able to prevent those changes in glucose and K. The tendency of increase in Na and Cl levels in serum of growing pigs fed diets with YCWE may be due to its composition. One of the components in the YCWE product is hydrated sodium calcium aluminosilicate, justifying the increase of Na in serum and the concomitant increase in Cl to maintain the electrolytic balance in serum.

The mycotoxin challenge can modulate the immune function of pigs and potentially increase animal susceptibility to infectious diseases or morbidity [34]. In the current study, mycotoxins reduced neutrophils blood levels for growing pigs in experiment 1. In growing pigs, the increased duodenal IgG concentration in animals fed mycotoxin compared to pigs without a mycotoxin challenge may indicate a late immune response, characterizing a specialized response by the adaptive immune system. In previous study carried out by our group, pigs challenged with DON and zearalenone did not show any alteration in white blood cells and IgG in comparison to animals fed a control diet [1]. In a different study, DON-challenged pigs have shown decreased serum IgG [33]. A combination of fermented media by *S. cerevisiae* and hydrolyzed yeast cell wall from *S. cerevisiae* have been shown to increase IgG and IgM levels in serum and IgA level in the gut [25]. In experiment 1, IgG levels in jejunum and serum, and lymphocyte count were increased by YCWE when pigs were fed diets without mycotoxins, suggesting YCWE's ability to stimulate an immune response. In experiment 2, it was possible to notice a reduction of albumin-to-globulin ratio in pigs fed diets with YCWE and no mycotoxins, reinforcing YCWE's effect as an immune stimulator. In experiment 1, equivalent IgG levels in jejunum were observed between pigs fed diets with YCWE and pigs fed diets with mycotoxins, indicating that YCWE could stimulate the immune system as much as mycotoxins but without the latter's toxic effects. On the other hand, IgG concentration in serum in experiments 1 and 2 did not follow the same behavior as observed for the jejunal IgG described. Indeed, there was a reduction when YCWE was added to diets of pigs fed diets with mycotoxins, indicating a protective role of YCWE at the gut level with a possible reduction of systemic immune response.

The hypothesis of late response by the adaptive immune system is supported by no differences in TNF-α and MDA in gut mucosa and blood serum, which are related to early inflammatory response and cell damage, respectively. The absence of difference between pigs fed mycotoxin diets and control pigs for TNF-α and MDA were also observed in pigs challenged with *Fusarium* toxins [1]. A mixture of YCWE, clay, and organic acids was able to reduce TLR-4 expression and improve gut barrier function in deoxynivalenol-challenged nursery pigs [15]. Regarding cytokines, IFN-γ, IL-6, IL-12B, TNF-α, and PTGS2 were over expressed in pigs fed diets with DON [33]. The inclusion of YCWE in diets decreased 8-OHdG, molecule that indicates nucleic acid injury, suggesting reduced oxidative stress and improved cell viability [1]. Furthermore, the inclusion of YCWE in diets with mycotoxins successfully overcame the increase in protein carbonyl in jejunum mucosa observed in nursery pigs fed diets with mycotoxins.

Despite the effects observed for immune and oxidative stress markers, there were no noticeable effects on tight junction expression for claudin, occludin, or zona occludens-1 protein in experiment 2. Tight junctions are responsible for the juxtaposition of enterocytes and thus, are indicative of intestinal wall integrity [35]. The absence of effect of mycotoxins, YCWE, or interaction suggest that both the challenge with mycotoxins and the YCWE supplementation could not alter gut wall structure regarding tight junction constitution. Even still, there are other immune-related structures present on enterocyte surface that seem to have be altered in current study. The immune system can be modulated by the interaction of molecules present in the intestinal lumen with receptors along the intestinal wall. One such receptor is the TLR2, which can be stimulated by both yeast components as well as bacterial lipopolysaccharide [36,37]. The supplementation with YCWE could have enhanced the expression of TLR2 which promoted the survivability of Spirochaetes [36], as observed in experiment 2. The supplementation with the yeast cell wall has previously shown to reduce the proportion of disease-related bacteria [38]. In the current study, similar results were observed with the decrease of the proportion of Erysipellotrichaceae and Prevotellaceae families in pigs fed diets with YCWE, despite the increase in specific species within the family (*P. copri* and *P. stercorea*), suggesting an improvement in intestinal health of pigs fed diets with YCWE. This line of thought can also be used to explain the decrase in *Lactobacillus equicursoris* observed in pigs fed diets with YCWE. The *L. equicursoris* has demonstrated antagonistic ability against pathogenic bacteria in pigs [39], indicating that the supplementation with YCWE could have a role in reducing the load of pathogenic bacteria in the intestinal tract of pigs. The species *Trabulsiella odontotermitis* is found in the gastrointestinal tract of termites that are able to digest fungi cell wall [40]. The reduction of *T. odontotermitis* in pigs fed diets with mycotoxins was unexpected, since the ingestion of mycotoxins should have enhanced pigs' ability to handle fungi presence in the feed. At the same time, pigs fed diets with mycotoxins had an increased proportion of Lactobalicaceae family and of *Lactobacillus kitasatonis*, which is known to play a probiotic role in pig intestine [41]. The *Lactobacillus* sp. have previously shown the ability to reduce mycotoxicity by binding to mycotoxins extracellularly [42,43] and, as gram-positive bacteria, can be considered as "native DON-degraders" [44]. Thus, the increase of Lactobacilaceae family proportion in the intestinal microbiome of mycotoxin-fed pigs as well as the increase of gram-positive bacteria as *Turicibacter sanguinis* and *Clostridium* sp. in pigs fed diets with YCWE can be indicative of an induced adaptation of the microbiome and of the pig itself to handle better mycotoxin challenge.

Cells from the intestinal crypts are responsible for enterocyte renewal and crypt depth is positively related with proliferative rate that can be measured by Ki-67 staining [45]. The tendency in reducing duodenal crypt depth in animals fed YCWE may indicate that the additive was able to enhance enterocyte survivability, thus reducing crypt cells' proliferative rate. Indeed, YCWE tended to increase villus height as previously reported in pigs fed YCWE in comparison to pigs fed a basal diet without *S. cerevisiae* cell wall [26]. On the other hand, feeding diets with mycotoxins reduced villus height and tended to reduce the percentage of cells positive to Ki-67. Such outcomes suggest that mycotoxins reduced the villus height by impairing crypt cell proliferation. At the same time, the tendency to increase in villus width may be an adaptation strategy to increase the absorptive surface area after mycotoxins damage.

Collectively, the current study suggests that susceptibility of pigs to AFB1 180 µg/kg, DON 1 mg/kg, and FB1 9 mg/kg is higher in nursery pigs (6 to 29 kg, challenged for 48 days) than in growing pigs (56 to 89 kg, challenged for 35 days) to AFB1 180 µg/kg and FB1 14 mg/kg, depending on the health status of gastrointestinal and immune systems. The YCWE at 0.2% showed a protective role against the aforementioned mycotoxins, improving pig growth and health mainly in nursery pigs in comparison to growing pigs.

4. Materials and Methods

A protocol of these experiments was reviewed and approved by the Institutional Animal Care and Use Committee (IACUC) at North Carolina State University (NCSU; Raleigh, NC, USA).

4.1. Animals and Experimental Diets

In experiment 1, one hundred and twenty pigs (60 barrows and 60 gilts at 55.58 ± 3.13 kg, crossbred pigs, Smithfield Premium Genetics, Rose Hill, NC, USA) were used. Pigs were housed in solid concrete floor indoor pens (1.42 × 3.86 m) at the North Carolina State University Swine Evaluation Station (Clayton, NC, USA). Pigs were grouped by body weight (BW) and randomly assigned to four treatments within a BW group. Each treatment had ten replicates and three pigs per pen.

In experiment 2, forty-eight newly weaned pigs at 3 weeks of age (24 barrows and 24 gilts at 5.98 ± 0.24 kg, PIC 337 × Camborough 22) were used. This study was conducted at the North Carolina State University Metabolism Evaluation Unit (Raleigh, NC, USA). Pigs were housed in a pen (0.74 × 1.5 m) equipped with a polyethylene feeder attached to the front of the pen, nipple water next to the feeder, and slatted flooring. Pigs were grouped by body weight (BW) and randomly assigned to four treatments within a BW group. Each treatment had twelve replicates and one pig per pen.

Corn and wheat naturally contaminated with mycotoxins were identified and the mycotoxin concentrations were confirmed. Corn was analyzed by the Alltech 37+ program at Alltech (Nicholasville, KY, USA) for 16 mycotoxins including AFB1 and FB1, and wheat was analyzed for 11 mycotoxins including DON. Quantification of AFB1 and FB1 was conducted using UPLC-MS/MS. Corn contained

AF (2.8 mg/kg for experiments 1 and 2) and FUM (170.2 mg/kg for experiments 1 and 2) and wheat contained DON (7.3 mg/kg, for experiment 2) and these were used to make experimental diets (Tables 16 and 17). This contaminated corn and wheat were blended with corn and wheat without mycotoxins in order to reach the desired levels of 180 µg/kg AFB1 and 14 mg/kg FB1 (experiment 1) and 180 µg/kg AFB1, 1 mg/kg DON, and 9 mg/kg FB1 (experiment 2) in the final diets. Non-contaminated corn and wheat were also used to formulate a control without mycotoxins. Mycotoxin analysis in corn and wheat was completed by collecting 10 samples from different locations to obtain a representative mixture. Ten samples were combined and thoroughly blended together before two subsamples were collected for analysis of mycotoxin content measured by the Alltech 37+ program using UPLC-MS/MS (Table 18).

Table 16. Composition of experimental diets in experiment 1 (%, as-fed basis)[1].

Item	Basal Diet
Ingredients, %	
Ground yellow corn	75.60
Soybean meal, dehulled	21.00
L-Lys HCl	0.18
Poultry fat	1.00
Salt	0.22
Vitamin premix[2]	0.03
Trace mineral premix[3]	0.15
Dicalcium P	1.12
Ground limestone	0.70
Calculated composition	
Dry matter, %	89.06
Metabolizable energy, Mcal/kg	3.35
Crude protein, %	16.49
Standardized ileal digestible Lys, %	0.85
Ca, %	0.60
Available P, %	0.27

[1] Basal diet (MT-YC 0%) without aflatoxin B1 and fumonisin B1; MT-YC 0.2%: MT-YC 0% + 2 g/kg of a yeast cell wall extract (Mycosorb A+, Alltech, Nicholasville, KY, USA); MT+YC 0%: 180 µg/kg aflatoxin B1 and 14 mg/kg fumonisin B1 by the use of naturally contaminated corn replacing clean corn used in MT-YC 0%; and MT+YC 0.2%: MT+YC 0% + 2 g/kg of a yeast cell wall extract; Naturally contaminated corn contained aflatoxins (2.8 mg/kg) and fumonisins (170.2 mg/kg); [2] The vitamin premix provided the following per kilogram of complete diet: 6613.8 IU of vitamin A as vitamin A acetate; 992.07 IU of vitamin D3; 19.84 IU of vitamin E; 0.026 mg of vitamin B12; 4.63 mg of riboflavin; 26.46 mg of niacin; 18.52 mg of d-pnatothenic acid; 2.65 mg of Vitamin K as menadione sodium bisulfate; 0.66 mg of biotin; [3] The trace mineral premix provided the following per kilogram of complete diet: 39.6 mg of Mn as manganous oxide; 165 mg of Fe as ferrous sulfate; 165 mg of Zn as Zinc sulfate; 15.15 mg of Cu as copper sulfate; 0.30 mg of I as ethyenediamine dihydroiodide; and 0.30 mg of Se as sodium selenite.

Four treatments were based on a 2 × 2 factorial arrangement with mycotoxin (180 µg/kg AFB1 and 14 mg/kg FB1 or 180 ug/kg AFB1, 1 mg/kg DON, and 9 mg/kg FB1 for experiments 1 or 2, respectively) and yeast cell wall extract (YCWE; Mycosorb A+, Alltech Inc., Nicholasville, KY, USA: 2 g/kg diet) as two factors. Thus, the 4 treatments were: (1) MT-YC 0%: corn-soybean meal-based diet without detectable AFB1 and FB1, (2) MT-YC 0.2%: MT-YC 0% + YCWE, (3) MT+YC 0%: MT-YC 0% + 180 µg/kg AFB1 and 14 mg/kg FB1 or 180 µg/kg AFB1, 1 mg/kg DON, and 9 mg/kg FB1 (respectively for experiments 1 or 2) by the use of naturally contaminated corn and wheat replacing clean corn and wheat used in MT-YC 0%, and (4) MT+YC 0.2%: MT+YC + YCWE. The YCWE-based MT-YC 0.2% and MT+YC 0.2% is composed of hydrolyzed yeast, which includes the cell wall fraction of the organism. Pigs were fed the experimental diets for a 5-week period based on the phase 5 diet for experiment 1, and were fed the experimental diets for 48 days based on a 2-phase feeding program (phase 1: 20 days and phase 2: 28 days). Feed intake and body weight were recorded weekly. During the entire experimental period, all pigs had free access to feed and water. Concentrations of essential nutrients met requirements suggested by the National Research Council [46]. All diets were free of antimicrobial growth promoter and ZnO. Titanium dioxide (0.4%) was added to experimental diets from day 43 of experiment 2 as an indigestible external marker to measure apparent ileal digestibility (AID).

Table 17. Composition of experimental diets in experiment 2 (%, as-fed basis)[1].

Item	Phase 1	Phase 2
Ingredient, %		
Ground yellow corn	37.5	48.82
Soybean meal, dehulled	22.0	27.0
Wheat, soft red	15.0	15.0
Whey permeate	12.0	2.0
Poultry meal	5.0	3.0
Blood plasma	3.3	–
L-Lys HCl	0.45	0.41
DL-Met	0.17	0.12
L-Thr	0.13	0.12
Salt	0.22	0.22
Vitamin and mineral premix[2]	0.18	0.18
Dicalcium P	0.45	0.79
Ground limestone	1.10	0.84
Poultry fat	2.5	1.50
Calculated composition:		
Metabolizable energy, Mcal/kg	3.4	3.4
Crude protein, %	22.09	21.12
Standardized ileal digestible Lys, %	1.35	1.23
Standardized ileal digestible Met + Cys	0.75	0.68
Standardized ileal digestible Thr, %	0.79	0.73
Standardized ileal digestible Trp, %	0.23	0.22
Standardized total tract digestible P, %	0.40	0.33

[1] Basal diet (MT-YC 0%) without aflatoxin B1 and fumonisin B1; MT-YC 0.2%: MT-YC 0% + 2 g/kg of a yeast cell wall extract (Mycosorb A+, Alltech, Nicholasville, KY, USA); MT+YC 0%: 180 µg/kg aflatoxin B1, 1 mg/kg DON, and 9 mg/kg fumonisin B1 by the use of naturally contaminated corn and wheat replacing clean corn and wheat used in MT-YC 0%; and MT+YC 0.2%: MT+YC 0% + 2 g/kg of a yeast cell wall extract; Naturally contaminated corn contained aflatoxins (2.8 mg/kg) and fumonisins (170.2 mg/kg) and naturally contaminated wheat contained deoxynivalenol (7.3 mg/kg); [2] The vitamin premix provided the following per kilogram of complete diet: 6613.8 IU of vitamin A as vitamin A acetate; 992.07 IU of vitamin D3; 19.84 IU of vitamin E; 0.026 mg of vitamin B12; 4.63 mg of riboflavin; 26.46 mg of niacin; 18.52 mg of d-pnatothenic acid; 2.65 mg of Vitamin K as menadione sodium bisulfate; 0.66 mg of biotin; [2] The trace mineral premix provided the following per kilogram of complete diet: 39.6 mg of Mn as manganous oxide; 165 mg of Fe as ferrous sulfate; 165 mg of Zn as Zinc sulfate; 15.15 mg of Cu as copper sulfate; 0.30 mg of I as ethyenediamine dihydroioidide; and 0.30 mg of Se as sodium selenite.

Table 18. Mycotoxin levels in corn and wheat used in Experiments 1 and 2 analyzed by UPLC-MS/MS[1].

Mycotoxin	Corn	Wheat
Aflatoxin B1, mg/kg	2.5	ND
Aflatoxin B2, mg/kg	0.1	ND
Aflatoxin G1, mg/kg	0.2	ND
Deoxynivalenol (DON), mg/kg	ND	5.5
DON-3-glucoside, mg/kg	ND	0.9
15-acetyl-DON, mg/kg	ND	0.5
3-acetyl- DON, mg/kg	ND	0.3
Fumonisin B1, mg/kg	142.9	0.1
Fumonisin B2, mg/kg	13.9	ND
Fumonisin B3, mg/kg	13.4	ND
Fusarenon X, mg/kg	ND	ND
Gliotoxin, mg/kg	ND	ND
Neosolaniol, mg/kg	ND	ND
Nivalenol, mg/kg	0.2	ND
Ochratoxin A, mg/kg	0.1	ND
Ochratoxin B, mg/kg	ND	ND
Zearalenone, mg/kg	1.1	1.8

[1] Mycotoxin analysis was performed by UPLC-MS/MS using the Alltech 37+ program at Alltech (Nicholasville, KY, USA).

Challenge periods and inclusion levels of mycotoxins in this study were based on previous studies where pigs at similar body weights were challenged with AF, FUM, and DON (isolated or in combination) for equivalent periods of time to enable comparison of results [2,4,16]. The inclusion level of 0.2% for YCWE was chosen based on the recommended level by the manufacturer, which was previously tested and showed the ability to reduce mycotoxin toxicity [3,47].

4.2. Sampling and Laboratory Analyses

4.2.1. Blood Sampling

In experiment 1, the pig with median BW from each pen was bled at the end of 4 weeks of feeding, whereas in experiment 2, pigs were bled on days 14 and 45 for hematological, biochemical, anti-oxidative, and immunological analysis. Blood was collected in Vacutainer tubes (BD Biosciences, San Jose, CA, USA) without anticoagulant to obtain serum for serum biochemistry as indicators of overall physiological status, TNF-α as an indicator of inflammatory status, IgA (only for experiment 2) and IgG as indicators of humoral immune status, MDA as an indicator of lipid peroxidation, protein carbonyl (only for experiment 2) as an indicator of oxidative protein damage, and 8-hydroxydeoxyguanosine (8-OHdG, only for experiment 1) as an indicator of oxidative DNA damage. Blood was allowed to clot before centrifuging for 15 min at 3000 × g (4 °C) to collect serum, and samples were stored at −80 °C until analyzed. Blood samples were also collected in tubes containing EDTA to obtain whole blood for hematological measurements.

4.2.2. Tissue, Mucosa, and Digesta Collection

At the last day of feeding, from each treatment, a pig representing an average body weight of each of the 8 pens (4 gilt pens and 4 barrow pens) were selected, excluding one of the heaviest and one of the lightest pens for experiment 1, and all pigs for experiment 2. Pigs were euthanized to collect mucosa tissue samples from duodenum (a portion of 20 cm, only for experiment 1) and distal jejunum (a portion of 20 cm prior to ileum). Duodenum and distal jejunum were isolated and flushed with saline solution. About 10 cm of their section was fixed in 10% formaldehyde phosphate buffer and kept for microscopic assessment of mucosal morphology, such as villus height and crypt depth. Mucosa from the left duodenum and jejunum were also stored in liquid nitrogen immediately after collection and moved to −80 °C until analysis. The mucosa was used to measure TNF-α, IgG, and MDA for both experiments and IgA and protein carbonyl only for experiment 2. In experiment 2, ileal portion (a portion of 20 cm prior to ileocecal valve) was used to obtain ileal digesta for apparent ileal digestibility. The ileal digesta was collected by gently squeezing. The ileal digesta were stored in sterile containers and kept frozen at −20 °C. The ileal digesta was freeze-dried (24D × 48, Virtis, Gardiner, NY) for storage and chemical analysis. Freeze-dried digesta was used for measuring apparent ileal digestibility of dry matter, crude protein, growth energy, and ether extract. In experiment 2, jejunal tissues were used to measure tight junction proteins (claudin-1, occludin, and zona occludens-1 protein) as indicators of gut integrity using Western Blot.

4.2.3. Hematological and Biochemical Assays

Whole blood with EDTA was sent to Antech Diagnostics (Cary, NC, USA) for complete blood counting. Measurements included hematocrit, hemoglobin, mean corpuscular hemoglobin, mean corpuscular hemoglobin concentration, mean corpuscular volume, platelet number, red blood cell count, white blood cell count, basophils, eosinophils, lymphocytes, monocytes, and neutrophils.

Concentrations of serum alanine aminotransferase, albumin, alkaline phosphatase, aspartate aminotransferase, bilirubin, BUN-to-creatinine ratio, calcium, chloride, cholesterol, creatinine, creatine phosphokinase, globulin, glucose, phosphorus, potassium, sodium, and BUN were measured (Antech Diagnostics, Cary, NC, USA) for determination of serum biochemistry.

4.2.4. Tumor Necrosis Factor-α

Tumor necrosis factor-α was measured in duodenal and jejunal mucosa as well as in serum by enzyme-linked immunosorbent assay (ELISA), as described by Weaver et al. [48]. Determination of TNF-α was completed following the manufacturer's procedure (PTA00; R and D System, Minneapolis, MN, USA). Mucosa samples (500 mg) of duodenum and jejunum were weighed and suspended into 1.0 mL PBS. Mucosa samples were homogenized (Tissuemiser; Thermo Fisher Scientific Inc., Rockford, IL, USA) on ice. The homogenate was centrifuged for 30 min at $10,000 \times g$ (4 °C) to collect supernatant, which was used to determine concentrations of TNF-α and protein concentrations. Protein concentrations of mucosa supernatant in duodenum and jejunum were measured using a BCA protein assay (23225; Thermo Fisher Scientific, Rockford, IL, USA). Briefly, 50 μL of standard plus dilute or 100 μL of sample was added to microplate wells coated with capture antibody in conjunction with biotinylated antibody reagent. Detection occurred by the use of horseradish peroxidase, TMB substrate, and a stop solution of 2 M sulfuric acid (H_2SO_4). Absorbance was read at 450 nm and 550 nm by an ELISA plate reader (Synergy HT, Biotek Inc. Winooski, VT, USA) and the Gen 5 data analysis software (Biotek Inc. Winooski, VT, USA). Concentrations of TNF-α in mucosa and serum were expressed as ng/g of protein and pg/mL, respectively. The detection limit for TNF-α was 5 pg/mL. Unless otherwise defined, all processes of sample extraction and protein measurements used herein have the same method.

4.2.5. Immunoglobulins A and G

Concentrations of porcine IgA and IgG in duodenal and jejunal mucosa as well as in serum were measured via ELISA, as described by Weaver et al. [4]. Goat anti-pig IgA or IgG was used to capture antibodies by coating wells. Horseradish peroxidase conjugated to goat anti-pig IgA or IgG were used as the detection antibody in combination with the TMB (3,3',5,5'-tetramethylbenzidene) enzyme substrate (E100-102 or E100-104; Bethyl Laboratories Inc., Montgomery, TX, USA). A solution of 0.18 M H_2SO_4 was used to stop the enzyme-substrate reaction. Absorbance was read at 450 nm using an ELISA plate reader and Gen 5 data analysis software. Concentrations of IgA and IgG in mucosa and serum were expressed as mg/g of protein and mg/mL, respectively. Detection limits were 15.6 to 1000 ng/mL or 7.8 to 500 ng/mL for IgA and IgG, respectively.

4.2.6. Malondialdehydes

Concentrations of MDA in duodenal and jejunal mucosa as well as in serum were analyzed using a TBARS assay (STA-330; Cell Biolabs, San Diego, CA, USA) as described by Shen et al. [49]. Concentrations of MDA in mucosa and serum were expressed as μmol/mg protein and nmol/mL, respectively. The assay range for MDA was 0 to 125 μM.

4.2.7. 8-Hydroxy-Deoxyguanosine

Production of 8-OHdG in serum was determined by ELISA (STA-320; Cell Biolabs, San Diego, CA, USA) as described by Weaver et al [48]. Undiluted samples were added to an 8-OHdG conjugate-coated microplate, followed by diluted anti-8-OHdG antibody, and finally diluted secondary antibody enzyme conjugate. After incubation, the provided stop solution was added to each well, and allowed to incubate for 8–10 min before being stopped with a stop solution in order to achieve a color change which was not over-saturated. Samples were then measured at 450 nm and concentration was determined based on the standard curve.

4.2.8. Protein Carbonyl

Concentration of protein carbonyl in jejunal mucosa and serum as an index of oxidative protein was analyzed using an ELISA kit (STA 310; Cell Biolabs, San Diego, CA, USA) as described by Shen et al. [49]. Concentrations of protein carbonyl in mucosa and plasma were expressed as µmol/g protein. The assay range for protein carbonyl was 0 to 7.5 nmol/mg protein.

4.2.9. Chemical Analysis

In experiment 2, dry matter of digesta was quantified by weighing digesta samples prior to and after freeze-drying, as described in Passos et al. [50]. Nitrogen was quantified in ground feed and digesta samples using TruSpec N Nitrogen Determinator (LECO Corp., St. Joseph, MI, USA) to calculate crude protein (method 992.15; [51]). Gross energy was quantified in ground feed and digesta samples using a Parr 6200 Calorimeter (Parr Instrument Co., Moline, IL). Ether extract was quantified in ground feed and digesta samples using ether extraction method (method 920.39; [51]).

4.2.10. Apparent Ileal Digestibility

In experiment 2, apparent ileal digestibility (%) of dry matter, crude protein, gross energy, and ether extract was calculated using the titanium dioxide concentration in digesta and feed by using the equation: AID = 100 − ((ND/NF) × (TiF/TiD) × 100), where, AID is the apparent nutrient digestibility, ND is the nutrient concentration present in the ileal digesta, NF is the nutrient concentration in the feed, TiF is the titanium dioxide concentration in the feed, and TiD is the titanium dioxide concentration in the ileal digesta. Titanium dioxide was measured and calculated using a standard curve based on the methods described by Myers et al. [52].

4.2.11. Immunohistochemistry for Ki-67 and Morphometry on Duodenum and Jejunum

In experiment 1, duodenal and jejunal samples were embedded in paraffin, cut cross-section to 5 µm thick, and mounted on polylysine-coated slides. Slides were then stained (hematoxylin and eosin) and examined under a Sony Van–Ox S microscope (Opelco, Washington, DC). Villus height (from the tip of the villi to the villus-crypt junction), villus width (width of the villus at one-half of the villus height), and crypt depth (from villus junction to the base of the crypt) were determined according to Weaver et al. [48]. Lengths of 10 well-oriented intact villi and their associated crypt were measured in each slide. The same person executed all the analyses of intestinal morphology.

In experiment 2, jejunal samples were embedded in paraffin. Epitope retrieval was performed using 10 mM citrate buffer, pH 6.0 in a pressure cooker (Dako, Carpinteria, CA). Endogenous peroxidase was quenched with 3% hydrogen peroxide and sections were blocked using protein block reagent (Dako, Carpinteria, CA). Primary monoclonal antibody of Ki-67 (Dako, Carpinteria, CA) was used after 1:500 dilutions. Secondary antibody was attached using Vector ImmPRESS anti-mouse polymer reagent (Vector Laboratories, Burlingame, CA) after 1:2 dilutions. Diaminobenzamine reagent (Vector Laboratories, Burlingame, CA) was used as the chromogen. Image JS software [53] was used for calculating the Ki-67-positive cell. Simultaneously, jejunal morphometry can be available with the immunohistochemistry.

4.2.12. Microbiome Analysis of Jejunal Mucosa

In experiment 2, mucosa-associated microbiome was sequenced. DNA was extracted from jejual mucosa with QIAGEN's QIAamp® DNA Stool MiniKit (Qiagen, Crawley, UK). Samples were prepared for template preparation on the Ion Chef TM instrument and sequencing on the Ion S5 TM system (ThermoFisher Scientific, Inc., Wilmington, DE, USA). Variable regions V2, V3, V4, V6, V7, V8, and V9 of the 16S rRNA gene were amplified with the Ion 16S Metagenomics Kit (ThermoFisher Scientific, Inc., Wilmington, DE). Sequences (hypervariable regions) were processed using the Torrent Suite TM Software (version 5.2.2; ThermoFisher Scientific, Inc., Wilmington, DE) to produce ".bam" files for further analysis. Sequence data analysis, alignment to GreenGenes (anybody) and MicroSeq (experts) databases, alpha and beta diversity plot generation, and OTU table generation were performed by the Ion Reporter TM Software Suite of bioinformatics analysis tools (version 5.2.2; ThermoFisher Scientific,

Inc., Wilmington, DE). Samples were analyzed using Ion Reporter's Metagenomics 16S workflow powered by Qiime (version w1.1).

4.2.13. Tight Junction Proteins in Jejunal Tissue

In experiment 2, four samples of jejunal tissue in each treatment were used to measure tight junction protein, as described by Yang et al. [37]. Tissue samples (50 mg) of jejunum were weighed and suspended into 0.5 mL RIPA lysis and extraction buffer containing 5 µL protease inhibitor cocktail. Tissue samples were homogenized on ice. The homogenate was centrifuged at 10,000 × g at 4 °C for 10 min to collect supernatant. Protein concentration of the supernatant was adjusted to 2 µg/µL by using a BCA protein assay, as mentioned above. The adjusted supernatant was denatured at 100 °C for 5 min in the water bath and was loaded in each well for SDS-PAGE. After SDS-PAGE, the gel was moved on polyvinylidene difluoride membrane for transferring a target protein to the membrane. Protein was electrophoretically transferred at 90 mV for 1 h. This was then blocked in 5% skim milk, and incubated (overnight at 4 °C) with primary antibodies against claudin, occluding, zona occludens-1 protein, and β-actin. The membrane was subsequently washed and incubated (1 h at room temperature) with horseradish-conjugated secondary antibodies. The immunoblot was developed with the DAB substrate kit (34002; Pierce, Rockford, IL). The density of bands was identified by using image analyzer software (LI-COR Biosciences, Lincoln, NE).

4.3. Data Analysis and Interpretation

In both experiment 1 and experiment 2, data from this study were analyzed based on a randomized complete block design by the Mixed model of SAS Software (Cary, NC, USA). The experimental unit was a pen. Factors were mycotoxin and YCWE. Factors, interaction between factors, and sex were the fixed effects and initial BW block was a random effect. Diets with or without mycotoxins were compared with the PDIFF option to evaluate if the mycotoxin effect was mitigated by YCWE once an interaction between mycotoxin and YCWE was found. Statistical differences among treatment means were considered significant with $p < 0.05$, whereas $0.05 \leq p < 0.10$ was used as the criteria for tendency.

Author Contributions: Conceptualization, S.W.K. and A.Y.; methodology, S.W.K. and A.Y.; formal analysis, I.P. and X.G.; investigation, I.P. and X.G.; resources, S.W.K. and A.Y.; data curation, S.W.K. and I.P.; writing—original draft preparation, D.M.H., S.W.K. and X.G.; writing—review and editing, S.W.K., D.M.H, and A.Y.; supervision, S.W.K.; project administration, S.W.K.; funding acquisition, S.W.K.

Funding: This research was funded by North Carolina Agricultural Foundation and Alltech Inc.

Acknowledgments: Financial supports from Alltech Inc., and North Carolina Agricultural Foundation

Conflicts of Interest: The authors declare no conflict of interest.

References

1. Weaver, A.; See, M.; Kim, S. Protective effect of two yeast based feed additives on pigs chronically exposed to deoxynivalenol and zearalenone. *Toxins* **2014**, *6*, 3336–3353. [CrossRef] [PubMed]
2. Chaytor, A.C.; See, M.T.; Hansen, J.A.; de Souza, A.L.P.; Middleton, T.F.; Kim, S.W. Effects of chronic exposure of diets with reduced concentrations of aflatoxin and deoxynivalenol on growth and immune status of pigs. *J. Anim. Sci.* **2011**, *89*, 124–135. [CrossRef] [PubMed]
3. Sun, Y.; Park, I.; Guo, J.; Weaver, A.C.; Kim, S.W. Impacts of low level aflatoxin in feed and the use of modified yeast cell wall extract on growth and health of nursery pigs. *Anim. Nutr.* **2015**, *1*, 177–183. [CrossRef] [PubMed]
4. Weaver, A.; See, M.; Hansen, J.; Kim, Y.; De Souza, A.; Middleton, T.; Kim, S. The use of feed additives to reduce the effects of aflatoxin and deoxynivalenol on pig growth, organ health and immune status during chronic exposure. *Toxins* **2013**, *5*, 1261–1281. [CrossRef] [PubMed]
5. Jouany, J.P. Methods for preventing, decontaminating and minimizing the toxicity of mycotoxins in feeds. *Anim. Feed Sci. Technol.* **2007**, *137*, 342–362. [CrossRef]

6. Yiannikouris, A.; André, G.; Buléon, A.; Jeminet, G.; Canet, I.; François, J.; Bertin, G.; Jouany, J.-P. Comprehensive conformational study of key interactions involved in zearalenone complexation with β-D-glucans. *Biomacromolecules* **2004**, *5*, 2176–2185. [CrossRef]
7. Yiannikouris, A.; François, J.; Poughon, L.; Dussap, C.-G.; Bertin, G.; Jeminet, G.; Jouany, J.-P. Adsorption of zearalenone by b-D-glucans in the Saccharomyces cerevisiae cell wall. *J. Food Prot.* **2004**, *67*, 1195–1200. [CrossRef]
8. Yiannikouris, A.; Francois, J.; Poughon, L.; Dussap, C.-G.; Rard Bertin, G.Ä.; Jeminet, G.; Jouany, J.-P. Alkali extraction of β-D-glucans from Saccharomyces cerevisiae cell wall and study of their adsorptive properties toward zearalenone. *J. Agric. Food Chem.* **2004**, *52*, 3666–3673. [CrossRef]
9. Yiannikouris, A.; André, G.; Poughon, L.; François, J.; Dussap, C.-G.; Jeminet, G.; Bertin, G.; Jouany, J.-P. Chemical and conformational study of the interactions involved in mycotoxin complexation with β-d-glucans. *Biomacromolecules* **2006**, *7*, 1147–1155. [CrossRef]
10. Yiannikouris, A.; Kettunen, H.; Apajalahti, J.; Pennala, E.; Moran, C.A. Comparison of the sequestering properties of yeast cell wall extract and hydrated sodium calcium aluminosilicate in three in vitro models accounting for the animal physiological bioavailability of zearalenone. *Food Addit. Contam. Part A* **2013**, *30*, 1641–1650. [CrossRef]
11. Firmin, S.; Gandia, P.; Morgavi, D.P.; Houin, G.; Jouany, J.P.; Bertin, G.; Boudra, H. Modification of aflatoxin B$_1$ and ochratoxin A toxicokinetics in rats administered a yeast cell wall preparation. *Food Addit. Contam. Part A* **2010**, *27*, 1153–1160. [CrossRef] [PubMed]
12. Prelusky, D.B.; Gerdes, R.G.; Underhill, K.L.; Rotter, B.A.; Jui, P.Y.; Trenholm, H.L. Effects of low-level dietary deoxynivalenol on haematological and clinical parameters of the pig. *Nat. Toxins* **1994**, *2*, 97–104. [CrossRef] [PubMed]
13. Harvey, R.B.; Edrington, T.S.; Kubena, L.F.; Elissalde, M.H.; Rottinghaus, G.E. Influence of aflatoxin and fumonisin B1-containing culture material on growing barrows. *Am. J. Vet. Res.* **1995**, *56*, 1668–1672. [PubMed]
14. Moeser, A.J.; Pohl, C.S.; Rajput, M. Weaning stress and gastrointestinal barrier development: Implications for lifelong gut health in pigs. *Anim. Nutr.* **2017**, *3*, 313–321. [CrossRef]
15. Linghong, J.; Wang, W.; Degroote, J.; Van Noten, N.; Yan, H.; Majdeddin, M.; Van Poucke, M.; Peelman, L.; Goderis, A.; Van De Mierop, K.; et al. Mycotoxin binder improves growth rate in piglets associated with reduction of toll-like receptor-4 and increase of tight junction protein gene expression in gut mucosa. *J. Anim. Sci. Biotechnol.* **2017**, *8*, 80.
16. Dersjant-Li, Y.; Verstegen, M.W.A.; Gerrits, W.J.J. The impact of low concentrations of aflatoxin, deoxynivalenol or fumonisin in diets on growing pigs and poultry. *Nutr. Res. Rev.* **2003**, *16*, 223–239. [CrossRef]
17. Pestka, J.J. Deoxynivalenol: Mechanisms of action, human exposure, and toxicological relevance. *Arch. Toxicol.* **2010**, *84*, 663–679. [CrossRef]
18. Pasternak, J.A.; Aiyer, V.I.A.; Hamonic, G.; Beaulieu, A.D.; Columbus, D.A.; Wilson, H.L. Molecular and physiological effects on the small intestine of weaner pigs following feeding with deoxynivalenol-contaminated feed. *Toxins* **2018**, *10*, 40. [CrossRef]
19. Flannery, B.M.; Clark, E.S.; Pestka, J.J. Anorexia induction by the trichothecene deoxynivalenol (vomitoxin) is mediated by the release of the gut satiety hormone peptide YY. *Toxicol. Sci.* **2012**, *130*, 289–297. [CrossRef]
20. Fioramonti, J.; Dupuy, C.; Dupuy, J.; Bueno, L. The mycotoxin, deoxynivalenol, delays gastric emptying through serotonin-3 receptors in rodents. *J. Pharmacol. Exp. Ther.* **1993**, *266*, 1255–1260.
21. Flannery, B.M.; Wu, W.; Pestka, J.J. Characterization of deoxynivalenol-induced anorexia using mouse bioassay. *Food Chem. Toxicol.* **2011**, *49*, 1863–1869. [CrossRef] [PubMed]
22. Wu, W.; Bates, M.A.; Bursian, S.J.; Flannery, B.; Zhou, H.-R.; Link, J.E.; Zhang, H.; Pestka, J.J. Peptide YY 3-36 and 5-hydroxytryptamine mediate emesis induction by trichothecene deoxynivalenol (vomitoxin). *Toxicol. Sci.* **2013**, *133*, 186–195. [CrossRef]
23. Manners, D.J.; Masson, A.J.; Patterson, J.C. The structure of a beta-(1-3)-D-glucan from yeast cell walls. *Biochem. J.* **1973**, *135*, 19–30. [CrossRef] [PubMed]
24. Yiannikouris, A.; Poughon, L.; Cameleyre, X.; Dussap, C.-G.; François, J.; Bertin, G.; Jouany, J.-P. A novel technique to evaluate interactions between Saccharomyces cerevisiae cell wall and mycotoxins: Application to zearalenone. *Biotechnol. Lett.* **2003**, *25*, 783–789. [CrossRef] [PubMed]

25. Xiong, X.; Yang, H.; Li, B.; Liu, G.; Huang, R.; Li, F.; Liao, P.; Zhang, Y.; Martin Nyachoti, C.; Deng, D. Dietary supplementation with yeast product improves intestinal function, and serum and ileal amino acid contents in weaned piglets. *Livest. Sci.* **2015**, *171*, 20–27. [CrossRef]
26. Shen, Y.B.; Piao, X.S.; Kim, S.W.; Wang, L.; Liu, P.; Yoon, I.; Zhen, Y.G. Effects of yeast culture supplementation on growth performance, intestinal health, and immune response of nursery pigs. *J. Anim. Sci.* **2009**, *87*, 2614–2624. [CrossRef]
27. Sweeney, T.; Collins, C.B.; Reilly, P.; Pierce, K.M.; Ryan, M.; O'Doherty, J.V. Effect of purified β-glucans derived from Laminaria digitata, Laminaria hyperborea and Saccharomyces cerevisiae on piglet performance, selected bacterial populations, volatile fatty acids and pro-inflammatory cytokines in the gastrointestinal tract of pig. *Br. J. Nutr.* **2012**, *108*, 1226–1234. [CrossRef]
28. Freire, L.; Sant'Ana, A.S. Modified mycotoxins: An updated review on their formation, detection, occurrence, and toxic effects. *Food Chem. Toxicol.* **2018**, *111*, 189–205. [CrossRef]
29. Anraku, M.; Chuang, V.T.G.; Maruyama, T.; Otagiri, M. Redox properties of serum albumin. *Biochim. Biophys. Acta Gen. Subj.* **2013**, *1830*, 5465–5472. [CrossRef]
30. Latimer, K.S. (Ed.) *Duncan and Prasse's Veterinary Laboratory Medicine: Clinical Pathology*, 5th ed.; John Wiley & Sons: Ames, IA, USA, 2011.
31. Ruiz, M.-J.; Macáková, P.; Juan-García, A.; Font, G. Cytotoxic effects of mycotoxin combinations in mammalian kidney cells. *Food Chem. Toxicol.* **2011**, *49*, 2718–2724. [CrossRef]
32. Hou, Y.-J.; Zhao, Y.-Y.; Xiong, B.; Cui, X.-S.; Kim, N.-H.; Xu, Y.-X.; Sun, S.-C. Mycotoxin-containing diet causes oxidative stress in the mouse. *PLoS ONE* **2013**, *8*, e60374. [CrossRef] [PubMed]
33. Reddy, K.; Song, J.; Lee, H.-J.; Kim, M.; Kim, D.-W.; Jung, H.; Kim, B.; Lee, Y.; Yu, D.; Kim, D.-W.; et al. Effects of high levels of deoxynivalenol and zearalenone on growth performance, and hematological and immunological parameters in pigs. *Toxins* **2018**, *10*, 114. [CrossRef] [PubMed]
34. Pierron, A.; Alassane-Kpembi, I.; Oswald, I.P. Impact of mycotoxin on immune response and consequences for pig health. *Anim. Nutr.* **2016**, *2*, 63–68. [CrossRef] [PubMed]
35. Garas, L.C.; Feltrin, C.; Kristina Hamilton, M.; Hagey, J.V.; Murray, J.D.; Bertolini, L.R.; Bertolini, M.; Raybould, H.E.; Maga, E.A. Milk with and without lactoferrin can influence intestinal damage in a pig model of malnutrition. *Food Funct.* **2016**, *7*, 665–678. [CrossRef]
36. Aderem, A.; Ulevitch, R.J. Toll-like receptors in the induction of the innate immune response. *Nature* **2000**, *406*, 782–787. [CrossRef]
37. Yang, F.; Wang, A.; Zeng, X.; Hou, C.; Liu, H.; Qiao, S. Lactobacillus reuteri I5007 modulates tight junction protein expression in IPEC-J2 cells with LPS stimulation and in newborn piglets under normal conditions. *BMC Microbiol.* **2015**, *15*, 32. [CrossRef]
38. Vaahtovuo, J.; Korkeamäki, M.; Munukka, E.; Hämeenoja, P.; Vuorenmaa, J. Microbial balance index—A view on the intestinal microbiota. *Livest. Sci.* **2007**, *109*, 174–178. [CrossRef]
39. Almeida, L.R.; Costa, P.S.; Nascimento, A.M.A.; Reis, M.d.P.; Barros, K.O.; Alvim, L.B.; Nunes, Á.C.; Queiroz, D.M.M.; Rocha, G.A.; Nicoli, J.R.; et al. Porcine stomachs with and without gastric ulcer differ in Lactobacillus load and strain characteristics. *Can. J. Microbiol.* **2018**, *64*, 493–499. [CrossRef]
40. Sapountzis, P.; Gruntjes, T.; Otani, S.; Estevez, J.; da Costa, R.R.; Plunkett, G., 3rd; Perna, N.T.; Poulsen, M. The Enterobacterium Trabulsiella odontotermitis presents novel adaptations related to its association with fungus-growing termites. *Appl. Environ. Microbiol.* **2015**, *81*, 6577–6588. [CrossRef]
41. De Angelis, M.; Siragusa, S.; Berloco, M.; Caputo, L.; Settanni, L.; Alfonsi, G.; Amerio, M.; Grandi, A.; Ragni, A.; Gobbetti, M. Selection of potential probiotic lactobacilli from pig feces to be used as additives in pelleted feeding. *Res. Microbiol.* **2006**, *157*, 792–801. [CrossRef]
42. Zou, Z.-Y.; He, Z.-F.; Li, H.-J.; Han, P.-F.; Meng, X.; Zhang, Y.; Zhou, F.; Ouyang, K.-P.; Chen, X.-Y.; Tang, J. In vitro removal of deoxynivalenol and T-2 toxin by lactic acid bacteria. *Food Sci. Biotechnol.* **2012**, *21*, 1677–1683. [CrossRef]
43. Haskard, C.A.; El-Nezami, H.S.; Kankaanpää, P.E.; Salminen, S.; Ahokas, J.T. Surface binding of aflatoxin B(1) by lactic acid bacteria. *Appl. Environ. Microbiol.* **2001**, *67*, 3086–3091. [CrossRef] [PubMed]
44. Sato, I.; Ito, M.; Ishizaka, M.; Ikunaga, Y.; Sato, Y.; Yoshida, S.; Koitabashi, M.; Tsushima, S. Thirteen novel deoxynivalenol-degrading bacteria are classified within two genera with distinct degradation mechanisms. *FEMS Microbiol. Lett.* **2012**, *327*, 110–117. [CrossRef] [PubMed]

45. Willing, B.P.; Van Kessel, A.G. Enterocyte proliferation and apoptosis in the caudal small intestine is influenced by the composition of colonizing commensal bacteria in the neonatal gnotobiotic pig. *J. Anim. Sci.* **2007**, *85*, 3256–3266. [CrossRef]
46. (NRC) National Research Council. *Nutrition Requirements of Swine*, 11th ed.; National Academy Press: Washington, DC, USA, 2012.
47. Swamy, H.V.L.N.; Smith, T.K.; MacDonald, E.J.; Karrow, N.A.; Woodward, B.; Boermans, H.J. Effects of feeding a blend of grains naturally contaminated with Fusarium mycotoxins on growth and immunological measurements of starter pigs, and the efficacy of a polymeric glucomannan mycotoxin adsorbent. *J. Anim. Sci.* **2003**, *81*, 2792–2803. [CrossRef]
48. Weaver, A.C.; Kim, S.W.; Campbell, J.M.; Crenshaw, J.D.; Polo, J. Efficacy of dietary spray dried plasma protein to mitigate the negative effects on performance of pigs fed diets with corn naturally contaminated with multiple mycotoxins. *J. Anim. Sci.* **2014**, *92*, 3878–3886. [CrossRef]
49. Shen, Y.B.; Weaver, A.C.; Kim, S.W. Effect of feed grade L-methionine on growth performance and gut health in nursery pigs compared with conventional DL-methionine. *J. Anim. Sci.* **2014**, *92*, 5530–5539. [CrossRef]
50. Passos, A.A.; Park, I.; Ferket, P.; von Heimendahl, E.; Kim, S.W. Effect of dietary supplementation of xylanase on apparent ileal digestibility of nutrients, viscosity of digesta, and intestinal morphology of growing pigs fed corn and soybean meal based diet. *Anim. Nutr.* **2015**, *1*, 19–23. [CrossRef]
51. AOAC International. *AOAC International Guidelines for Laboratories Performing Microbiological and Chemical Analyses of Food and Pharmaceuticals: An Aid to Interpretation of ISO/IEC 17025: 2005*; AOAC: Frederick, MD, USA, 2006.
52. Myers, W.D.; Ludden, P.A.; Nayigihugu, V.; Hess, B.W. Technical Note: A procedure for the preparation and quantitative analysis of samples for titanium dioxide. *J. Anim. Sci.* **2004**, *82*, 179–183. [CrossRef]
53. Almeida, J.S.; Iriabho, E.E.; Gorrepati, V.L.; Wilkinson, S.R.; Hackney, J.R.; Grüneberg, A.; Robbins, D.E. ImageJS: Personalized, participated, pervasive, and reproducible image bioinformatics in the web browser. *J. Pathol. Inform.* **2012**, *3*, 25. [CrossRef]

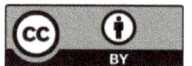

© 2019 by the authors. Licensee MDPI, Basel, Switzerland. This article is an open access article distributed under the terms and conditions of the Creative Commons Attribution (CC BY) license (http://creativecommons.org/licenses/by/4.0/).

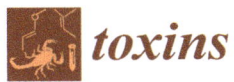

Article

Calcination Enhances the Aflatoxin and Zearalenone Binding Efficiency of a Tunisian Clay

Roua Rejeb [1,2,*], Gunther Antonissen [2,3], Marthe De Boevre [4], Christ'l Detavernier [4], Mario Van de Velde [4], Sarah De Saeger [4], Richard Ducatelle [2], Madiha Hadj Ayed [1] and Achraf Ghorbal [5]

1. Université de Sousse, Institut Supérieur Agronomique de Chott-Mariem, LR18AG01, ISA-CM-BP, 47, Sousse 4042, Tunisia; mediha.ayed@yahoo.fr
2. Department of Pathology, Bacteriology and Avian Diseases, Faculty of veterinary medicine, Ghent University, Salisburylaan 133, 9820 Merelbeke, Belgium; Gunther.Antonissen@UGent.be (G.A.); Richard.Ducatelle@UGent.be (R.D.)
3. Department of Pharmacology, Toxicology and Biochemistry, Faculty of Veterinary Medicine, Ghent University, Salisburylaan 133, 9820 Merelbeke, Belgium
4. Department of Bioanalysis, Centre of Excellence in Mycotoxicology and Public Health, Faculty of Pharmaceutical Sciences, Ghent University, Ottergemsesteenweg 460, 9000 Ghent, Belgium; Marthe.DeBoevre@UGent.be (M.D.B.); Christel.Detavernier@UGent.be (C.D.); Mario.VandeVelde@UGent.be (M.V.d.V.); Sarah.DeSaeger@UGent.be (S.D.S)
5. Research Laboratory LR18ES33, National Engineering School of Gabes, University of Gabes, Avenue Omar Ibn El Khattab, Gabes 6029, Tunisia; achraf.ghorbal.issat@gmail.com
* Correspondence: Roua.Rejeb@UGent.be or rouaa.rejeb@gmail.com; Tel.: +216-5293-9154

Received: 3 September 2019; Accepted: 14 October 2019; Published: 16 October 2019

Abstract: Clays are known to have promising adsorbing characteristics, and are used as feed additives to overcome the negative effects of mycotoxicosis in livestock farming. Modification of clay minerals by heat treatment, also called calcination, can alter their adsorption characteristics. Little information, however, is available on the effect of calcination with respect to mycotoxin binding. The purpose of this study was to characterize a Tunisian clay before and after calcination (at 550 °C), and to investigate the effectiveness of the thermal treatment of this clay on its aflatoxin B1 (AFB1), G1 (AFG1), B2 (AFB2), G2 (AFG2), and zearalenone (ZEN) adsorption capacity. Firstly, the purified clay (CP) and calcined clay (CC) were characterized with X-ray Fluorescence (XRF), X-ray Diffraction (XRD), Fourier transform infrared spectroscopy (FTIR-IR), cation exchange capacity (CEC), specific surface area (S_{BET}), and point of zero charge (pH_{PZC}) measurements. Secondly, an in vitro model that simulated the pH conditions of the monogastric gastrointestinal tract was used to evaluate the binding efficiency of the tested clays when artificially mixed with aflatoxins and zearalenone. The tested clay consisted mainly of smectite and illite. Purified and calcined clay had similar chemical compositions. After heat treatment, however, some changes in the mineralogical and textural properties were observed. The calcination decreased the cation exchange capacity and the specific surface, whereas the pore size was increased. Both purified and calcined clay had a binding efficacy of over 90% for AFB1 under simulated poultry GI tract conditions. Heat treatment of the clay increased the adsorption of AFB2, AFG1, and AFG2 related to the increase in pore size of the clay by the calcination process. ZEN adsorption also increased by calcination, albeit to a more stable level at pH 3 rather than at pH 7. In conclusion, calcination of clay minerals enhanced the adsorption of aflatoxins and mostly of AFG1 and AFG2 at neutral pH of the gastrointestinal tract, and thus are associated with protection against the toxic effects of aflatoxins.

Keywords: aflatoxins; zearalenone; clay; purified; calcined; adsorption; pH

Key Contribution: In vitro binding capacity of purified and calcined clay was determined for AFB1, AFB2, AFG1, AFG2 and ZEN in the pH of the poults gastrointestinal tract. The calcined clay has successfully improved the binding efficiency of AFB2, AFG1, AFG2 and ZEN.

1. Introduction

Mycotoxins are secondary metabolites produced by toxigenic fungi growing on a wide range of agricultural products [1]. The Food and Agriculture Organization (FAO) of the United Nations stated that nearly 25% of the cereal products is contaminated with mycotoxins [2].

Aflatoxins (AFs) are considered as the most important mycotoxins in food and feed because of their carcinogenicity (IARC monograph class I) and their high prevalence, especially in Southern regions [3,4]. AFs are a group of heterocyclic metabolites that are mainly produced by members of the genus *Aspergillus*, contaminating agricultural commodities. *Aspergillus* fungi are both found in the field as storage pathogens, therefore the AFs' content is omnipresent, but with a tendency to increase during storage [5,6]. AFs cause serious health problems, economic losses, and deleterious effects on performance in a variety of farm animals including pigs, poultry, and cattle [7]. More specifically in poultry, AFs reduce the growth rate, decrease egg production, induce changes in organ weight, and increase the risk of disease [4]. In young chicks, AFs reduce immune competence and cause liver damage [8–10]. Aflatoxin B1 (AFB1) is the most potent of the aflatoxins, followed by AFG1, AFB2, and AFG2 [11]. AFB1 comprise a greater potency associated with the cyclopentenone ring of the B series, when compared with the six-membered lactone ring of the G series [12].

Zearalenone (ZEN) is a phenolic resorcyclic acid lactone mycotoxin produced by *Fusarium* fungi growing on cereal grains and derived products worldwide. *Fusarium* mycotoxins are primarily produced before harvest, on the field. ZEN is a potent estrogenic metabolite as it has the ability to bind to estrogen receptors and induces estrogenic alterations including uterine enlargement, swelling of the vulva and mammary glands, and pseudopregnancy [13,14].

To offset the negative effects of mycotoxins on animal health, a wide range of mycotoxin decontamination strategies has been reported in the literature [15–17]. Adding mycotoxin binders to the feed is probably the most common post-harvest mitigation approach [18–20]. Binders decrease the absorption of mycotoxins from the gastrointestinal (GI) tract into the blood circulation and target organs by adsorbing them on their surface [21], forming a binder-toxin complex which is eliminated through the fecal material [22]. Inclusion of mycotoxin binders improves the average daily gain and the average daily feed intake in pigs and reduced the injurious effect of AFs on body weight, feed conversion ratio (FCR), serum alanine aminotransferase (ALT), and urea concentration in broiler chickens [8,23]. However, it should be noted that adding a high dose of clay in the feed might cause nutrient deficiency by adsorbing micronutrients, vitamins and organic compounds, while also having negative effects on the bioavailability of minerals and trace elements [15,24]. In addition, the risk of the contamination of raw clays with metals and dioxins has to be considered [25]. Among mycotoxin binders, clay minerals are the largest group. Several aluminosilicate clays such as hydrated sodium calcium aluminosilicate (HSCAS), bentonite, montmorillonite, smectite, and zeolite have good binding efficiency to mycotoxins [26,27]. These clays mostly bind small mycotoxins, such as AFs and ochratoxin A, but have less binding affinity for the larger molecules of certain *Fusarium* toxins. ZEN can be adsorbed by only a limited number of binders with a large variation in binding capacity [28]. Effectiveness of binding also depends on the type, and the dosage of the binders. A Brazilian study showed that about 64% of the products on the market were ineffective in binding AFs [29,30].

Clays are used in their natural state or treated through various processes such as calcination, acid activation, pillaring, organic modification with polymers, or cation and anion exchange. These modified clays can be more effective in binding some mycotoxins than the untreated clay [31–34]. Calcination is a process in which clay minerals are heated to different temperatures [33].

It removes the water located in intra-crystalline tunnels, which changes the pore structure and surface proprieties [35,36]. Consequently, heat treatment has an impact on the specific surface area of clay, which is responsible for the adsorption capacity [37]. Calcined clays have been used in numerous studies as adsorbents to eliminate heavy metals and cationic dyes [38,39].

To the best of the authors' knowledge, only one study investigated the effect of calcination on mycotoxin binding [40]. In this paper it was reported that the adsorption of AFB1 was reduced after calcination of a bentonite clay. It is questionable whether this observation can be extrapolated to other types of clay and other mycotoxins. Therefore, the purpose of the present study was to analyze the physical characteristics and to evaluate the binding of different mycotoxins before and after calcination of a montmorillonite type of clay from Tunisia.

2. Results

2.1. Chemical Characterization

XRF analyses revealed that purified native clay (CP) and its calcined form (CC) were mainly composed of silicon dioxide (SiO2), aluminum oxide (Al_2O_3), calcium oxide (CaO) and iron oxide (Fe_2O_3) (Table 1). In addition, the occurrence of magnesium oxide in both samples can be due to the presence of smectite, and also to a small amount of dolomite, which is confirmed by the results of XRD and FTIR-IR [41].

Table 1. Chemical composition of clays.

	Oxide Composition of the Clays (%)	
	CP	CC
SiO_2	42.04	43.62
Al_2O_3	14.60	15.67
CaO	13.34	13.78
Fe_2O_3	11.03	9.69
K_2O	1.12	1.17
MgO	1.74	1.78
Na_2O	0.18	0.18
SO_3	0.18	0.16

CP: purified clay, CC: calcined clay.

2.2. Infrared Spectroscopy Characterization (FTIR-ATR)

The FTIR patterns of the CP (Figure 1) exhibits several characteristic bands corresponding to the stretching vibrations of the surface hydroxyl groups (Si–Si–OH, or Al–Al–OH) at 3695 cm^{-1} which indicates the presence of kaolinite [40–44]. The spectrum shows a characteristic band of montmorillonite at 3620 cm^{-1} [43]. The band at 1432 cm^{-1} corresponds to carbonate [calcite (Ca CO_3) or dolomite (Ca, Mg $(CO_3)_2$)] [44–46]. The band at 711 cm^{-1} corresponds to calcite [44,45]. The band at 518 cm^{-1} is due to Si–O–Al (octahedral) bending vibration [46,47]. Vibration at 1635 cm^{-1} was attributed to the bending of adsorbed water. The band of deformation near to 873 cm^{-1} indicates that the clay is octahedral [48], while the band near 910 cm^{-1} corresponds to an Al-O-H deformation characteristic of dioctahedral smectite [49].

After calcination, the water OH-bending (1635 cm^{-1}) mode totally disappeared. This is a consequence of dehydroxylation and dehydration by the thermal treatment.

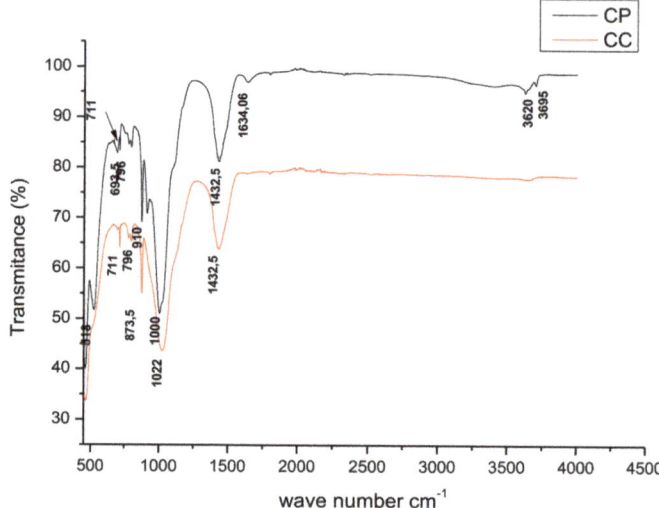

Figure 1. Infrared spectra of purified clay (CP) and calcinated clay (CC).

2.3. X-Ray Diffraction (XRD)

XRD characterization as presented in Figure 2 showed that CP and CC consisted mainly of calcic smectite, as demonstrated by the main peak near 14.10 Å and the additional peaks at 4.48 Å and 2.56 Å [50]. The XRD patterns confirmed the presence of kaolinite by the basal spacing at 7.16 Å, 3.84 Å, and 3.57 Å [45,50,51]. The characteristic reflection of dolomite was observed at 2.89 Å [45], while that of calcite was observed at 3.03 Å and 1.90 Å [45,50,52]. Both clays were also characterized by the presence of quartz, indicated by several peaks at 4.25 Å, 3.34 Å, 2.28 Å, 2.09 Å, and 1.87 Å [47,48,53,54]. Following calcination, the characteristic peaks of kaolinite at 7.16 Å and 3.57 Å disappeared, while a new peak appeared at 9.91 Å.

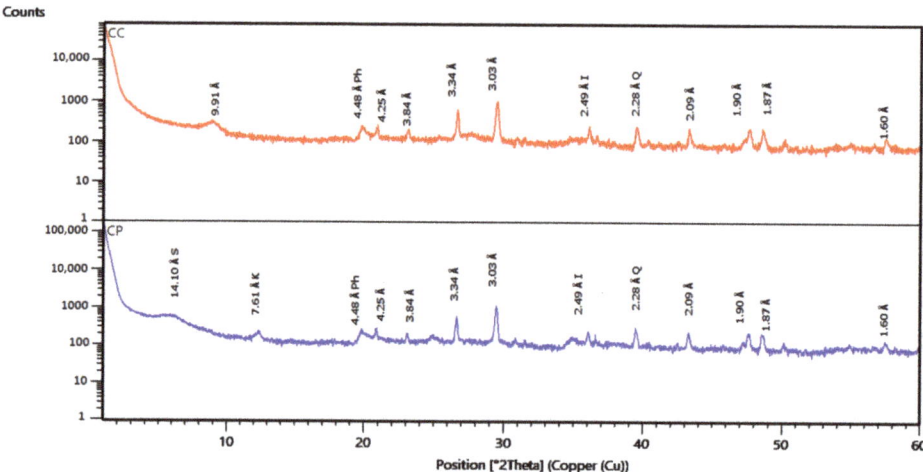

Figure 2. X-ray diffractograms of purified and calcined clay (S: smectite, I: illite, K: kaolinite, Q: quartz, C: calcite, D: dolomite), CP: purified clay, CC: calcined clay.

2.4. Cation Exchange Capacity (CEC)

The thermal treatment resulted in a decreased CEC (9.28 $Cmol_{(+)}$ (kg^{-1}) for CC) and a reduction in Ca, Mg and Na after calcination (Table 2).

Table 2. Cation exchange capacity of purified clay (CP) and calcined clay (CC).

Clay Samples	Ca (mg/L)	K (mg/L)	Mg (mg/L)	Na (mg/L)	CEC ($Cmol_{(+)}(kg^{-1})$)
CP	126.18	14.1	24.44	17.94	12.266
CC	88.56	25.56	19	11.54	9.287

CP: purified clay, CC: calcined clay, CEC: cation exchange capacity.

2.5. BET Surface Analysis

Brauner-Emmett-Teller (BET) N_2 adsorption/desorption analysis showed a surface area of CP 64.06 m^2/g. Thermal treatment resulted in a decreased surface area: 44.42 m^2/g for CC (Table 3) and an increase in pore size from 57.03 Å for CP to 66.72 Å for CC.

Table 3. Textural characteristic of clay minerals.

Clay Samples	S_{BET} (m^2/g)	Pore Volume (cm^3/g)	Pore Size (Å)
CP	64.06	0.05	57.03
CC	44.42	0.05	66.72

S_{BET}: BET Surface Area, CP: purified clay, CC: calcined clay.

2.6. Point of Zero Charge (PZC)

As can be seen in Figure 3, the pH_{PZC} of CP was 9.94, while it was 10.03 for the CC.

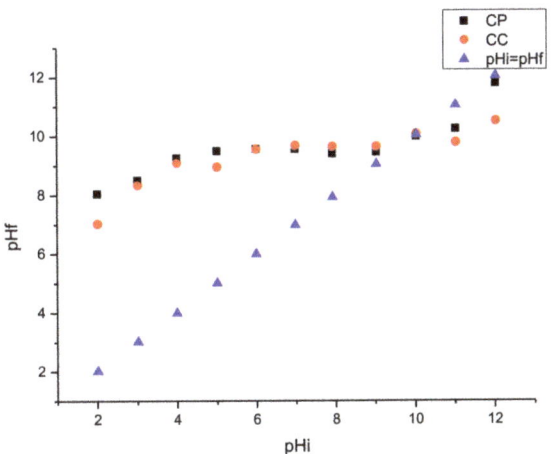

Figure 3. Determination of point of zero charge of purified clay (CP) and calcined clay (CC).

2.7. Mycotoxin Binding Efficiency

At pH of 3, CC and CP were able to bind 100% of AFB1. However, compared to CP, CC had a higher ($p < 0.05$) adsorption capacity for AFB2, AFG1 and AFG2 (Table 4). Moreover, CP was not able to bind ZEN at pH 3, while the calcinated clay did adsorb ZEN ($p < 0.05$). Table 5 contains the results of mycotoxin adsorption of the CP and CC at pH 7. The adsorption of AFB1, AFB2, AFG1, and AFG2 at pH 7 was significantly higher ($p < 0.05$) for CC compared to CP. As almost no ZEN was bound to CP, the adsorption of ZEN at pH 7 was significantly higher ($p < 0.05$) for the CC (41 ± 12%) than the CP (1 ± 1%).

Table 4. In vitro adsorption of AFB1, AFB2, AFG1, AFG2 and ZEN by purified clay (CP) and calcined clay (CC) at pH 3. Results are presented as mean ± SD. Means of CC indicated with * are significantly different compared to CP ($p < 0.05$). (NS: not significantly different).

	Binding Capacity (%)		
Mycotoxins	CP	CC	p-Value
AFB1	100 ± 0	100 ± 0	NS
AFB2	88 ± 1	100 ± 0 *	<0.001
AFG1	96 ± 1	100 ± 0 *	<0.001
AFG2	76 ± 2	99 ± 1 *	<0.001
ZEN	0 ± 0	75 ± 3 *	<0.001

Table 5. In vitro adsorption of AFB1, AFB2, AFG1, AFG2 and ZEN by purified clay (CP) and calcined clay (CC) at pH 7. Results are presented as mean ± SD. Means of CC indicated with * are significantly different compared to CP ($p < 0.05$).

	Binding Capacity (%)		
Mycotoxins	CP	CC	p-Value
AFB1	94 ± 3	99 ± 0 *	0.031
AFB2	86 ± 8	99 ± 1 *	0.048
AFG1	60 ± 17	98 ± 2 *	0.019
AFG2	30 ± 29	96 ± 2 *	0.017
ZEN	1 ± 1	41 ± 12 *	0.026

Based on these in vitro adsorption data, the in vitro binding efficiency of AFs and ZEN of the purified and calcined clay was predicted (Figure 4). The results show that both clays exhibited a strong in vitro binding affinity to AFs. Heat treatment of the clay improved the binding efficiency of ZEN (29 ± 18%) compared to the CP (0 ± 0%). The binding efficiency of AFB1 was 94 ± 3% and 99 ± 0% for the CP and CC, respectively. The effectiveness of CP and CC in binding AFB2 was 86 ± 9% and 99 ± 1%, respectively. The in vitro binding efficiency of AFG1 and AFG2 was significantly higher ($p < 0.05$) for the CC than the CP. AFG1 binding efficiency was 59 ± 18% for CP and 98 ± 2% for CC ($p < 0.05$). Furthermore, the binding efficiency of AFG2 was 15 ± 38% for the CP and 96 ± 2% for the CC. These results demonstrate that the thermal treatment of the clay enhances the binding efficiency of AFG1 and AFG2.

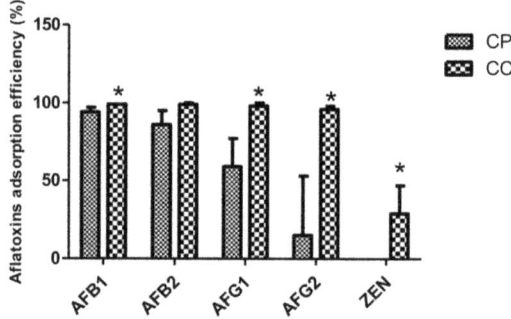

Figure 4. In vitro binding efficiency (%) of AFB1 (5 ng/mL), AFB2 (5 ng/mL), AFG1 (5 ng/mL), AFG2 (5 ng/mL) and ZEN (25 ng/mL) of purified clay (CP) and calcined clay (CC). Data are represented as mean values ± SD. Means of CC indicated with * are significantly different compared to CP ($p < 0.05$)

3. Discussion

Several reports have shown that adding phyllosilicate clay supplements to animal feed represents one of the most powerful prevention strategies for aflatoxicosis in livestock [21,55–57]. Heat treatment may alter the adsorbing properties of the clays, however, this has not been investigated much with respect to mycotoxins so far.

Our results show that the chemical composition of the studied clay was not affected after heat treatment. Similar results were found in another study with a different type of clay [40]. Indeed, there is no change in bentonite composition before and after calcination. The chemical composition of the studied clay is a typical composition of south-eastern Tunisian clays [45]. CP and CC were also characterized by a high calcium oxide content and a low percentage of sodium oxide which are in accordance with previous work [48].

Disappearance of the characteristic peaks of kaolinite following calcination, as observed by XRD, is probably due to the dehydroxylation of the kaolinite structure, leading to the collapse of clay mineral structure [40,50,58]. Aluminosilicate minerals are characterized by a CEC varying from 10 (meq/100 g) for kaolinite minerals to 100 (meq/100 g) for illite and smectite minerals [59]. The tested clay showed a low value of CEC which can be due to the poor crystallinity of smectite and to the presence of kaolinite, illite, and some impurities (calcite, quartz, dolomite, etc.). The decrease in CEC is due to the dehydration and dehydroxylation of smectite which results in a collapse of the interlayer [53,60]. This result is in agreement with previous reports [34,61] stating that the thermal treatment reduces the cation exchange capacity of clays. The surface area is an important property for clay adsorption capacity. Previous work reported that the surface area decreases with increasing temperatures of thermal treatment [33,46,54]. Calcination of clay at 560 °C causes an agglomeration of the particles leading to a 15% decrease in the surface area and an increase in the pore size [62]. According to the literature [35], the increase in the diameter of pores is due to a reduction of the basal spacing through dehydration of the interlayer spaces which is a consequence of a first collapse of smectite layers. Similar research observed that calcination of clay affects the interlayer space [63,64]. The pH_{PZC} is an important characteristic of minerals and usually used to define the state of the surface of a dispersed solid phase at the solid-electrolyte solution surface and may indicate the ionization of functional groups and their possible interaction with the mycotoxin molecules [65]. In addition, low-charge montmorillonites or other low-charge smectites would be more effective feed additives than higher-charge clays [34]. The surface is negative at $pH>pH_{PZC}$, positive at $pH<pH_{PZC}$ and neutral at $pH=pH_{PZC}$ [66]. The obtained results for pH_{PZC} in our study indicated that the surface of the studied clays is positive at pH3 and pH7 and are moderately higher than the pH_{PZC} reported in the literature for Tunisian smectitec clays (8.2) [67]. The use of adsorbents mixed with food and feed is one of the prominent post-harvest approaches to protect against mycotoxins toxicity, which are supposed to bind efficiently mycotoxins in the gastrointestinal tract. In the current study, we evaluate the binding capacity of AFs and ZEN of purified and calcined clay. The in vitro ZEN and AFs adsorption is assessed at pH 3 and pH 7 which are representative for the GI tract of the monogastric animals. Similar models were successfully applied in previous in vitro experiments [21,59,68]. Regarding adsorption and desorption of ZEN, the adsorption of ZEN by clay is usually lower than aflatoxins [21]. This could be because of the low polarity of ZEN compared to AFs [19]. Furthermore, ZEN has a more spherical molecular geometry than the planar structure of AFs [18]. Moreover, in a recent study [21], it was reported that ZEN is significantly less adsorbed in alkaline than in acid and neutral conditions. De Mil et al. [18] suggested that the pH may influence the phenolic hydroxyl group of ZEN or the ionization-state of the functional groups of the mycotoxin binders, and thereby alter the adsorption by the ionic interactions.

Our findings confirmed a better adsorption capacity for ZEN for the calcined clay than the purified native clay. It has been reported that modified clays have been developed to improve ZEN adsorption, which provide sufficient space between the layers to react with mycotoxin with a relatively less polarity with the appropriate electrical charging [69–72]. These modified surface properties lead to greater hydrophobicity by exchanging the structural load balance cations with high molecular weight quaternary amines [27]. Feng et al. [73] have concluded that the modified clays have led to low desorption rates, with higher ZEN adsorption than the non-modified clay. The increase in adsorption capacity of AFs and ZEN with calcined clay in our study might be related to the increase in pore size (Table 3), and the decrease in CEC (Table 2) of clay after heat treatment at 550 °C. Chen et al. [35] reported that calcination of palygorskite at high temperatures improves dye adsorption efficiency, which is basically associated with a larger size and a wider size distribution of pores. In addition to the pore size, CEC play an important role in the adsorption phenomenon [18]. Exchangeable cations neutralize the interlayer charges in phyllosilicates, and are involved in the binding of AFB1 [7,74]. Deng et al. [75] suggested that layer charge density and the type of exchange cations have a distinct influence on the adsorption of AF. Recent research [43] demonstrated that heating of bentonite improves the clays' adsorption affinity and capacity of AFB1, which is mainly because of the reduction of cation exchange capacity. Furthermore, AFB1 is a polar mycotoxin and contains ß-carbonyl, which is involved in the adsorption process [55]. According to Prapapanpong et al. [21], the adsorption process involves the exchange of electrons of the metallic cation on the surface of the adsorbent, especially the positive charge of calcium ions on each layer of clay. A hypothesis proposed by Jaynes et al. [76] discussed the possibility that aflatoxins can be captured at multiple locations on hydrated sodium calcium aluminosilicate (HSCAS) surfaces, as well as between HSCAS inter-layers.

4. Conclusions

In this study, calcination improved the adsorption efficacy of the clay for AFB2, AFG1, AFG2, and ZEN. The adsorption-desorption rate showed that the pH condition in the GI tract might influence ZEN adsorption rate. The authors conclude that this specific clay has the potential to be used as a mycotoxin binder in poultry and probably for other animal species.

Unraveling the exact binding-mechanism, including the verification of the kinetics of mycotoxin binders has to this day remained largely uninvestigated. However, these data are of crucial importance to further ameliorate mycotoxin binders' efficacies, and to aim for a wider adaption of these mitigation strategies in both animals and humans.

5. Materials and Methods

5.1. Chemical Products and Reagents

Methanol (LC-MS/MS grade) and glacial acetic acid (LC-MS/MS grade were procured from Biosolve B.V. (Valkenswaard, The Netherlands). Acetic acid and ammonium acetate (analytical grade) were supplied by Merck (Darmstadt, Germany). A Milli-Q® SP Reagent water apparatus (Millipore; Brussels, Belgium) was used for water purification. For the mycotoxin standards, AFB1, AFB2, AFG1, AFG2 and ZEN were purchased from Sigma-Aldrich (Bornem, Belgium). Disinfectol® (denatured ethanol + 5% ether) was supplied by Chem-Lab (Belgium). Mycotoxin standards were dissolved in methanol (1 mg/mL), and were storable for a minimum of 1 year at −18 °C. Other chemicals and reagents were of analytical grade.

5.2. Source and Preparation of Clay

The raw clay sample was collected from Jebel Aïdoudi (El Hamma, Gabes) in the southern part of Tunisia. To purify the clay, the sample was ground and wet-sieved with an electromagnetic sieve shaker (Matest S.p.A., Triviolo, Italy) in order to eliminate all the impurities. Next, they were dried in an oven (Memmert GmbH + Co.KG, Schwabach, Germany) at 105 °C. The obtained clay was subsequently washed with distilled water until separation of the liquid/solid phases became difficult, and were dried again in an oven at 105 °C. The thermally-treated clay was obtained by a calcination process of the purified clay in a muffle furnace (Sirio Dentel Srl, Meldola, Italy) at 550 °C for 5h. Subsequently, purified clay (CP) and calcined clay (CC) samples were ground and sieved into fine powder (≈100 μm).

5.3. Physico-Chemical Characterization of Clays

5.3.1. X-Ray Fluorescence (XRF)

The chemical composition of the minerals present in the two clays was performed using the XRF spectrometer model Thermo OASIS 9900 (Thermo Fisher Scientific (Schweiz) AG, Bâle, Suisse). It was performed in order to know the elemental oxides that are present in the clays.

5.3.2. X-Ray Diffraction (XRD)

XRD was performed to identify the mineral composition of clays and the crystal line phases. It was conducted by an X-ray diffractometer « PANALYTICAL X'PERT PROMPD » using Cu Kα radiation ($\lambda = 0.154$ nm) with the voltage of 45 kV, 40 mA. Then the basal spacing of samples was determined from Bragg's law ($n \lambda = 2\, d \sin \theta$), where 'n' is the path difference between the reflected waves, equal to an integral number of wavelengths (λ), 'λ' the wavelength (nm), 'd' the interlayer spacing (nm), and 'θ' the diffraction angle (°).

5.3.3. Fourier Transformed Infrared Spectroscopy (FTIR-ATR)

FTIR-IR helps in the identification of various forms of the minerals present in the clay. The vibrational spectra were performed with FTIR with a Spectrum Two PerkinElmer spectrometer, in the attenuated total reflection (ATR) mode, with a highly sensitive Deuterated Triglycine Sulfate (DTGS) detector. The samples were scanned 10 times in the range of 500–4000 cm^{-1}, with a 2 cm^{-1} spectral resolution.

5.3.4. Point of Zero Charge (PZC)

The Chemistry surface characterization was performed according to the solid addition method described by Noridine et al. [77] with slight modifications. A series of 50 mL of 0.01 mol/mL of NaCl (0.1 M) solutions were poured in beakers. The pH was adjusted in the range of 2–12 with 0.1 M HCl or 0.1 M NaOH solutions. Then, 0.2 g of clay was soaked in each solution under agitation at room temperature, and the final pH was measured after 24 h. The pH$_{PZC}$ is the point in the curve when the pH$_{initial}$ (pHi) verses pH$_{final}$ (pHf) intersects the line (pHi = pHf).

5.3.5. Cation Exchange Capacity (CEC)

CEC of clays was conducted using the barium chloride method [78]. Briefly, samples between 1 g and 5 g, depending on their probable CEC, were weighed into 50 mL centrifuge tubes. Then, 30 mL of 0.1 M BaCl$_2$ was added, and the tubes were shaken slowly on a reciprocal shaker for 2 h. The samples were then centrifuged at 2500 rpm for 10 min and the supernatant solution were filtered through Whatman 42 filter paper. The solution was collected in polyethylene bottles for analysis.

5.3.6. BET Surface Analysis

The textural properties of the clays (specific surface area, porosity) were determined by nitrogen adsorption using the multipoint Brunauer-Emmet-Teller (BET) method (ASAP 2020 Micromeritics Instruments, Norcross, GA, USA). The specific surface area was measured at 77 K and the pore size distribution was calculated in the radius range from 2000 to 100,000 nm by the BJH method using the adsorption isotherm.

5.4. Mycotoxin Adsorption

In vitro evaluation of the adsorption capacity of both clays for AFB1, AFB2, AFG1, AFG2, and ZEN was adopted from Di Mavungu et al. [79] with slight modifications. To determine the effect of pH on the mycotoxin binding capacity within the pH range of the gastrointestinal tract of poults, tests were performed at pH 3 and 7. In brief, 50 mg of clay sample was shaken and incubated for 3 h in 10 mL citrate buffer (pH 3) or phosphate buffer (pH 7) together with AFB1, AFB2, AFG1, and AFG2 at a concentration of 5 ng/mL, or with ZEN at a concentration of 25 ng/mL.

The mycotoxins were determined by LC-MS/MS using previously described methods [80]. A Waters Acquity UPLC system coupled to a Quattro Premier XE mass spectrometer (Waters, Milford, MA, USA) equipped with a Z-spray electrospray ionization (ESI) interface was used for the determination and quantification of mycotoxins. Chromatographic separation was achieved using a Symmetry C_{18} column (5 µm, 150 × 2.1 mm i.d.) with a Sentry guard column (3.5 µm, 10 × 2.1 mm i.d.) both supplied by Waters (Zellik, Belgium). The column was kept at room temperature. A mobile phase consisting of eluents A [water/methanol/acetic acid (94/5/1, $v/v/v$) containing 5 mM ammonium acetate] and B [methanol/water/acetic acid (97/2/1, $v/v/v$) containing 5 mM ammonium acetate] was used at a flow rate of 0.3 mL min^{-1}. A gradient elution was applied as follows: 0–7 min, 95% A/5% B –35% A/65% B; 7–11 min, 35% A/65% B–25% A/75% B; 11–13 min, 25% A/75% B–0% A/ 100% B; 13–15 min, 0% A/100% B; 15–16 min, 0% A/ 100% B–40% A/60% B; 16–22min, 40% A/60% B–60% A/40% B; 22–23 min, 60% A/40% B–95% A/5% B; 23–25 min 95% A/5% B. The injection volume was 20 µL.

5.5. Calculation of Mycotoxin Adsorption Rate (%)

The percentage of adsorption rate was calculated according to the following equation:

$$\% \text{ binding capacity} = 100 \times (C_i - C_f)/C_i \quad (1)$$

where

C_i is the initial concentration of mycotoxin

C_f is the concentration of unbound mycotoxin after incubation period

5.6. Calculation of the Binding Efficiency

The binding efficiency of the clays was determined according to the obtained results of the adsorption and desorption rate ((1) and (2))

$$\% \text{ Desorption} = ((\% \text{ Adsorption pH3} - \% \text{ Adsorption pH7})/\% \text{ Adsorption pH3}) \times 100 \quad (2)$$

with

$$\% \text{ binding efficiency} = \% \text{ Adsorption} - \% \text{ Desorption} \quad (3)$$

5.7. Statistical Analysis

Data were analyzed using the statistical software SPSS version 24 (IBM, New York, NY, USA) and results are presented as means ± SD. All analyses were performed in triplicate, and the significance of the means value was performed with the student's t-test after determination of normality. Results were considered statistically significant at $p \leq 0.05$.

Author Contributions: R.R. perform the extraction, preparation, and characterization of clays, contribute in the mycotoxin binding experiment and was involved in all aspect of this study. G.A. secured, premise and set the mycotoxin binding experiment and reviewed the paper. M.D.B. and S.D.S. reviewed data of the mycotoxin binding experiment and reviewed the paper. M.V.d.V. performed the experiment of the mycotoxin binding capacity. C.D. collected the data of the mycotoxin binding experiment. R.D. supervised editing and reviewed the entire work. M.H.A. who proposed the initial idea of studying the characteristics of the Tunisian clays and their efficiency in poultry feeds, helped in performing the characterization of clays and reviewed the paper. A.G. supervised the preparation and a part of the characterization of clays.

Funding: This research received no external funding.

Acknowledgments: We would like to express our sincere appreciation and gratitude to Professor Maher Radaoui and Sana Ncib who helped us in doing the BET and DRX analyses of clays. We would like to thank Imen Yehmed for doing the XRF analyses of clays. The authors acknowledge the support of MYTOX-SOUTH (https://mytoxsouth.org).

Conflicts of Interest: The authors declare no conflict of interest.

References

1. Bryden, W.L. Mycotoxins in the food chain: Human health implications. *Asia Pac. J. Clin. Nutr.* **2007**, *16* (Suppl. 1), 95–101.
2. Jard, G.; Liboz, T.; Mathieu, F.; Guyonvarch, A.; Lebrihi, A. Review of mycotoxin reduction in food and feed: From prevention in the field to detoxification by adsorption or transformation. *Food Addit. Contam. Part A* **2011**, *28*, 1590–1609. [CrossRef] [PubMed]
3. Peng, W.X.; Marchal, J.L.M.; Van der Poel, A.F.B. Strategies to prevent and reduce mycotoxins for compound feed manufacturing. *Anim. Feed Sci. Technol.* **2018**, *237*, 129–153. [CrossRef]
4. Rawal, S.; Kim, J.E.; Coulombe, R., Jr. Research in Veterinary Science Aflatoxin B 1 in poultry: Toxicology, metabolism and prevention. *Res. Vet. Sci.* **2010**, *89*, 325–331. [CrossRef] [PubMed]
5. Wacoo, A.P.; Wendiro, D.; Vuzi, P.C.; Hawumba, J.F. Methods for Detection of Aflatoxins in Agricultural Food Crops. *J. Appl. Chem.* **2014**, *12*, 1–15. [CrossRef]
6. Scheidegger, K.A.; Payne, G.A. Unlocking the Secrets Behind Secondary Metabolism: A Review of Aspergillus flavus from Pathogenicity to Functional Genomics. *J. Toxicol. Toxin Rev.* **2003**, *22*, 423–459. [CrossRef]
7. Phillips, T.D.; Williams, J.; Huebner, H.; Ankrah, N.; Jolly, P.; Johnson, N.; Taylor, J.; Xu, L.; Wang, J. Reducing human exposure to aflatoxin through the use of clay: A review. *Food Addit. Contam. Part A* **2008**, *25*, 134–145. [CrossRef]
8. Bhatti, S.A.; Khan, M.; Kashif, M.; Saqib, M. Aflatoxicosis and Ochratoxicosis in Broiler Chicks and their Amelioration with Locally Available Bentonite Clay. *Pak. Vet. J.* **2016**, *36*, 68–72.
9. Khanian, M.; Allameh, A. Alleviation of aflatoxin-related oxidative damage to liver and improvement of growth performance in broiler chickens consumed Lactobacillus plantarum 299v for entire growth period. *Toxicon* **2018**, *158*, 57–62. [CrossRef]
10. Ma, Q.; Li, Y.; Fan, Y.; Zhao, L.; Wei, H.; Ji, C.; Zhang, J. Molecular Mechanisms of Lipoic Acid Protection against Aflatoxin B 1 -Induced Liver Oxidative Damage and Inflammatory Responses in Broilers. *Toxins* **2015**, *7*, 5435–5447. [CrossRef]
11. Wogan, G.N. Chemical Nature and Biological Effects of the Aflatoxins. *Am. Soc. Microbiol.* **1966**, *30*, 460–470.
12. Dutton, F. Cellular Interactions and Metabolism of Aflatoxin: An Update. *Pharmacol. Ther.* **1995**, *65*, 163–192.
13. Antonissen, G.; Martel, A.; Pasmans, F.; Ducatelle, R.; Verbrugghe, E.; Vandenbroucke, V.; Li, S.; Haesebrouck, F.; Van Immerseel, F.; Croubels, S. The impact of Fusarium Mycotoxins on human and animal host susceptibility to infectious diseases. *Toxins* **2014**, *6*, 430–452. [CrossRef] [PubMed]
14. Tamura, M.; Mochizuki, N.; Nagatomi, Y.; Harayama, K.; Toriba, A.; Hayakawa, K. A method for simultaneous determination of 20 fusarium toxins in cereals by high-resolution liquid chromatography-orbitrap mass spectrometry with a pentafluorophenyl column. *Toxins* **2015**, *7*, 1664–1682. [CrossRef]
15. Kolosova, A.; Stroka, J. Substances for reduction of the contamination of feed by mycotoxins: A review. *World Mycotoxin J.* **2011**, *4*, 225–256. [CrossRef]
16. Aiko, V.; Mehta, A. Occurrence, detection and detoxification of mycotoxins. *J. Biosci.* **2015**, *40*, 943–954. [CrossRef]
17. Kabak, B.; Dobson, A.D.W.; Var, I. Strategies to prevent mycotoxin contamination of food and animal feed: A review. *Crit. Rev. Food Sci. Nutr.* **2006**, *46*, 593–619. [CrossRef]
18. De Mil, T.; Devreese, M.; Bagane, M.; Van Ranst, E.; Eeckhout, M.; De Backer, P.; Croubels, S. Characterization of 27 Mycotoxin Binders and the Relation with in Vitro Zearalenone Adsorption at a Single Concentration. *Toxins* **2015**, *7*, 21–33. [CrossRef]
19. Huwig, A.; Freimund, S.; Käppeli, O.; Dutler, H. Mycotoxin detoxication of animal feed by different adsorbents. *Toxicol. Lett.* **2001**, *122*, 179–188. [CrossRef]
20. Bocarov-Stancic, A.; Adamovic, M.; Salma, N.; Bodroza-Solarov, M.; Vuckovic, J.; Pantic, V. In vitro efficacy of mycotoxins adsorption by natural mineral adsorbents. *Biotechnol. Anim. Husb.* **2011**, *27*, 1241–1251. [CrossRef]
21. Prapapanpong, J.; Udomkusonsri, P.; Mahavorasirikul, W.; Choochuay, S.; Tansakul, N. In Vitro Studies on Gastrointestinal Monogastric and Avian Models to Evaluate the Binding Efficacy of Mycotoxin adsorbents by Liquid Chromatography-Tandem Mass Spectrometry. *J. Adv. Vet. Anim. Res.* **2019**, *6*, 125–132. [CrossRef] [PubMed]

22. Mutua, F.; Lindahl, J.; Grace, D. Availability and use of mycotoxin binders in selected urban and Peri-urban areas of Kenya. *Food Secur.* **2019**, *11*, 359–369. [CrossRef]
23. Clarke, L.C.; Sweeney, T.; Curley, E.; Duffy, S.K.; Vigors, S.; Rajauria, G.; O'Doherty, J.V. Mycotoxin binder increases growth performance, nutrient digestibility and digestive health of finisher pigs offered wheat based diets grown under different agronomical conditions. *Anim. Feed Sci. Technol.* **2018**, *240*, 52–65. [CrossRef]
24. Barrientos-velázquez, A.L.; Arteaga, S.; Dixon, J.B.; Deng, Y. The effects of pH, pepsin, exchange cation, and vitamins on a fl atoxin adsorption on smectite in simulated gastric fl uids. *Appl. Clay Sci.* **2016**, *120*, 17–23. [CrossRef]
25. Jouany, J.P. Methods for preventing, decontaminating and minimizing the toxicity of mycotoxins in feeds. *Anim. Feed Sci. Technol.* **2007**, *137*, 342–362. [CrossRef]
26. Kang'Ethe, E.K.; Sirma, A.J.; Murithi, G.; Mburugu-Mosoti, C.K.; Ouko, E.O.; Korhonen, H.J.; Nduhiu, G.J.; Mungatu, J.K.; Joutsjoki, V.; Lindfors, E.; et al. Occurrence of mycotoxins in food, feed, and milk in two counties from different agro-ecological zones and with historical outbreak of aflatoxins and fumonisins poisonings in Kenya. *Food Qual. Saf.* **2017**, *1*, 161–169. [CrossRef]
27. Papaioannou, D.; Katsoulos, P.D.; Panousis, N.; Karatzias, H. The role of natural and synthetic zeolites as feed additives on the prevention and/or the treatment of certain farm animal diseases: A review. *Microporous Mesoporous Mater.* **2005**, *84*, 161–170. [CrossRef]
28. Avantaggiato, G.; Solfrizzo, M.; Visconti, A. Recent advances on the use of adsorbent materials for detoxification of Fusarium mycotoxins. *Food Addit. Contam.* **2005**, *22*, 379–388. [CrossRef]
29. Mallmann, C.A.; Dilkin, P. Brazilian mycotoxin experiences. *Int. Pig Top.* **2002**, *27*, 28–30.
30. Zaviezo, D. Brazilian experiences with mycotoxins. *Int. Poult. Prod.* **2009**, *17*, 2–3.
31. Cheknane, B.; Bouras, O.; Baudu, M.; Basly, J.P.; Cherguielaine, A. Granular inorgano-organo pillared clays (GIOCs): Preparation by wet granulation, characterization and application to the removal of a Basic dye (BY28) from aqueous solutions. *Chem. Eng. J.* **2010**, *158*, 528–534. [CrossRef]
32. Sassi, H.; Lafaye, G.; Ben Amor, H.; Gannouni, A.; Jeday, M.R. Wastewater treatment by catalytic wet air oxidation process over Al-Fe pillared clays synthesized using microwave irradiation. *Front. Environ. Sci. Eng.* **2018**, *12*, 2. [CrossRef]
33. Tlili, A.; Saidi, R.; Fourati, A.; Ammar, N.; Jamoussi, F. Mineralogical study and properties of natural and flux calcined porcelanite from Gafsa-Metlaoui basin compared to diatomaceous filtration aids. *Appl. Clay Sci.* **2012**, *62*, 47–57. [CrossRef]
34. Jaynes, W.F.; Zartman, R.E. Aflatoxin Toxicity Reduction in Feed by Enhanced Binding to Surface-Modified Clay Additives. *Toxin* **2011**, *3*, 551–565. [CrossRef] [PubMed]
35. Chen, H.; Zhao, J.; Zhong, A.; Jin, Y. Removal capacity and adsorption mechanism of heat-treated palygorskite clay for methylene blue. *Chem. Eng. J.* **2011**, *174*, 143–150. [CrossRef]
36. Kuang, W.; Facey, G.A.; Detellier, C. Dehydration and rehydration of palygorskite and the influence of water on the nanopores. *Clays Clay Miner.* **2004**, *52*, 635–642. [CrossRef]
37. Wang, W.; Chen, H.; Wang, A. Adsorption characteristics of Cd(II) from aqueous solution onto activated palygorskite. *Sep. Purif. Technol.* **2007**, *55*, 157–164. [CrossRef]
38. Chen, T.; Liu, H.; Li, J.; Chen, D.; Chang, D.; Kong, D.; Frost, R.L. Effect of thermal treatment on adsorption-desorption of ammonia and sulfur dioxide on palygorskite: Change of surface acid-alkali properties. *Chem. Eng. J.* **2011**, *166*, 1017–1021. [CrossRef]
39. Vieira, M.G.A.; Neto, A.F.A.; Gimenes, M.L.; da Silva, M.G.C. Removal of nickel on Bofe bentonite calcined clay in porous bed. *J. Hazard. Mater.* **2010**, *176*, 109–118. [CrossRef]
40. Nones, J.; Nones, J.; Gracher, H.; Poli, A.; Gonçalves, A.; Cabral, N. Thermal treatment of bentonite reduces aflatoxin b1 adsorption and affects stem cell death. *Mater. Sci. Eng. C* **2015**, *55*, 530–537. [CrossRef]
41. Felhi, M.; Tlili, A.; Gaied, M.E.; Montacer, M. Mineralogical study of kaolinitic clays from Sidi El Bader in the far north of Tunisia. *Appl. Clay Sci.* **2008**, *39*, 208–217. [CrossRef]
42. Hajjaji, M.; Kacim, S.; Alami, A.; El Bouadili, A.; El Mountassir, M. Chemical and mineralogical characterization of a clay taken from the Moroccan Meseta and a study of the interaction between its fine fraction and methylene blue. *Appl. Clay Sci.* **2001**, *20*, 1–12. [CrossRef]
43. Gan, F.; Hang, X.; Huang, Q.; Deng, Y. Assessing and modifying China bentonites for aflatoxin adsorption. *Appl. Clay Sci.* **2019**, *168*, 348–354. [CrossRef]

44. Sdiri, A.; Higashi, T.; Hatta, T. Mineralogical and spectroscopic characterization, and potential environmental use of limestone from the Abiod formation, Tunisia. *Environ. Earth Sci.* **2010**, *61*, 1275–1287. [CrossRef]
45. Sdiri, A.; Higashi, T.; Hatta, T.; Jamoussi, F.; Tase, N. Evaluating the adsorptive capacity of montmorillonitic and calcareous clays on the removal of several heavy metals in aqueous systems. *Chem. Eng. J.* **2011**, *172*, 37–46. [CrossRef]
46. Chaari, I.; Fakhfakh, E.; Chakroun, S.; Bouzid, J.; Boujelben, N. Lead removal from aqueous solutions by a Tunisian smectitic clay. *J. Hazard. Mater.* **2008**, *156*, 545–551. [CrossRef]
47. Temuujin, J.; Jadambaa, T.; Burmaa, G.; Erdenechimeg, S.; Amarsanaa, J. Characterisation of acid activated montmorillonite clay from Tuulant (Mongolia). *Ceram. Int.* **2004**, *30*, 251–255. [CrossRef]
48. Bouguerra, S.; Neji Mahmoud Trabelsi, M.H.F. Activation d'une argile smectite Tunisienne à l'acide sulfurique: Catalytique de l'acide adsorbé par l'argile. *J. De La Société Chim. De Tunis.* **2009**, *11*, 191–203.
49. Madejová, J. FTIR techniques in clay mineral studies. *Vib. Spectrosc.* **2003**, *31*, 1–10. [CrossRef]
50. Gannouni, A.; Amari, A.; Bellagi, A. Activation acide de quelques argiles du sud tunisien: II. Préparation de terres décolorantes pour huiles minérales usagées. *J. Société Chim. Tunis.* **2011**, *13*, 157–171.
51. Khalfa, L.; Cervera, M.L.; Souissi-Najjar, S.; Bagane, M. Removal of Fe(III) from synthetic wastewater into raw and modified clay: Experiments and models fitting. *Sep. Sci. Technol.* **2017**, *52*, 1–11. [CrossRef]
52. Eloussaief, M.; Hamza, W.; Kallel, N.; Benzina, M. Wastewaters Decontamination: Mechanisms of Pb (II), Zn (II), and Cd (II) Competitive Adsorption on Tunisian Smectite in Single and Multi-Solute Systems. *Environ. Prog. Sustain. Energy* **2012**, *32*, 229–238. [CrossRef]
53. Önal, M. Swelling and cation exchange capacity relationship for the samples obtained from a bentonite by acid activations and heat treatments. *Appl. Clay Sci.* **2007**, *37*, 74–80. [CrossRef]
54. Bojemueller, E.; Nennemann, A.; Lagaly, G. Enhanced pesticide adsorption by thermally modified bentonites. *Appl. Clay Sci.* **2001**, *18*, 277–284. [CrossRef]
55. Phillips, T.D. Dietary Clay in the Chemoprevention of Aflatoxin-Induced Disease. *Toxicol. Sci.* **1999**, *52*, 118–126. [CrossRef] [PubMed]
56. Valchev, I.; Marutsova, V.; Zarkov, I.; Ganchev, A.; Nikolov, Y. Effects of aflatoxin B1 alone or co-administered with mycotox NG on performance and humoral immunity of Turkey broilers. *Bulg. J. Vet. Med.* **2017**, *20*, 38–50. [CrossRef]
57. Bhatti, S.A.; Khan, M.Z.; Kashif, M.; Saqib, M.; Khan, A. Protective role of bentonite against aflatoxin B1- and ochratoxin A-induced immunotoxicity in broilers. *J. Immunotoxicol.* **2017**, *14*, 66–76. [CrossRef]
58. Danner, T.; Norden, G.; Justnes, H. Characterisation of calcined raw clays suitable as supplementary cementitious materials. *Appl. Clay Sci.* **2018**, *162*, 391–402. [CrossRef]
59. Ayo, E.M.; Matemu, A.; Laswai, G.H.; Kimanya, M.E. An In Vitro Evaluation of the Capacity of Local Tanzanian Crude Clay and Ash-Based Materials in Binding Aflatoxins in Solution. *Toxins* **2018**, *10*, 510. [CrossRef]
60. Gu, B.X.; Wang, L.M.; Minc, L.D.; Ewing, R.C. Temperature effects on the radiation stability and ion exchange capacity of smectites. *J. Nucl. Mater.* **2001**, *297*, 345–354. [CrossRef]
61. Gurgel, M. Cu (II) Adsorption on Modified Bentonitic Clays: Different Isotherm Behaviors in Static and Dynamic Systems. *Mater. Res.* **2012**, *15*, 114–124.
62. He, C.; Makovicky, E.; Osbæck, B. Thermal stability and pozzolanic activity of raw and calcined mixed-layer mica/smectite. *Appl. Clay Sci.* **2000**, *17*, 141–161. [CrossRef]
63. Cótica, L.F.; Freitas, V.F.; Santos, I.A.; Barabach, M.; Anaissi, F.J.; Miyahara, R.Y.; Sarvezuk, P.W.C. Cobalt-modified Brazilian bentonites: Preparation, characterisation, and thermal stability. *Appl. Clay Sci.* **2011**, *51*, 187–191. [CrossRef]
64. Li, L.; Dong, J.; Lee, R. Preparation of α-alumina-supported mesoporous bentonite membranes for reverse osmosis desalination of aqueous solutions. *J. Colloid Interface Sci.* **2004**, *273*, 540–546. [CrossRef] [PubMed]
65. Daković, A.; Kragović, M.; Rottinghaus, G.E.; Sekulić, Ž.; Milićević, S.; Milonjić, S.K.; Zarić, S. Influence of natural zeolitic tuff and organozeolites surface charge on sorption of ionizable fumonisin B1. *Colloids Surf. B Biointerfaces* **2010**, *76*, 272–278. [CrossRef]
66. Gulicovski, J.J.; Čerović, L.S.; Milonjić, S.K. Point of zero charge and isoelectric point of alumina. *Mater. Manuf. Process.* **2008**, *23*, 615–619. [CrossRef]
67. Arfaouia, S.; Hamdia, N.; Frini-Srasrab, N.; Srasra, E. Determination of point of zero charge of PILCS with single and mixed oxide pillars prepared from Tunisian smectite. *Geochem. Int.* **2012**, *50*, 447–454. [CrossRef]

68. Daković, A.; Tomašević-Čanović, M.; Dondur, V.; Rottinghaus, G.E.; Medaković, V.; Zarić, S. Adsorption of mycotoxins by organozeolites. *Colloids Surf. B Biointerfaces* **2005**, *46*, 20–25. [CrossRef]
69. Sabater-vilar, M.; Malekinejad, H.; Selman, M.H.J.; Fink-gremmels, J. In vitro assessment of adsorbents aiming to prevent deoxynivalenol and zearalenone mycotoxicoses. *Mycopathologia* **2007**, *163*, 81–90. [CrossRef]
70. Denli, M.; Blandon, J.C.; Guynot, M.E.; Salado, S.; Pérez, J.F. Efficacy of activated diatomaceous clay in reducing the toxicity of zearalenone in rats and piglets. *J. Anim. Sci.* **2015**, *93*, 637–645. [CrossRef]
71. Jiang, S.Z.; Yang, Z.B.; Yang, W.R.; Wang, S.J.; Liu, F.X.; Johnston, L.A.; Chi, F.; Wang, Y. Effect of purified zearalenone with or without modified montmorillonite on nutrient availability, genital organs and serum hormones in post-weaning piglets. *Livest. Sci.* **2012**, *144*, 110–118. [CrossRef]
72. Zhang, Y.; Gao, R.; Liu, M.; Yan, C.; Shan, A. Adsorption of modified halloysite nanotubes in vitro and the protective effect in rats exposed to zearalenone. *Arch. Anim. Nutr.* **2014**, *68*, 320–335. [CrossRef] [PubMed]
73. Feng, J.; Shan, M.; Du, H.; Han, X.; Xu, Z. In vitro adsorption of zearalenone by cetyltrimethyl ammonium bromide-modified montmorillonite nanocomposites. *Microporous Mesoporous Mater.* **2008**, *113*, 99–105. [CrossRef]
74. Deng, Y.; Velázquez, A.L.B.; Billes, F.; Dixon, J.B. Bonding mechanisms between aflatoxin B1 and smectite. *Appl. Clay Sci.* **2010**, *50*, 92–98. [CrossRef]
75. Deng, Y.; Liu, L.; Velá Zquez, A.L.B.; Dixon, J.B. The determinative role of the exchange cation and layer-charge density of smectite on aflatoxin adsorption. *Clays Clay Miner.* **2012**, *60*, 374–386. [CrossRef]
76. Jaynes, W.F.; Zartman, R.E.; Hudnall, W.H. Aflatoxin B1 adsorption by clays from water and corn meal. *Appl. Clay Sci.* **2007**, *36*, 197–205. [CrossRef]
77. Nordine, N.; El Bahri, Z.; Sehil, H.; Fertout, R.I.; Rais, Z.; Bengharez, Z. Lead removal kinetics from synthetic effluents using Algerian pine, beech and fir sawdust's: Optimization and adsorption mechanism. *Appl. Water Sci.* **2016**, 349–358. [CrossRef]
78. Hendershot, W.H.; Duquette, M. A Simple Barium Chloride Method for Determining Cation Exchange Capacity and Exchangeable Cations. *Soil Sci. Soc. Am. J.* **1986**, *50*, 605–608. [CrossRef]
79. di Mavungu, J.D.; Monbaliu, S.; Scippo, M.L.; Maghuin-Rogister, G.; Schneider, Y.J.; Larondelle, Y.; Callebaut, A.; Robbens, J.; van Peteghem, C.; de Saeger, S. LC-MS/MS multi-analyte method for mycotoxin determination in food supplements. *Food Addit. Contam. Part A* **2009**, *26*, 885–895. [CrossRef]
80. Monbaliu, S.; Van Poucke, C.; Van Peteghem, C.; Van Poucke, K.; Heungens, K.; De Saeger, S. Development of a multi-mycotoxin liquid chromatography/tandem mass spectrometry method for sweet pepper analysis. *Rapid Commun. Mass Spectrom.* **2009**, *23*, 3–11. [CrossRef]

© 2019 by the authors. Licensee MDPI, Basel, Switzerland. This article is an open access article distributed under the terms and conditions of the Creative Commons Attribution (CC BY) license (http://creativecommons.org/licenses/by/4.0/).

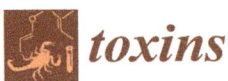

Article

In Vitro Activity of Neem (*Azadirachta indica*) Oil on Growth and Ochratoxin A Production by *Aspergillus carbonarius* Isolates

Mariana Paiva Rodrigues [1], Andrea Luciana Astoreca [2], Águida Aparecida de Oliveira [3], Lauranne Alves Salvato [1], Gabriela Lago Biscoto [1], Luiz Antonio Moura Keller [4], Carlos Alberto da Rocha Rosa [3], Lilia Renée Cavaglieri [5], Maria Isabel de Azevedo [6] and Kelly Moura Keller [6,*]

[1] Programa de Pós-Graduação em Ciência Animal, Escola de Veterinária, Universidade Federal de Minas Gerais, Belo Horizonte, Minas Gerais 31270-901, Brazil; rodrigues.mpaiva@gmail.com (M.P.R.); lausalvato@gmail.com (L.A.S.); gabrielabiscoto@gmail.com (G.L.B.)

[2] Centro de Investigación y Desarrollo en Fermentaciones Industriales, Consejo Nacional de Investigaciones Científicas y Técnicas, Facultad de Ciencias Exactas, Universidad Nacional de La Plata, La Plata, Buenos Aires B1900ASH, Argentina; astoreca@biotec.quimica.unlp.edu.ar

[3] Departamento de Microbiologia e Imunologia Veterinária, Instituto de Veterinária, Universidade Federal Rural do Rio de Janeiro, Seropédica, Rio de Janeiro 23890-000, Brazil; aguidaoliveira@gmail.com (Á.A.d.O.); shalako1953@gmail.com (C.A.d.R.R.)

[4] Departamento de Zootecnia e Desenvolvimento Agrossocioambiental Sustentável, Faculdade de Veterinária, Universidade Federal Fluminense, Niterói, Rio de Janeiro 24230-340, Brazil; kellers@bol.com.br

[5] Consejo Nacional de Investigaciones Científicas y Técnicas, Departamento de Microbiología e Inmunología, Facultad de Ciencias Exactas, Físico Químicas y Naturales, Universidad Nacional de Río Cuarto, Río Cuarto, Córdoba X5804BYA, Argentina; lcavaglieri247@gmail.com

[6] Departamento de Medicina Veterinária Preventiva, Escola de Veterinária, Universidade Federal de Minas Gerais, Belo Horizonte, Minas Gerais 31270-901, Brazil; beelazevedo@gmail.com

* Correspondence: kelly.medvet@gmail.com

Received: 1 August 2019; Accepted: 30 September 2019; Published: 5 October 2019

Abstract: *Aspergillus carbonarius* is a saprobic filamentous fungus, food spoiling fungus and a producer of ochratoxin A (OTA) mycotoxin. In this study, the in vitro antifungal activity of neem oil (0.12% p/p of azadirachtin) was evaluated against the growth of six strains of *A. carbonarius* and the production of OTA. Four different concentrations of neem oil were tested in addition to three incubation times. Only the concentration of 0.3% of neem oil inhibited more than 95% of the strain's growth (97.6% ± 0.5%), while the use of 0.5% and 1.0% of neem oil showed lower antifungal activity, 40.2% ± 3.1 and 64.7% ± 1.1, respectively. There was a complete inhibition of OTA production with 0.1% and 0.3% neem oil in the four strains isolated in the laboratory from grapes. The present study shows that neem essential oil can be further evaluated as an auxiliary method for the reduction of mycelial growth and OTA production.

Keywords: mycotoxins; essential oils; ecophysiology

Key Contribution: Neem oil was an effective inhibitor of mycelial growth of the assayed *Aspergillus carbonarius* strains and ochratoxin A production in vitro.

1. Introduction

Members of the *Aspergillus* spp., among many other toxigenic fungi, have been found to have a strong ecological link with human food supplies [1]. They are often associated with food and animal feed during drying and storage but may also occur as plant pathogens. Black aspergilli, *Aspergillus* classified into the section *Nigri* [2], have been isolated from a wide variety of food and are distributed worldwide (animal feed, cereals, cocoa, coffee, dried fruits, fruits, garlic, olives, onions) and are considered as common fungi causing food spoilage and biodeterioration of other materials [3,4]. Furthermore, they are important producers of ochratoxin A (OTA), the main species involved in OTA biosynthesis is *Aspergillus carbonarius*, commonly isolated from tropical regions as a contaminant of vineyards [5].

OTA can result in toxic effects to human and animal species. This toxicity may be acute or chronic, and varies depending on the amount of OTA absorbed, the exposure time, species affected, age and sex [6]. Among the toxic effects it is possible to highlight nephrotoxicity (tubular necrosis), hepatotoxicity, teratogenicity, enteritis and carcinogenesis [7]. OTA is also classified as Group 2B, possibly carcinogenic to humans, according to the International Agency for Research on Cancer [8]. OTA has also been correlated to Balkan endemic nephropathy (BEN) [9]. Due to all the economic, human and animal health damages that the contamination of *A. carbonarius* and OTA can cause, the prevention and control of these fungi and mycotoxin are of extreme importance.

Essential oils (EO) are a complex mixture of volatile, odoriferous, aromatic compounds that have antioxidant and antimicrobial components [10,11]. In addition, studies have already shown that EOs improve the flavor and palatability of feed, thus increasing voluntary feed intake by animals [12,13]. This could make these substances good for biological control against fungi and mycotoxins. The physical nature of essential oils (i.e., low molecular weight combined with pronounced lipophilic tendencies) allow them to penetrate the cell membrane more quickly than other substances [14]. Moreover, several studies have focused on the possible use of different essential oils as biological drivers against aflatoxigenic fungi [15–18].

Neem oil is an EO extracted from different parts of the neem tree *(Azadirachta indica)*, a native tree from the drier regions of Asia and Africa that is considered a very important medicinal plant. So far, more than 300 phytochemicals, chemically diverse and structurally complex, have been extracted and isolated from different parts of this tree [19]: from leaves—azadirachtin (AZ), nimonol, nimocinol and nimocinolide; from barks—gallic acid, gallocatechin and epicatechin; from seeds—azadirachtin (AZ), azadiradione, nimbin, salannin and epoxyazadiradione [20–24]. These chemical compounds have demonstrated a wide range of unusual effects against a wide spectrum of pests (insects, fungi, and viruses) [25]. Neem EO is commonly used as an antipyretic, natural insecticide, antimicrobial, antimalarial agent, antibacterial, antifungal, antiviral and for the treatment of leptospirosis [26–30]. Neem leaf extract (NLE) also has anti-fertility effects, by NLE–induced oocyte apoptosis [31]. Even though they are effective against a wide spectrum of insects, fungi and viruses, these compounds have low toxicity to mammals [25], which reveals the great potential of this oil for use a possible biological control of fungi and mycotoxins. There are no values of reference for the use of neem oils and extracts but based on the "lead compound concept" the European Commission, Health and Consumers Directorate-General established 0.1 mg/kg body weight/day as the acceptable daily intake (ADI) for the lead compound AZ [32].

Thus, the aims of the present work were to evaluate: (i) the efficacy of different concentration levels of neem oil on growth parameters: lag phase and growth rate of six ochratoxigenic *Aspergillus carbonarius* strains; (ii) the potential to control ochratoxin A production by these strains grown on Czapek yeast extract agar (CYA) at different incubation times.

2. Results

The effects of different concentrations of neem oil on the percentage of growth inhibition of six *Aspergillus carbonarius* strains assayed on a CYA medium are shown in Table 1.

Among the four concentrations of neem oil screened, 0.1% and 0.3% inhibited more than 82% and 97%, respectively, of the growth of *A. carbonarius* strains, which indicate a high antifungal activity (>80%). The 0.5% concentration had a poor anti-fungal effect (<50%), whereas the application of 1.0%

of neem oil had a medium effect (59–71%). Although the regression analysis indicated significant linear dose-responses (Table 2), the data fit a more cubic polynomial model (Figure 1).

Table 1. Percentage of growth inhibition of six *A. carbonarius* strains produced by different concentrations of neem oil on a Czapek yeast extract agar (CYA) medium.

Strains	Concentration Levels of Neem Oil (%)			
	0.1	0.3	0.5	1.0
FRR5690	73.7 ± 8.5	96.3 ± 0.3	45.1 ± 1.7	58.5 ± 1.7
A2034	91.1 ± 1.1	98.8 ± 0	34.5 ± 2.8	70.8 ± 3.1
RCG1	97.8 ± 2.2	100 ± 0	47.3 ± 9.3	62.2 ± 4.0
RCG2	87.1 ± 0.6	98.9 ± 0	36.4 ± 4.4	65.6 ± 4.9
RCG3	96.3 ± 2.3	98.2 ± 0.6	40.9 ± 1.1	61.5 ± 3.6
RCG4	49.2 ± 4.5	93.7 ± 1.3	37.1 ± 1.7	69.5 ± 2.9
Means ± SD	82.5 ± 17.7 [b]	97.6 ± 2.2 [a]	40.2 ± 6.1 [d]	64.7 ± 5.4 [c]

SD: standard deviation. [a–d] Means with different letters are significantly different ($p < 0.001$).

Table 2. Outputs of the ANOVA with single-degree-of-freedom orthogonal polynomial contrasts for the effects of different concentrations (C) of neem oil on growth inhibition of six *A. carbonarius* strains (ST).

Source	df	Type III SS	MS	F	*p*-Value
(C)	3	32,923.07	10,974.36	118.79	<0.0001*
Covariate: (ST)	1	340.49	340.49	3.69	0.0591
Error	67	6189.78	92.38		
Contrast	df	Contrast SS	MS	F	*p*-value
(C)-linear	1	11,077.80	11,077.80	119.91	<0.0001*
(C)-quadratic	1	392.93	392.93	4.25	0.0431*
(C)-cubic	1	21,452.34	21,452.34	232.21	<0.0001*
Parameter			Estimate	SE	*p*-value
(C)-linear			−110.94	10.13	<0.0001*
(C)-quadratic			9.34	4.53	0.0431*
(C)-cubic			154.39	10.13	<0.0001*

"Strains" was not a significant covariate. Overall model $R^2 = 0.84$. df: degrees of freedom; SS: sum of squares; MS: mean squares; F: Fisher–Snedecor test. * Significant $p < 0.001$.

Mean lag phase (h) of six *A. carbonarius* strains at different concentration levels of neem oil are shown in Table 3.

Table 3. Lag phase (h) of six *A. carbonarius* strains at five different concentration levels of neem oil.

Strains	Concentration Levels of Neem Oil (%)				
	0 (Control)	0.1	0.3	0.5	1.0
FRR5690	7.4 ± 3.8	101.7 ± 27.0	≥540	29.6 ± 1.3	52.5 ± 2.6
A2034	5.6 ± 1.7	53.2 ± 8.2	≥540	16.6 ± 4.2	40.7 ± 4.5
RCG1	13.1 ± 0.8	531.7 ± 14.4	≥540	31.9 ± 6.2	40.5 ± 6.7
RCG2	8.4 ± 2.0	87.6 ± 4.1	≥540	26.5 ± 2.0	45.8 ± 3.3
RCG3	2.9 ± 2.6	≥540	≥540	18.0 ± 3.7	41.3 ± 2.8
RCG4	6.5 ± 0.5	154.0 ± 15.4	36.0 ± 6.9	15.7 ± 3.6	47.9 ± 0.6
Means ± SD	7.5 ± 3.7 [c]	226.6 ± 207.5 [b]	456.2 ± 193.3 [a]	23.2 ± 7.4 [c]	44.9 ± 5.6 [c]

SD: standard deviation. [a–c] Means with different letters are significantly different ($p < 0.001$).

Neem oil concentrations of 0.3% and 0.1% had a significant effect on lag phase, increasing the time needed for each strain to reach the exponential phase. The regression analysis showed a significant polynomial trend model correlation of different neem oil concentrations with the lag phase (Table 4), and the cubic trend seemed to better fit the model (Figure 1).

Table 4. Outputs of the ANOVA with single-degree-of-freedom orthogonal polynomial contrasts for the effects of different concentrations (C) of neem oil on lag phase of six *A. carbonarius* strains (ST).

Source	df	Type III SS	MS	F	*p*-Value
(C)	4	2,640,845.40	660,211.35	42.09	<0.0001*
Covariate: (ST)	1	23,815.89	23,815.89	1.52	0.2213
Error	83	1,301,845.28	15,684.88		
Contrast	df	Contrast SS	MS	F	*p*-value
(C)-linear	1	29,536.64	29,536.64	1.88	0.1737
(C)-quadratic	1	1,431,427.76	1,431,427.76	91.26	<0.0001*
(C)-cubic	1	347,184.26	347,184.26	22.13	<0.0001*
Parameter			Estimate	SE	*p*-value
(C)-linear			−128.48	93.62	0.1737
(C)-quadratic			−1057.38	110.68	<0.0001*
(C)-cubic			444.36	94.45	<0.0001*

"Strains" was not a significant covariate. Overall model $R^2 = 0.67$. df: degrees of freedom; SS: sum of squares; MS: mean squares; F: Fisher–Snedecor test. * Significant $p < 0.001$.

The effect of neem oil treatments on OTA production by six *A. carbonarius* strains assayed after 2, 7 and 10 days of incubation is shown in Table 5.

Table 5. Ochratoxin A (OTA) concentration (ng/g) produced by six *A. carbonarius* strains at five different concentration levels of neem oil at the incubation times assayed.

Strains	Incubation Time (Days)	OTA Concentration (ng/g)				
		0	0.1	0.3	0.5	1.0
FRR5690	2	62.5 ± 4.7	Nd	Nd	368.8 ± 34.3	Nd
	7	267.9 ± 46.5	Nd	Nd	637.7 ± 35.4	2817.2 ± 219.9
	10	334.3 ± 7.4	Nd	28.2 ± 3.2	986.3 ± 86.1	2954.7 ± 54.4
A2034	2	117.9 ± 2.1	Nd	Nd	468.2 ± 12.1	110.5 ± 4.0
	7	225.5 ± 10.0	13.8 ± 0.0	Nd	624.4 ± 18.4	454.5 ± 4.5
	10	325.7 ± 20.3	22.2 ± 2.2	Nd	741.3 ± 21.6	720.2 ± 1.3
RCG1	2	201.6 ± 2.2	Nd	NG	232.2 ± 25.9	168.0 ± 12.2
	7	278.8 ± 10.8	Nd	NG	358.0 ± 8.0	268.3 ± 0.6
	10	396.3 ± 7.8	Nd	NG	432.9 ± 2.0	258.5 ± 26.5
RCG2	2	102.6 ± 6.4	Nd	Nd	512.7 ± 30.7	160.2 ± 11.0
	7	573.2 ± 19.2	Nd	Nd	2281.2 ± 79.2	1808.3 ± 50.4
	10	758.6 ± 58.6	Nd	Nd	1785.0 ± 10.2	6164.4 ± 329.4
RCG3	2	227.8 ± 49.8	Nd	Nd	232.5 ± 56.6	280.1 ± 81.4
	7	384.3 ± 25.8	Nd	Nd	2232.6 ± 273.4	1904.2 ± 155.8
	10	528.6 ± 33.0	Nd	Nd	1403.5 ± 300.7	3054.8 ± 199.9
RCG4	2	86.4 ± 7.5	Nd	Nd	542.9 ± 41.1	Nd
	7	160.7 ± 6.1	Nd	Nd	183.5 ± 5.5	1507.4 ± 9.4
	10	203.8 ± 6.8	Nd	Nd	278.5 ± 16.5	2103.7 ± 102.9
Means ± SD	2	122.3 ± 68.8 [cC]	Nd [dC]	0.8 ± 0.4 [dC]	392.9 ± 132.8 [bC]	120.1 ± 105.1 [aC]
	7	309.6 ± 142.2 [cB]	3.13 ± 4.9 [dB]	0.8 ± 0.4 [dB]	1025.2 ± 869.7 [bB]	1460.0 ± 905.3 [aB]
	10	424.6 ± 184.7 [cA]	4.5 ± 8.2 [dA]	5.4 ± 10.6 [dA]	965.7 ± 597.7 [bA]	2542.7 ± 1987.7 [aA]

SD: standard deviation; NG: not growth; Nd: not detected (limit of detection 1ng/g). [a–d] Means with different lowercase letters in the row are significantly different ($p < 0.001$). [A–C] Means with different capital letters in column are significantly different ($p < 0.001$).

There was a complete inhibition in OTA production with the addition of 0.1% and 0.3% of neem oil for the four strains isolated from grapes whereas the two reference strains assayed (FRR5690 and A2034) produced low levels of OTA (28.2 and 22.2 ng/g, respectively) at 10 days of incubation. The absence of OTA production was also observed at two days of incubation and 1% of neem oil for FRR5690 and RCG4 strains.

The overall treatment time showed an increase in OTA production as incubation time increased and the regression analysis indicated significant linear dose-responses (Table 6; Figure 1).

An increase in OTA production was observed at 0.5% and 1% of neem oil. These two concentrations stimulated the OTA production at the end of the incubation period in 116.8 ± 78.8% and 498.8 ± 385.4%, respectively.

Single factors (concentration of neem oil and incubation time) as well as two-way interaction had a significant effect on OTA production by *A. carbonarius* strains studied ($p < 0.001$) (Table 6).

Table 6. Outputs of the ANOVA with single-degree-of-freedom orthogonal polynomial contrasts for the effects of different concentrations (C) of neem oil on ochratoxin A (OTA) production of six *A. carbonarius* strains (ST) at three incubation times (T).

Source	df	Type III SS	MS	F	*p*-Value
(C)	4	75,146,241.75	18,786,560.44	47.27	<0.0001*
(T)	2	20,290,698.84	10,145,349.42	25.52	<0.0001*
Covariate: (ST)	1	569,135.62	569,135.62	1.43	0.2326
(C)* (T)	8	37,954,380.17	4,744,297.52	11.94	<0.0001*
Error	254	100,956,999.01			
Contrast	df	Contrast SS	MS	F	*p*-value
(C)-linear	1	47,609,459.27	47,609,459.27	119.78	<0.0001*
(C)-quadratic	1	24,443,018.97	24,443,018.97	61.50	<0.0001*
(C)-cubic	1	1,320,779.85	1,320,779.85	3.32	0.0695
Parameter			Estimate	SE	*p*-value
(C)-linear			2969.27	271.30	<0.0001*
(C)-quadratic			2517.36	321.01	<0.0001*
(C)-cubic			−494.56	271.30	0.0695
Contrast	df	Contrast SS	MS	F	*p*-value
(T)-linear	1	19,669,576.14	19,669,576.14	49.49	<0.0001*
(T)-quadratic	1	621,122.70	621,122.70	1.56	0.2124
Parameter			Estimate	SE	*p*-value
(T)-linear			661.14	93.98	<0.0001*
(T)-quadratic			−203.49	162.78	0.2124

"Strains" was not a significant covariate. Overall model $R^2 = 0.57$. df: degrees of freedom; SS: sum of squares; MS: mean squares; F: Fisher–Snedecor test. * Significant $p < 0.001$.

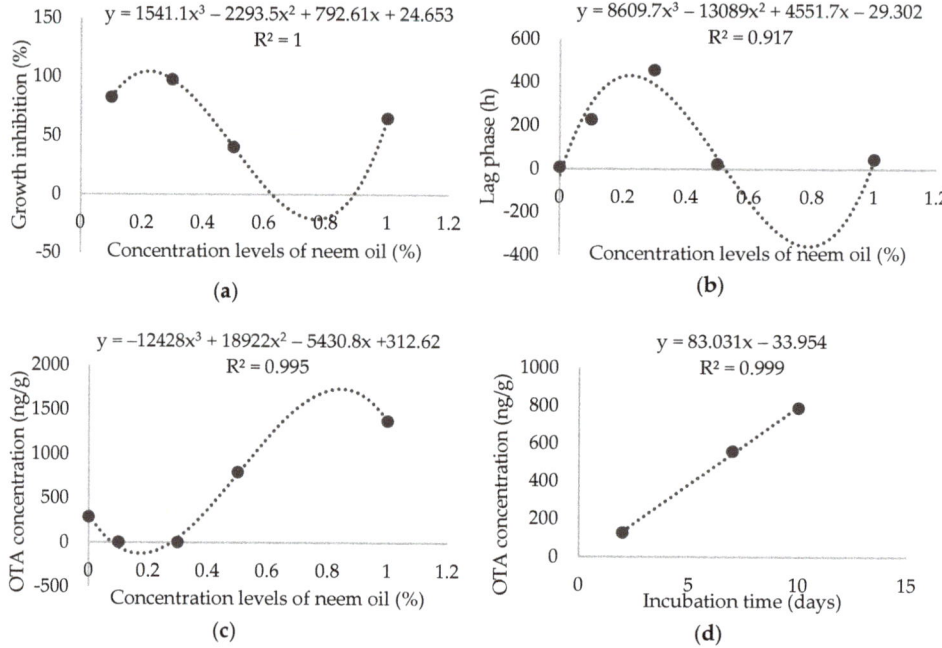

Figure 1. (**a**) The cubic polynomial fitting curve for percentage of growth inhibition of *A. carbonarius* strains against different concentrations of neem oil; (**b**) fitted regression curve using non-linear cubic splines for lag phase vs. different concentrations of neem oil; (**c**) the fitted cubic spline model to the OTA concentration data; (**d**) the linear curve fitting of incubation time vs. OTA concentration.

3. Discussion

The effect of natural or synthetic compounds on *Aspergillus* section *Flavi* species growth and aflatoxin production has already been described by some authors. Gowda, Malathi and Suganthi [33] studied the effect of some chemical and herbal compounds on the growth of other toxicogenic specie, *Aspergillus parasiticus*, and it was observed that neem oil at 0.5% had moderate anti-fungal activity (84% reduction vs. control), and at 0.2% and 0.1% a low antifungal activity, 52% and 36%, respectively. A lower percentage of reduction in fungal biomass (51%) was obtained by Zeringue and Bhatnagar [34] who studied the effects of neem leaf volatiles on submerged cultures of the same species. The contradictions between these results and the present study can possibly be explained by the different biochemical pathways that regulate the synthesis of the different mycotoxins produced by studied *Aspergillus* species and by the differences in the composition and therefore, the properties of each oil fraction. Razzaghi-Abyaneh et al. [35] agreed with those authors previously mentioned since they reported that neem leaf and seed extract can cause morphological alterations in the exposed mycelia, and then lead to cellular destruction.

Sitara et al. [36] concluded that the ideal concentrations for the reduction of the *Alternaria alternata* growth was 0.1% and 0.15% of neem oil extracted from seeds. These results corroborate the ideal concentrations of 0.1% and 0.3% found in this study. On the other hand, Bhatnagar and McCormick [37], studied the effects of the neem leaf extracts at 1%, 5%, 10%, 20% and 50% (*v/v*) on growth of *A. parasiticus* and concluded that it had no significant alterations at the mycelial growth. These results were very similar to Zeringue and Bhatnagar [38], that evaluated the effects of neem leaf extract on *Aspergillus flavus* and found only 4–7% of growth reduction.

On the other hand, Zeringue, Shih and Bhatnagar [39] studied the effects of clarified neem oil on growth in submerged and plated cultures of aflatoxigenic *Aspergillus* spp. which resulted in an increase of 11–31% measured by mycelia mass. Garcia and Garcia [40] agreed with those authors previously mentioned since they reported that neem did not inhibit either growth or aflatoxin production by *A. flavus* and *A. parasiticus*.

The 0.1% and 0.3% concentrations of neem oil completely inhibited the production of OTA for the four strains isolated from grapes. This can be explained since none of the four wild strains at 0.1% and three strains (RCG1, RCG2 and RCG3) at 0.3% had reached the exponential growth phase. However, at 0.5% and 1.0% concentrations, all the strains, except RCG1, showed increased production of OTA; this possibly occurred because these concentrations inhibited less of the mycelial growth in all of the six strains assayed. Another possibility is that the presence of the neem oil and the AZ compound in high concentrations could lead to an exacerbated oxidative stress situation by the fungus and an increase in OTA production.

According to the previous data in literature [41] the sensitivity of *Aspergillus* spp. to oxidative status perturbations is closely related to the production of mycotoxins. Several publications [41,42] addressed the exact mechanisms included in regulating the development and secondary metabolism of many *Aspergillus* spp. The production of mycotoxins is triggered by oxidative stress; an increase in reactive oxygen species (ROS) levels can increase mycotoxins levels, noting this phenomenon as one of the defense mechanisms of fungal cells. The tolerance of *A. flavus* and *A. parasiticus* isolates to oxidative stress has also been shown to be correlated with their levels of aflatoxin production. Roze et al. [43] showed that conidia of isolates with higher levels of aflatoxin production also exhibited greater viability when cultured in ROS-amended medium.

Finally, another possibility is that higher concentrations (0.5% and 1.0%) of neem oil could have exceeded the solubility limits of the tested medium and the effective compounds did not have the same activity as in the lower concentrations [44,45].

These results are divergent to Bhatnagar and McCormick [37] who found that using 10% concentration of neem leaf extract reduces 98% of *A. parasiticus* aflatoxins production even if there is no inhibition of the mycelial growth. Allameh et al. [46] concluded that the concentration needed to reduce 90% of the aflatoxin production from *A. parasiticus* was 50% of neem leaf extract (v/v). This concentration was 150 times greater than the ideal concentration of neem oil found in this study. Razzaghi-Abyaneh et al. [35] also found a high reduction (91.3%) of aflatoxin production per µg of mycelia by *A. parasiticus* using 1.56% of neem extracts from seeds and leaf.

While many compounds and substances have been found to effectively inhibit fungal growth and aflatoxin production, others have stimulatory properties and affect the biosynthesis or bioregulation of aflatoxins, just like what happened with the utilization of 0.5% and 1.0% concentration of neem oil [47]. Nowadays, the information about action mechanisms of these compounds on *Aspergillus* species is limited, however it is possible to assure that the neem oil has important antifungal properties against *A. carbonarius*.

4. Conclusions

These findings clearly indicate the use of neem oil in low concentrations, such as 0.1% and 0.3%, is a good possibility as an auxiliary control method for mycelial growth reduction in *Aspergillus carbonarius* strains and the inhibition of ochratoxin A production. Mycotoxin contamination in food poses serious health hazards to animals and humans. Very few scattered reports are available on the effects of plant oils on growth of ochratoxigenic fungi. This study can contribute to the knowledge to develop effective anti-mycotoxigenic natural products for reduction of mycotoxigenic fungi and mycotoxins in foods.

5. Materials and Methods

5.1. Fungal Strains

Six *Aspergillus carbonarius* strains were evaluated as follows: two reference strains (FRR5690 and A2034) from the CSIRO Collection Centre, Australia and four *A. carbonarius* strains (RCG1, RCG2, RCG3 and RCG4) isolated from dry grapes in Argentina [48]; all of them were OTA producers on yeast extract sucrose (YES, HiMedia Laboratories Pvt. Ltd., Mumbai, India) medium (2% yeast extract, 15% sucrose).

5.2. Culture Medium

Commercial neem oil (Base Fértil Agrícola, Cravinhos, SP, Brazil) was used in this study. According to the manufacturer's certificate of analysis, neem oil was extracted from seeds and contained 0.12% p/p of azadirachtin (= 1200 ppm). Neem oil was added to the Czapek yeast extract agar (CYA, HiMedia Laboratories Pvt. Ltd., Mumbai, India) at final concentrations of 0.1%, 0.3%, 0.5% or 1.0% (v/v) at 45 °C. Plates containing CYA media without neem oil were used as control.

5.3. Inoculation and Incubation Conditions

Spore suspensions of the six *A. carbonarius* strains were obtained by scraping the surface of a 7-day-old colony cultured in 2% malt extract agar (MEA, HiMedia Laboratories Pvt. Ltd., Mumbai, India) and transferring the conidia to a tube containing 10 mL of sterile distilled water supplemented with 0.1% Tween 20. The solution was homogenized and read in a spectrophotometer (530 nm) to obtain a transmittance between 80% and 82%, which corresponds to $1-5 \times 10^6$ colony forming units per milliliter (CFU/mL). Then the Petri plates were needle-inoculated centrally with 10 µL of the spore suspension. The plates were incubated at 25 °C ± 2 for a maximum of two weeks.

5.4. Growth Assessment

Two perpendicular diameters of the growing colonies were measured daily until the colony reached the edge of the plate or for a maximum of two weeks. The percentage inhibition of diameter growth (PIDG) values were determined according to the equation as below:

$$\text{PIDG (\%)} = \frac{\text{Diameter of sample} - \text{Diameter of control}}{\text{Diameter of control}} \times 100$$

Growth rate (mm day^{-1}) was calculated by linear regression of colony diameter against time for each strain at each set of conditions tested, and the time at which the line intercepted the x-axis was used to calculate the lag phase (h) in relation to isolate and essential oil. In all cases, the experiments were carried out with three replicates per treatment. The growth of fungal cultures containing different concentrations of neem oil was compared with that of the control culture that was grown with no EO.

5.5. Ochratoxin A Extraction from Culture

Ochratoxin A production was analyzed after 2, 7 and 10 days of incubation. The methodology proposed by Bragulat, Abarca and Cabañes [49] with some modifications was used. On each sampling occasion, three agar plugs were removed from different points of the colony and extracted with 1 mL of methanol. The mixture was centrifuged at 14,000 rpm for 10 min. The solutions were filtered (syringe filters, 17 mm, 0.45 µm, nylon membranes), evaporated to dryness, and re-dissolved in 200 µL of mobile phase (acetonitrile:water:acetic acid, 57:41:2) and the extracts injected into the high-performance liquid chromatography system.

5.6. OTA Detection and Quantification

The OTA production was detected and quantified by reversed phase in a high performance liquid chromatography system Hewlett Packard Serie 1100 (HP/Agilent, Santa Clara, CA, USA) with fluorescence detection (λ_{exc} 330 nm; λ_{em} 460 nm) using a C_{18} column (Supelcosil™ LC-ABZ, 150 × 4.6 mm, 5 µm particle size), connected to a precolumn (Supelguard™ LC-ABZ, 20 × 4.6 mm, 5 µm particle size). The mobile phase was pumped at 1.0 mL/min. The injection volume was 100 µL and the retention time was around 4 ± 1 min. The detection limit of the analyses was 1 ng/g [50].

5.7. Statistical Analyses

Statistical analyses were conducted using PROC GLM in SAS program (SAS Institute Inc., Cary, NC, USA). The differences between growth inhibition percentage, lag phase and OTA production at different concentration levels of neem oil by six *Aspergillus carbonarius* strains at 2, 7 and 10 days were analyzed statistically by analyses of variance (ANOVA). The statistical models used in ANOVA considered the effects of the dependent variables and "strains" as a covariate within the different concentration levels of neem oil. The independence of the covariate was formally checked. Means were compared by Fisher's LSD test to determine the influence of the neem oil on the ecophysiology of the strains assayed [51]. Orthogonal polynomial contrasts were used to determine linear, quadratic and cubic responses to neem oil. The OTA production data contained some results of "not detected" (ND). That is, the OTA concentration was not detected above the detection limit (DL) of the used method. The actual concentration represented by ND is some value below the DL, however, the analytical method cannot determine whether the ND is truly zero or some unquantifiable value between zero and the DL. For this situation we used the substitution method, replacing the ND with the DL value (1 ng/g). In the cases of "not growth" (NG) results, we performed the substitution with zero.

Author Contributions: Investigation, M.P.R., A.L.A. and Á.A.d.O.; formal analysis, K.M.K.; project administration, C.A.d.R.R. and K.M.K.; supervision, L.R.C. and M.I.d.A.; writing—original draft, M.P.R. and A.L.A.; writing—review and editing, M.P.R., A.L.A., Á.A.d.O., L.A.S., G.L.B., L.A.M.K. and K.M.K.

Funding: The authors would like to thank Coordenação de Aperfeiçoamento de Pessoal de Nível Superior (CAPES), Conselho Nacional de Desenvolvimento Científico e Tecnológico (CNPq), Consejo Nacional de Investigaciones Científicas y Técnicas (CONICET), Pró-Reitoria de Pesquisa da Universidade Federal de Minas Gerais (PRPq-UFMG), Secretaría de Ciencia y Técnica de la Universidad Nacional de Río Cuarto (SECYT-UNRC) and Fondo para la Investigación Científica y Tecnológica (FONCYT-PICTO).

Conflicts of Interest: The authors declare no conflicts of interest.

References

1. Pitt, J.I. Toxigenic fungi and mycotoxins. *Br. Med. Bull.* **2000**, *56*, 184–192. [CrossRef] [PubMed]
2. Gams, W.; Christensen, M.; Onions, A.H.S.; Pitt, J.I.; Samson, R.A. Infrageneric taxa of *Aspergillus*. In *Advances in Penicillium and Aspergillus Systematics*; Samson, R.A., Pitt, J.I., Eds.; Plenum: New York, NY, USA, 1985; pp. 55–61.
3. Varga, J.; Frisvad, J.C.; Kocsubé, S.; Brankovics, B.; Tóth, B.; Sziget, G.; Samson, R.A. New and revisited species in *Aspergillus* section *Nigri*. *Stud. Mycol.* **2011**, *69*, 1–17. [CrossRef] [PubMed]
4. Taniwaki, M.H.; Pitt, J.I.; Magan, N. *Aspergillus* species and mycotoxins: Occurrence and importance in major food commodities. *Curr. Opin. Food Sci.* **2018**, *23*, 38–43. [CrossRef]
5. Cabañes, F.J.; Bragulat, M.R. Black aspergilli and ochratoxin A-producing species in foods. *Curr. Opin. Food Sci.* **2018**, *23*, 1–10. [CrossRef]
6. CAST. *Mycotoxins: Risks in Plant, Animal, and Human Systems, n. 139*; CAST: Motor City, IA, USA, 2003; p. 199.
7. Tao, Y.; Xiea, S.; Xua, F.; Liub, A.; Wangb, Y.; Chenb, D.; Pana, Y.; Huangb, L.; Penga, D.; Wanga, X.; et al. Ochratoxin A: Toxicity, oxidative stress and metabolism. *Food Chem. Toxicol.* **2018**, *112*, 320–331. [CrossRef] [PubMed]

8. IARC. IARC Monographs on the Evaluation of Carcinogenic Risks to Humans, v. 56. 1993. Available online: https://monographs.iarc.fr/iarc-monographs-on-the-evaluation-of-carcinogenic-risks-to-humans-65/ (accessed on 4 April 2018).
9. Pfohl-Leszkowicz, A.; Petkova-Bocharova, T.; Chernozemsky, I.N.; Castegnaro, M. Balkan endemic nephropathy and associated urinary tract tumours: A review on aetiological causes and the potential role of mycotoxins. *Food Addit. Contam.* **2002**, *19*, 282–302. [CrossRef]
10. Tongnuanchan, P.; Benjakul, S. Essential Oils: Extraction, Bioactivities, and Their Uses for Food Preservation. *J. Food Sci.* **2014**, *79*, 1231–1249. [CrossRef] [PubMed]
11. Calo, J.R.; Crandall, P.G.; O'Bryan, C.; Ricke, A.S.C. Essential oils as antimicrobials in food systems—A review. *Food Control* **2015**, *54*, 111–119. [CrossRef]
12. Yang, C.; Chowdhury, M.A.K.; Huo, Y.; Gong, J. Phytogenic Compounds as Alternatives to In-Feed Antibiotics: Potentials and Challenges in Application. *Pathogens* **2015**, *4*, 137–156. [CrossRef]
13. Stevanović, Z.D.; Bošnjak-Neumüller, J.; Pajić-Lijaković, I.; Raj, J.; Vasiljević, M. Essential Oils as Feed Additives-Future Perspectives. *Molecules* **2018**, *23*, 1717. [CrossRef]
14. Pawar, V.C.; Thaker, V.S. In vitro efficacy of 75 essential oils against *Aspergillus niger*. *Mycoses* **2007**, *49*, 316–323. [CrossRef] [PubMed]
15. El-Nagerabi, S.A.F.; Al-Bahry, S.N.; Elshafie, A.E.; AlHilali, S. Effect of *Hibiscus sabdariffa* extract and *Nigella sativa* oil on the growth and aflatoxin B1 production of *Aspergillus flavus* and *Aspergillus parasiticus* strains. *Food Control* **2012**, *25*, 59–63. [CrossRef]
16. Ferreira, F.D.; Kemmelmeier, C.; Arrotéia, C.C.; Costa, C.L.; Mallmann, C.A.; Janeiro, V.; Ferreira, F.M.; Mossini, S.A.; Silva, E.L.; Machinski, M., Jr. Inhibitory effect of the essential oil of *Curcuma longa* L. and curcumin on aflatoxin production by *Aspergillus flavus* Link. *Food Chem.* **2013**, *136*, 789–793. [CrossRef] [PubMed]
17. Passone, M.A.; Girardi, N.S.; Etcheverry, M. Antifungal and antiaflatoxigenic activity by vapor contact of three essential oils, and effects of environmental factors on their efficacy. *LWT Food Sci. Technol.* **2013**, *53*, 434–444. [CrossRef]
18. Manso, S.; Pezo, D.; Gómez-Lus, R.; Nerín, C. Diminution of aflatoxin B1 production caused by an active packaging containing cinnamon essential oil. *Food Control* **2014**, *45*, 101–108. [CrossRef]
19. Gupta, S.C.; Prasad, S.; Tyagi, A.K.; Kunnumakkara, A.B.; Aggarwal, B. Neem (*Azadirachta indica*): An Indian traditional panacea with modern molecular basis. *Phytomedicine* **2017**, *34*, 14–20. [CrossRef] [PubMed]
20. Quelemes, P.V.; Perfeito, M.L.G.; Guimarães, M.A.; dos Santos, R.C.; Lima, D.F.; Nascimento, C.; Silva, M.P.N.; Soares, M.J.S.; Ropke, C.D.; Eaton, P.; et al. Effect of neem (*Azadirachta indica* A. Juss) leaf extract on resistant *Staphylococcus aureus* biofilm formation and *Schistosoma mansoni* worms. *J. Ethnopharmacol.* **2015**, *175*, 287–294. [CrossRef]
21. Suresh, G.; Narasimhan, N.S.; Masilamani, S.; Partho, R.D.; Gopalakrishnan, G. Antifungal Fractions and Compounds from Uncrushed Green Leaves of *Azadirachta indica*. *Phytoparasitica* **1997**, *25*, 33–39. [CrossRef]
22. Siddiqui, B.S.; Afshan, F.; Ghiasuddin, S.F.; Naqvi, S.N.H.; Tariq, R.M. New insect-growth-regulator meliacin butenolides from the leaves of *Azadirachta indica* A. Juss. *J. Chem. Soc. Perkin Trans.* **1999**, *16*, 2367–2370. [CrossRef]
23. Van der Nat, J.M.; van der Sluis, W.G.; Hart, L.A.; Dijk, H.V.; de Silva, K.T.D.; Labadie, R.P. Activity-Guided Isolation and Identification of *Azadirachta indica* Bark Extract Constituents which Specifically Inhibit Chemiluminescence Production by Activated Human Polymorphonuclear Leukocytes. *Planta Med.* **1991**, *57*, 65–68. [CrossRef]
24. Govindachari, T.R.; Suresh, G.; Gopalakrishnan, G.; Banumathy, B.; Masilamani, S. Identification of Antifungal Compounds from the Seed Oil of *Azadirachta indica*. *Phytoparasitica* **1998**, *26*, 109–116. [CrossRef]
25. Roychoudhury, R. Chapter 18—Neem Products. In *Ecofriendly Pest Management for Food Security*; Omkar, Ed.; Academic Press: Cambridge, MA, USA, 2016; pp. 545–562. [CrossRef]
26. Brahmachari, G. Neem–An Omnipotent Plant: A Retrospection. *ChemBioChem* **2004**, *5*, 408–421. [CrossRef] [PubMed]
27. Del Serrone, P.; Failla, S.; Nicoletti, M. Natural control of bacteria affecting meat quality by a neem (*Azadirachta indica* A. Juss) cake extract. *Nat. Prod. Res.* **2015**, *29*, 985–987. [CrossRef] [PubMed]

28. Al Akeel, R.; Mateen, A.; Janardhan, K.; Gupta, V.C. Analysis of anti-bacterial and anti oxidative activity of *Azadirachta indica* bark using various solvents extracts. *Saudi J. Biol. Sci.* **2017**, *24*, 11–14. [CrossRef]
29. Al Saiqali, M.; Tangutur, A.D.; Banoth, C.; Bhukya, B. Antimicrobial and anticancer potential of low molecular weight polypeptides extracted and characterized from leaves of *Azadirachta indica*. *Int. J. Biol. Macromol.* **2018**, *114*, 906–921. [CrossRef]
30. Parida, M.M.; Upadhyay, C.; Pandya, G.; Jana, A.M. Inhibitory potential of neem (*Azadirachta indica* Juss) leaves on Dengue virus type-2 replication. *J. Ethnopharmacol.* **2002**, *79*, 273–278. [CrossRef]
31. Chaube, S.K.; Shrivastav, T.G.; Tiwari, M.; Prasad, S.; Tripathi, A.; Pandey, A.K. Neem (*Azadirachta indica* L.) leaf extract deteriorates oocyte quality by inducing ROS-mediated apoptosis in mammals. *SpringerPlus* **2014**, *3*, 464. [CrossRef]
32. European Commission. Available online: http://ec.europa.eu/food/plant/pesticides/eu-pesticides-database/public/?event=activesubstance.ViewReview&id=721 (accessed on 13 August 2019).
33. Gowda, N.K.S.; Malathi, V.; Suganthi, R.U. Effect of some chemical and herbal compounds on growth of *Aspergillus parasiticus* and aflatoxin production. *Anim. Feed Sci. Tech.* **2004**, *116*, 281–291. [CrossRef]
34. Zeringue, H.J.; Bhatnagar, D. Effects of neem leaf volatiles on submerged cultures of aflatoxigenic *Aspergillus parasiticus*. *Appl. Environ. Microbiol.* **1994**, *60*, 3543–3547.
35. Razzaghi-Abyaneh, M.; Allameh, A.; Tiraihi, T.; Shams-Ghahfarokhi, M.; Ghorbanian, M. Morphological alterations in toxigenic *Aspergillus parasiticus* exposed to neem (*Azadirachta indica*) leaf and seed aqueous extracts. *Mycopathologia* **2005**, *159*, 565–570. [CrossRef]
36. Sitara, U.; Niaz, I.; Naseem, J. Antifungal effect of essential oils on in vitro growth of pathogenic fungi. *Pak. J. Bot.* **2008**, *40*, 409–414.
37. Bhatnagar, D.; McCormick, S.P. The Inhibitory Effect of Neem (*Azadirachta indica*) Leaf Extracts on Aflatoxin Synthesis in *Aspergillus parasiticus*. *J. Am. Oil Chem. Soc.* **1988**, *65*, 1166–1168. [CrossRef]
38. Zeringue, H.J.; Bhatnagar, D. Inhibition of Aflatoxin Production in *Aspergillus flavus* Infected Cotton Bolls After Treatment with Neem (*Azadirachta indica*) Leaf Extracts. *J. Am. Oil Chem. Soc.* **1990**, *67*, 215–216. [CrossRef]
39. Zeringue, H.J.; Shih, B.Y.; Bhatnagar, D. Effects of clarified neem oil on growth and aflatoxin B formation in submerged and plate cultures of aflatoxigenic *Aspergillus* spp. *Phytoparasitica* **2001**, *29*, 1–4. [CrossRef]
40. Garcia, R.P.; Garcia, M.I. Laboratory evaluation of neem derivatives against *Aspergillus* growth and aflatoxin formation. *Philipp. Agric. Sci.* **1990**, *73*, 333–342.
41. Bok, J.W.; Keller, N.P. LaeA, a Regulator of Secondary Metabolism in Aspergillus spp. *Eukaryot. Cell* **2004**, *3*, 527–535. [CrossRef] [PubMed]
42. Lind, A.L.; Smith, T.D.; Saterlee, T.; Calvo, A.M.; Rokas, A. Regulation of Secondary Metabolism by the Velvet Complex is Temperature-Responsive in *Aspergillus*. *Genes Genomes Genet.* **2016**, *6*, 4023–4033.
43. Roze, L.V.; Chanda, A.; Linz, J.E. Compartmentalization and molecular traffic in secondary metabolism: A new understanding of established cellular processes. *Fungal Genet. Biol.* **2011**, *48*, 35–48. [CrossRef]
44. Arroteia, C.C.; Kemmelmeier, C.; Junior, M.M. Effect of aqueous and oily extracts of Neem [*Azadirachta indica* A. Juss (*Meliaceae*)] on patulin production in apples contaminated with *Penicillium expansum*. *Ciência Rural.* **2007**, *37*, 1518–1523.
45. Burt, S. Essential oils: Their antibacterial properties and potential applications in foods—A review. *Int. J. Food Microbiol.* **2004**, *94*, 223–253. [CrossRef]
46. Allameh, A.; Razzaghi-abyane, M.; Shams, M.; Rezaee, M.B.; Jaimand, K. Effects of neem leaf extract on production of aflatoxins and activities of fatty acid synthetase, isocitrate dehydrogenase and glutathione S-transferase in *Aspergillus parasiticus*. *Mycopathologia* **2002**, *154*, 79–84. [CrossRef] [PubMed]
47. Zaika, L.L.; Buchanan, R.L. Review of compounds affecting the biosynthesis or bioregulation of aflatoxins. *J. Food Prot.* **1987**, *50*, 691–708. [CrossRef] [PubMed]
48. Magnoli, C.; Violante, M.; Combina, M.; Palacio, G.; Dalcero, A. Mycoflora and ochratoxin-producing strains of *Aspergillus* section *Nigri* in wine grapes in Argentina. *Lett. Appl. Microbiol.* **2004**, *39*, 326–331. [CrossRef] [PubMed]

49. Bragulat, M.R.; Abarca, M.L.; Cabañes, F.J. An easy screening method for fungi producing ochratoxin A in pure culture. *Int. J. Food Microbiol.* **2001**, *71*, 139–144. [CrossRef]
50. Scudamore, K.A.; MacDonald, S.J. A collaborative study of an HPLC method for determination of ochratoxin A in wheat using immunoaffinity column clean-up. *Food Addit. Contam.* **1998**, *15*, 401–410. [CrossRef] [PubMed]
51. Quinn, G.P.; Keough, M.J. (Eds.) *Experimental Design Data Analysis for Biologists*; Cambridge University Press: Cambridge, UK, 2002; pp. 1–537.

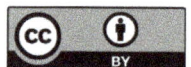

© 2019 by the authors. Licensee MDPI, Basel, Switzerland. This article is an open access article distributed under the terms and conditions of the Creative Commons Attribution (CC BY) license (http://creativecommons.org/licenses/by/4.0/).

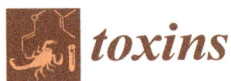

Article

Impact of Naturally Contaminated Substrates on *Alphitobius diaperinus* and *Hermetia illucens*: Uptake and Excretion of Mycotoxins

Giulia Leni [1], Martina Cirlini [1,*], Johan Jacobs [2], Stefaan Depraetere [2], Natasja Gianotten [3], Stefano Sforza [1] and Chiara Dall'Asta [1]

1. Department of Food and Drug, University of Parma, Parco Area delle Scienze 27/A, 43124 Parma, Italy
2. Circular Organics, Slachthuisstraat 120/6, 2300 Turnhout, Belgium
3. Protifarm, Harderwijkerweg 141B, 3852 AB Ermelo, The Netherlands
* Correspondence: martina.cirlini@unipr.it; Tel.: +39-05-2190-6079

Received: 23 July 2019; Accepted: 16 August 2019; Published: 18 August 2019

Abstract: Insects are considered a suitable alternative feed for livestock production and their use is nowadays regulated in the European Union by the European Commission Regulation No. 893/2017. Insects have the ability to grow on a different spectrum of substrates, which could be naturally contaminated by mycotoxins. In the present work, the mycotoxin uptake and/or excretion in two different insect species, *Alphitobius diaperinus* (Lesser Mealworm, LM) and *Hermetia illucens* (Black Soldier Fly, BSF), grown on naturally contaminated substrates, was evaluated. Among all the substrates of growth tested, the *Fusarium* toxins deoxynivalenol (DON), fumonisin 1 and 2 (FB1 and FB2) and zearalenone (ZEN) were found in those based on wheat and/or corn. No mycotoxins were detected in BSF larvae, while quantifiable amount of DON and FB1 were found in LM larvae, although in lower concentration than those detected in the growing substrates and in the residual fractions. Mass balance calculations indicated that BSF and LM metabolized mycotoxins in forms not yet known, accumulating them in their body or excreting in the faeces. Further studies are required in this direction due to the future employment of insects as feedstuff.

Keywords: *Alphitobius diaperinus*; *Hermetia illucens*; edible insects; mycotoxin; uptake; excretion; feed safety

Key Contribution: This study demonstrates that *Alphitobius diaperinus* and *Hermetia illucens*; two common edible insects; reared on naturally contaminated substrates; did not accumulate DON; FBs and ZEN in their body; but seemed to metabolize them in forms not yet known; excreting them in the faeces also by the hydrolysis of masked forms.

1. Introduction

Given the large growth of the World population expected in the coming years, it has been estimated that the demand for food will raise of about the 60% in 2050 [1]. Along the food chain, the meat production represents the field with the most impact, with serious consequences on the demand of feed supply. Edible insects have been explored as an alternative to common livestock, and their use is encouraged for their sustainability and the minimal environmental impact applied in their breeding [2,3]. Furthermore, edible insects have been proposed as a promising alternative nutrient source due to the high content and quality of their macronutrients [4]. In general, they have a well-balanced nutrient profile, high in polyunsaturated fatty acids and essential amino acids which meet the requirement for humans and livestock, rich in micronutrients and vitamins [5].

In the European Union, the use of insects in the feed and food sector is nowadays regulated by a package of legislative texts. Insects are included in the category of Novel Foods and the European Food Safety Authority (EFSA) authorization is mandatory before their marketing in the European Union (EU) [6]. As alternative source for feedstock, they may substitute the sources of protein and fat normally added in animal feed, as soy, maize, grain and fishmeal [7]. Insects can be used as whole or processed. Whole insects, alive or dried, and fat fraction can be employed for livestock feed, except for aquaculture [8]. Whereas, the protein fraction isolated from insects can be used to feed pet and fur animals, but not for ruminants and monogastrics [9]. Recently, the European Commission (EC) has expanded also to the aquaculture sector, the addition of processed proteins from seven insect species: Black Soldier Fly (*Hermetia illucens*), Common Housefly (*Musca domestica*), Yellow Mealworm (*Tenebrio molitor*), Lesser Mealworm (*Alphitobius diaperinus*), House Cricket (*Acheta domesticus*), Banded Cricket (*Gryllodes sigillatus*) and Field Cricket (*Gryllus assimilis*) [8].

One of the limitations in the use of insects as feed and food is certainly linked to safety aspects. The potential hazards are related to exogenous and endogenous factors, which could be influenced also by harvesting and processing methods, and which could be achieved during all the insect life-cycle [4,10]. Exogenous factors may occur from the behavior and from the substrate of growth which, as feed, must meet the requirements of the current regulation that fixed the maximum limits of undesirable substances in feedstock [11,12]. In particular, the potential hazards could be heavy metal residues, pesticides and mycotoxins.

Mycotoxins are a wide range of different substances, produced by the secondary metabolism of various species of fungi, that can infect cereal or vegetable crops at pre- or post-harvest [13]. Mycotoxins are characterized by a large chemical diversity and may exert a broad spectrum of adverse effects in animals and humans [14,15]. In addition, they can undergo biotransformation in plants, microbes and animals [16] leading to the uptake of modified forms which may account for a similar toxicity compared to parent compounds [14].

Although mycotoxin occurrence in food and feed is extensively covered by regulation/guidelines at EU level, their presence at concentration levels not exceeding the EU limits cannot be ruled out in rearing substrates obtained from vegetable waste. Therefore, insects are potentially exposed to mycotoxins when reared on a contaminated substrate and, at least from a theoretical point of view, they could accumulate mycotoxins (or modified forms) at levels exceeding the legal limits.

However, despite a growing interest, only few papers have addressed the possible uptake and biotransformation of mycotoxins in insects so far [17–22]. Although information on the possible biotransformation and/or excretion mechanisms are still scattered, all the studies performed to date consistently demonstrated that parent mycotoxins are not bioaccumulated by insects grown in contaminated substrates.

However, many of these studies were done on substrates artificially contaminated with mycotoxins, possibly not exactly describing the situation arising in the case of a natural contamination.

The aim of this research, in the framework of the EU project InDIRECT, was to investigate the possible uptake and excretion of mycotoxins in two species of insect larvae, Lesser Mealworm (LM) and Black Soldier Fly (BSF), produced on different naturally contaminated substrates, obtained from vegetable and cereals waste.

2. Results

Different feed materials were selected for the experiments, in order to ensure optimal growth of the larvae on the basis of preliminary trials. These wastes derived from the processing of cereals, as wheat, corn, rice, while others were chosen among vegetables, as olive and apple pomace, rapeseed and chopped carrots (Table 1).

Table 1. Substrates used for feed formulations with results about their mycotoxin contamination (deoxynivalenol (DON), fumonisins 1 and 2 (FB1 and FB2), zearalenone (ZEN)). Results showed the detected mycotoxins and are reported as mean of two different replicates ± standard deviation.

Substrate Samples		Mycotoxin Amount (µg/kg)			
Sample Code	Description	DON	FB1	FB2	ZEN
WM	Wheat middlings	938 ± 100	<LOD	<LOD	<LOD
CDR	Corn distillation residues	779 ± 5	573 ± 3	441 ± 3	<LOD
CG	Corn gluten feed	1207 ± 43	727 ± 6	294 ± 5	173 ± 4
RB	Rice Bran	<LOD	<LOD	<LOD	<LOD
RW	Rapeseed wastes	<LOD	<LOD	<LOD	<LOD
OP	Olive pomace	LOD	<LOD	<LOD	<LOD
AP	Apple pomace	<LOD	<LOD	<LOD	<LOD
CC	Chopped carrots	<LOD	<LOD	<LOD	<LOD

Samples were analysed for all the regulated mycotoxins, according to the possible occurrence. In particular, samples were analysed for *Fusarium* toxins (deoxynivalenol (DON), fumonisins 1 and 2 (FB1 and FB2), zearalenone (ZEN)) as well as aflatoxins, while the possible presence of patulin was checked in vegetable-based samples. All samples underwent ochratoxin (OTA) analysis, in consideration of its possible synthetisation postharvest in all the considered feed materials. As shown in Table 1, only *Fusarium* toxins were found in three out of eight matrices, at concentration levels in agreement with the EU limits for cereal-based feed. While only DON (938 ± 100 µg/kg) was found in wheat middlings, the contemporary presence of DON, FB1, FB2 and ZEN was detected in corn wastes. In order to optimize and promote the insect growth, 15 feed formulations were obtained by mixing these substrates (originated from the same batch) in different percentages. In particular, corn distillation residues were mixed with chopped carrots, olive and apple pomace, while wheat middlings with corn gluten feed, rice bran and rapeseed, as indicated in Table 2.

According to the contamination pattern observed in raw waste materials, BSF and LM larvae were analysed for the target mycotoxins and results are reported in Table 2. No mycotoxin uptake was observed in BSF larvae, while DON was detected in six out of 13 LM larvae samples, being one contaminated by FB1 as well.

Table 2. Larvae of Black Soldier Fly (*Hermetia illucens*, BSF) and Lesser Mealworm (*Alphitobius diaperinus*, LM) reared on the feed formulations with results about the target mycotoxins occurrence. Results are the mean of two different replicates and are reported as mean ± standard deviation. Abbreviations: deoxynivalenol, DON; fumonisins 1 and 2, FB1 and FB2; zearalenone, ZEN; corn distillation residues, CDR; olive pomace, OP; apple pomace, AP; wheat middlings, WM; corn gluten feed, CG; rice bran, RB; rapeseed wastes, RW.

Larvae Samples		Mycotoxin Amount (µg/kg)			
Sample Code	Description	DON	FB1	FB2	ZEN
BSF-100% CDR	BSF larvae grown on: 100% CDR	<LOD	<LOD	<LOD	<LOD
BSF-79% CDR-10.5% OP/AP	BSF larvae grown on: 79% CDR, 10.5% OP, 10.5% AP	<LOD	<LOD	<LOD	<LOD
LM-100% WM	LM larvae grown on: 100% WM, 0% CG	416 ± 28	<LOD	<LOD	<LOD
LM-75% WM-25% CG	LM larvae grown on: 75% WM, 25% CG	608 ± 59	<LOD	<LOD	<LOD
LM-50% WM-50% CG	LM larvae grown on: 50% WM, 50% CG	<LOD	<LOD	<LOD	<LOD
LM-100% CG	LM larvae grown on: 100% CG	726 ± 164	127 ± 6	<LOD	<LOD
LM-100% CDR *	LM larvae grown on: 100% CDR *	468 ± 181	<LOD	<LOD	<LOD
LM-95% WM-5% RB	LM larvae grown on: 95% WM, 5% RB	<LOD	<LOD	<LOD	<LOD
LM-90% WM-10% RB	LM larvae grown on: 90% WM, 10% RB	755 ± 134	<LOD	<LOD	<LOD
LM-85% WM-15% RB	LM larvae grown on: 85% WM, 15% RB	<LOD	<LOD	<LOD	<LOD
LM-80% WM-20% RB	LM larvae grown on: 80% WM, 20% RB	<LOD	<LOD	<LOD	<LOD
LM-95% WM-5% RW	LM larvae grown on: 95% WM, 5% RW	<LOD	<LOD	<LOD	<LOD
LM-90% WM-10% RW	LM larvae grown on: 90% WM, 10% RW	<LOD	<LOD	<LOD	<LOD
LM-85% WM-15% RW	LM larvae grown on: 85% WM, 15% RW	557 ± 237	<LOD	<LOD	<LOD
LM-80% WM-20% RW	LM larvae grown on: 80% WM, 20% RW	<LOD	<LOD	<LOD	<LOD

* A small amount of chopped carrots was arbitrarily added in order to get the desired water content for optimal insect growth.

In particular, DON was detected in samples of LM larvae grown on substrates prepared with high percentages of wheat and/or corn residues, and the amount of contamination ranged between 416 ± 28 µg/kg of larvae produced on 100% of wheat wastes and 755 ± 134 µg/kg of insects cultivated on wheat (90%) added with rice (10%). Low concentrations of FB1 (127 ± 6 µg/kg) were detected in LM larvae grown on a substrate composed of 100% of corn gluten feed.

In order to evaluate the uptake and possible excretion of mycotoxins, the residual fractions were also analysed. All the results are listed in Table 3. Interestingly, the contemporary presence of DON, FB1, FB2 and ZEN was observed in the residual fraction obtained from BSF larvae grown on 100% corn residues, while DON and FB1 were detected in residual fractions from LM corn-based growing substrates. No residual contamination was observed in wheat-based residual fractions, in spite of the DON occurrence detected in wheat waste.

Table 3. Residual fractions harvested from insects resulted positive to the presence of target mycotoxins and results about their concentration level expresses as µg/kg. Results are the mean of two different replicates and are reported as mean ± standard deviation. Abbreviations: black soldier fly, BSF; lesser mealworm, LM; deoxynivalenol, DON; fumonisins 1 and 2, FB1 and FB2; zearalenone, ZEN; corn distillation residues, CDR; olive pomace, OP; apple pomace, AP; wheat middlings, WM; corn gluten feed, CG; chopped carrots, CC; rice bran, RB; rapeseed wastes, RW.

Residual Fraction Samples		Mycotoxin Amount (µg/kg)			
Sample Code	Description	DON	FB1	FB2	ZEN
REST-BSF-100% CDR	Rests of BSF larvae grown on: 100% CDR	1473 ± 197	951 ± 152	344 ± 64	334 ± 44
REST-BSF-79% CDR-10.5% OP/AP	Rests of BSF larvae grown on: 79% CDR, 10.5% OP, 10.5% AP	<LOD	<LOD	<LOD	<LOD
REST-LM-100% WM	Rests of LM larvae grown on: 100% WM, 0% CG	<LOD	<LOD	<LOD	<LOD
REST-LM-75% WM-25% CG	LM larvae grown on: 75% WM, 25% CG	<LOD	<LOD	<LOD	<LOD
REST-LM-100% CG	Rests of LM larvae grown on: 100% CG	827 ± 61	728 ± 7	<LOD	<LOD
REST-LM-100% CDR *	Rests of LM larvae grown on: 100% CDR *	587 ± 73	224 ± 8	<LOD	<LOD
REST-LM-90% WM-10% RB	Rests of LM larvae grown on: 90% WM, 10% RB	<LOD	<LOD	<LOD	<LOD
REST-LM-85% WM-15% RW	Rests of LM larvae grown on: 85% WM, 15% RW	<LOD	<LOD	<LOD	<LOD

* A small amount of chopped carrots was arbitrarily added in order to get the desired water content for optimal insect growth.

In order to better investigate the amount of mycotoxins and its distribution in the larvae and in the residual fraction, the mass balance was calculated for larvae which had been resulted positive to the presence of mycotoxins, or grown on contaminated substrates, as in the case of BSF. This calculation was performed on the basis of the concentration of contaminants found in feed, in larvae and in the respective residual fractions. The samples for which the amount of mycotoxins resulted below the LOD were considered as equal to LOD values. Results are represented in Figure 1.

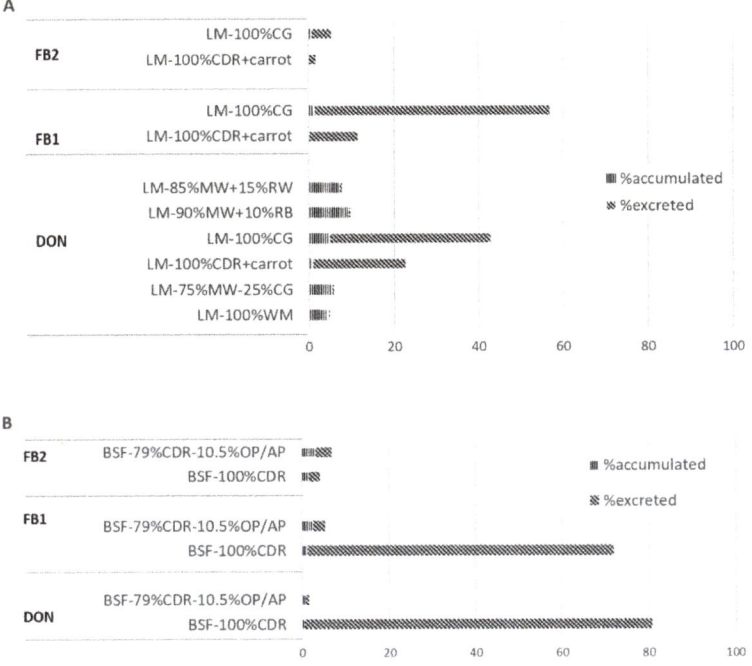

Figure 1. Mass balance of deoxynivalenol (DON), fumonisins 1 and 2 (FB1 and FB2) in Lesser Mealworm (*Alphitobius diaperinus*, LM) (**A**) and Black Soldier Fly (*Hermetia illucens*, BSF) (**B**) treatments. Abbreviations: corn distillation residues, CDR; olive pomace, OP; apple pomace, AP; wheat middlings, WM; corn gluten feed, CG; rice bran, RB; rapeseed wastes, RW.

As far as DON concerned, the mass balance ranged from 2 to 81% in BSF, while it was found to be between 1% and 43% in LM. The average mass balance of fumonisins in BSF ranged between 4% and 72%, and it was ranged from 1% to 57% in LM for FB2 and FB1 respectively. Almost the total amount of ZEN resulted excreted in BSF (data not shown in figure).

3. Discussion

This study is focused on the uptake of mycotoxins in BSF and LM larvae, grown on naturally contaminated substrates, obtained from residues of cereal and vegetable processing.

In particular, BSF were reared on two different substrates based on corn distillation residues, which had been found to be contaminated by DON, FB1 and FB2. In agreement with other studies from the literature [21], no uptake of mycotoxins in BSF larvae was observed for both trials, while DON, FB1 and FB2 were found only in the residual fractions collected from the BSF reared on 100% of pure substrate. In this case, the concentration of DON, FB1 and FB2 found in the rests were higher as compared to the concentrations detected in feed. Interestingly, ZEN, lower than LOD in the initial feed, was detected in the residual fraction at 334 ± 44 µg/kg. Since the insects were exclusively grown on the selected substrate, the occurrence of ZEN after harvesting suggested its possible cleavage from the matrix, due to a hydrolytic activity carried out by the insect. An overall increase of ZEN in BSF larvae growing substrates was already observed by Camenzuli et al. [20], although the authors measured the parent compound together with its major phase I metabolites, α- and β-ZEL.

It is well-known that *Fusarium* mycotoxins can be biotransformed by plants into phase I and phase II metabolites, being the glycosylation the most common pathway [16]. Conjugates mycotoxins can be however cleaved by microbial enzymes, as reported by several authors [16,23,24]. Although a hydrolytic activity in insects towards modified mycotoxins has never been described so far, it cannot be ruled out and can be a possible explanation for the observed data.

In addition, it is known that *Fusarium* mycotoxins are often associated to the matrix, and this binding strongly affect the extractability [25,26]. Therefore, taking into consideration the increase of mycotoxins from starting materials to post-growing residues, it can be argued that BSF larvae may induce the substrate degradation upon growing, thus increasing the overall extractability of mycotoxins.

In contrast with BSF larvae, DON was found in LM larvae grown on contaminated substrates, mainly in those containing wheat middlings in combination with corn gluten. When 100% corn gluten was used as growing substrate, DON, FB1 but not ZEN were transferred to LM larvae.

The lack of ZEN uptake in Lesser Mealworm is in agreement with the literature [19], while the possible transferal of DON and FB1 in LM larvae grown on naturally incurred substrates, was observed in this study for the first time.

In case of LM residual fractions, the overall mass balance never exceeded 60%, clearly indicating that mycotoxins are partially metabolised by the larvae to unknown compounds, in agreement with the literature [19,20]. It should be noticed that the occurrence of DON in residual fractions was lower than the one reported in previous studies performed on Yellow mealworm larvae under similar conditions [18]. However, uptake, biotransformation and excretion of mycotoxins in insects could be affected by a range of factors, among them the substrate, the species, and the dose, as well as the use of naturally incurred or spiked growing material [20].

Different from other studies, in which larvae were grown on a substrate artificially contaminated by mycotoxins, at higher concentrations than those found in the substrate samples considered in this study [18–20], the present work clearly demonstrated that DON and FB1 can be found in LM (but not in BSF) larvae. The amount of mycotoxins anyway never exceeds the starting levels, indicating that there is no active uptake in insects, and there is rather a degradation or an excretion.

In addition, the mass balance calculation clearly indicated that biotransformation is rather the operating mechanism instead of simple excretion. Further experiments will be needed in order to investigate the mycotoxin biotransformation pattern in insects.

4. Conclusions

The present study reported on the possible uptake and/or excretion of mycotoxins in two insect species, LM and BSF, reared on naturally contaminated substrates. As feed, organic side streams recovered from cereal and vegetable processing were considered under a circular economy perspective.

Collected data clearly indicated that transfer from the waste to the insect of mycotoxins is possible, but without uptake into insects, and rather with an overall decrease of their amount. LM larvae were found able to transfer DON and FB in low amounts from naturally incurred growing substrates. Data were consistent with the possible biotransformation of mycotoxins in unknown metabolites in insects. ZEN was detected in BSF residual fractions but not in starting materials, suggesting a possible hydrolytic activity carried out by larvae upon growing.

Taken all together, our results proved the urgency of better deciphering the ability of insects to uptake, transform, and excrete mycotoxins, in view of a safer use of insects as an alternative protein source.

5. Materials and Methods

5.1. Chemicals

Mycotoxin standard solutions of aflatoxins B1, B2, G1 and G2, fumonisin B1 and B2, A and B trichothecenes (nivalenol, deoxynivalenol, 3-acetyl-deoxynivalenol, fusarenone X, diacetoxyscirpenol, T-2 toxin, HT-2 toxin), zearalenone, ochratoxin A, and patulin were obtained from Romer Labs (Tulln, Austria). All the solvents applied for both the extraction and analysis steps, methanol, acetonitrile formic acid and acetic acid, were HPLC-grade and were purchased from Sigma-Aldrich (Milan, Italy), while Bi-distilled water was produced in-house by using a Milli-Q System (Millipore, Bedford, MA, USA). Salts used for extraction as for the preparation of the eluents as sodium chloride and ammonium acetate were obtained from Sigma-Aldrich (Milan, Italy).

5.2. Insect Treatments and Sampling

For the experiments described herein, two insect species were selected: *Alphitobius diaperinus* (Lesser Mealworm, LM) and *Hermetia illucens* (Black Soldier Fly, BSF). The larvae were grown on different substrates prepared using different feed materials, prevalently coming from the processing of cereals (wheat, corn, rice and rapeseed) and vegetable (apple and olive), as indicated in Table 1. The choice of these substrates was driven by the seasonality, the availability and the cost of different by-products of agriculture sector. The substrates were analysed previously for mycotoxins presence, then also larvae were extracted and analysed using the same protocol applied for feed samples. Moreover, rests of insects grown on substrates resulted positive to the presence of mycotoxins were also collected and analysed.

Insects were grown on naturally contaminated feed, and in particular 2 substrates were used for BSF cultivation, while 13 different feeds were prepared for LM production (Table 2). The insects rearing was conducted as indicated in a previous work by Leni et al. [27]. Briefly, BSF eggs were initially placed in a specific incubator at 28 °C for 2 days, then the eggs were transferred in the rearing bins and the new-born larvae treated for 2 days with a started feed composed of chicken feed, the feed materials selected for the experiment and water, with a total dry matter of about 30%. During this time the temperature was set at 28–32 °C and humidity at 60% minimum. After that, the growth substrate was removed and substituted with that selected for the experiment, provided ad libitum. The larvae were reared under these conditions for 15 days. After this period, larvae were removed and quantified, and samples of remaining fractions were also collected as listed in Table 3. Similarly, LM larvae were reared utilizing the selected feed materials chosen for the experiments, under the same controlled conditions of temperature and humidity used for BSF growth, providing feed daily ad libitum. In this case, larvae were harvested for 28 days and then collected. As for BSF, also samples of remaining fractions were recovered and weighted.

Larvae of BSF and LM were killed at −18 °C and stored at the same temperature before each analysis. At the same time, samples of growth substrates and remaining fraction were stored at −18 °C until analyses.

5.3. Mycotoxins Extraction and Purification

Mycotoxins class is represented by several organic compounds with different chemical and physical properties. For this reason, we decided to apply different extraction protocols, selected for a specific class of toxins. In addition, all the samples of insect larvae and samples of remaining fractions were subjected to a lyophilisation process (Freeze dryer Lio-5P, 5Pascal, Milano, Italy) for 48 h and milled using a laboratory miller. The dried powders obtained from these steps were stored at −20 °C until extraction and analysis.

For the extraction of aflatoxins, 1g of sample added with 0.2 g of NaCl was extracted using 4 mL of a mixture of methanol/bi-distilled water, 80/20 *v/v* on a shaker at room temperature, at 200 strokes/min for 90 min. After that, the extract was centrifuged at 10,621× *g*, at 25 °C for 10 min. 1 mL of the supernatant was transferred in a tube, diluted with 4 mL of bi-distilled water and submitted to a purification step using immuno-affinity columns (VICAM, Afla Test®, mycotoxin testing system; VICAM, Milford, MA, USA). The cartridges were conditioned with 10 mL of bi-distilled water and subsequently with 10 mL of pure methanol. The diluted extract was then eluted through the column and, after the elution, a washing step with 10 mL of bi-distilled water was performed. The analytes were recovered with 1 mL of pure methanol. The purified sample was dried under a gently nitrogen flow, suspended in 1 mL of bi-distilled water/methanol, 80/20 *v/v*, and analysed by HPLC-FLD technique.

The contemporary extraction of fumonisins, ochratoxin A, zearalenone, patulin and A and B trichothecenes was performed on the basis of different protocols with slight modifications [28,29]. Briefly, 1 g of sample was extracted adding 4 mL of a solution composed of bi-distilled water/acetonitrile/methanol 50/25/25 v/v. The sample was positioned on a shaker at room temperature, at 200 strokes/min for 90 min. After that, the extracts were centrifuged at $10,621\times g$, for 10 min at 25 °C. 1 mL of the supernatant was collected and dried under a gently nitrogen flow. The residue was then dissolved in 1 mL of bi-distilled water/methanol 80/20 v/v. The samples were then subjected to UHPLC-MS/MS analyses.

5.4. Mycotoxins Analysis

Aflatoxins B1, B2, G1 and G2 were analysed on a HPLC Waters Alliance 2695 separation module, coupled with a FLD detector (Waters, Multi λ Fluorescence detector 2475) and an UV detector (Waters, Dual λ Absorbance Detector 2489) (Waters, Milford, MA, USA). The analytes separation was achieved on a C18-RP XTerra (Waters, Milford, MA, USA; 250 × 2.1 mm, i.d. 5 mm) column using as eluents bi-distilled water (A) and methanol (B), in isocratic conditions (65% A and 35% B). The flow was set at 0.25 mL/min and the column oven temperature was kept at 30 °C. A volume of 10 µL was injected. For the detection of aflatoxins, the UV detector was set at $\lambda = 365$ nm, while for the FLD $\lambda = 365$ nm and $\lambda = 425$ nm were chosen as the typical wavelength of absorbance and of emission, respectively.

For the quantitative determination of aflatoxins, a calibration curve was prepared starting from the commercial standard which contained AFB1 and AFG1 at the concentration of 2 mg/kg and AFB2 and AFG2 at the concentration of 0.5 mg/kg. Starting from this solution, 5 different dilutions in pure methanol were performed obtaining AFB1 and AFG1 at 0.5, 0.75, 1, 1.5 and 2 µg/kg, while for AFB2 and AFG2 concentrations of 0.125, 0.187, 0.25, 0.375 and 0.5 µg/kg, obtaining a good linearity ($R^2 > 0.99$) for the both calibration ranges.

Fumonisins B1 and B2, ochratoxin A, zearalenone, patulin and A and B trichothecenes (nivalenol, deoxynivalenol, 3-acetyl-deoxinivalenol, fusarenone X, T2 toxin, HT2 toxin and deacetoxyscirpenol) were determined on an UHPLC–MS/MS apparatus consisted of an UHPLC Ultimate 3000 separation module (Dionex, Sunnyvale, CA, USA), coupled with a TSQ Vantage triple quadrupole (Thermo Fisher, Waltham, MA, USA) equipped with an ESI interface. The separation of the analytes was achieved on a RP-C18 EVO Kinetex column (2.6 µ, 100A; 100 × 2.10 mm) from Phenomenex (Torrance, CA, USA). Ammonium acetate 5 mM in bi-distilled water and methanol were used as eluent A and B respectively, both acidified with the 0.2% of acetic acid. A gradient was applied as follows: the elution started with 2% of B and these conditions were maintained for 1 min, then at 2 min the percentage of B was increased at 20% and kept for 6 min, at 17 min the column was flashed with the 90% of B for 3 min, then in 1 min the initial conditions were re-established and the column was re-equilibrated for 9 min, with a total run time of 30 min. During the analyses the column temperature was maintained at 40 °C while samples were maintained at 20 °C. The flow was 0.35 mL/min and for each sample 4 µL were injected into the system.

PAT, NIV, DON, 3ADON, FUSX, and ZEN were monitored in negative ion mode with a spray voltage of 3500 V, a capillary temperature of 270 °C, a vaporizer temperature of 200 °C, a sheath gas flow of 50 units and an auxiliary gas flow of 5 units. T2, HT2 toxins, DAS, FB1, FB2, and OTA were monitored applying a positive ionization mode, with the following parameters: spray voltage of 3000 V, a capillary temperature of 270 °C, a vaporizer temperature of 200 °C, a sheath gas flow of 50 units and an auxiliary gas flow of 5 units. All the other parameters as S-Lens RF amplitude values were obtained and set by tuning methanolic solutions of each considered molecule (1 mg/kg).

Detection of all the considered analytes was performed in SRM modality (Single Reaction Monitoring) monitoring the characteristic transitions for each considered mycotoxin (Table 4).

Table 4. Characteristic transitions monitored for the target mycotoxins: fumonisins B1 and B2 (FB1, FB2), ochratoxin A (OTA), zearalenone (ZEN), patulin (PAT) and A and B trichothecenes (nivalenol (NIV), deoxynivalenol (DON), 3-acetyl-deoxinivalenol (3ADON), fusarnone X (FUSX), T2 toxin, HT2 toxin and deacetoxyscirpenol (DAS)).

Compound	Ionization Mode	Precursor Ion (m/z)	Product Ions (m/z)	Collision Energy (V)	LOD (µg/kg)
PAT	Negative	152.9 [M − H]⁻	109/81	−12/−12	100
NIV	Negative	371.1 [M + CH3COO]⁻	311.1/281.1/59.1	−10/−32/−48	10
DON	Negative	355.1 [M + CH3COO]⁻	295.1/265.1	−13/−16	10
3ADON	Negative	397.1 [M + CH3COO]⁻	307.1/59	−18/−20	20
FUSX	Negative	413.3 [M + CH3COO]⁻	353.6/262.9/59.1	−14/−22/−10	20
OTA	Positive	404.5 [M + H]⁺	238.7/220.7/101.7	21/31/68	20
FB1	Positive	722.3 [M + H]⁺	704.7/352.1/334.1	26/35/38	25
FB2	Positive	706.5 [M + H]⁺	688.4/336.3	51/51	25
DAS	Positive	384.2 [M + NH4]⁺	307.2/105.1	17/61	10
T2	Positive	484.3 [M + NH4]⁺	215.0/185.0	19/22	10
HT2	Positive	442.0 [M + NH4]⁺	263.1	11	10
ZEN	Negative	317.0 [M − H]⁻	175.0/131.0	−26/−32	10

In order to quantify these mycotoxins, a calibration curve containing all the considered analytes was prepared starting from the commercial standard. For this purpose, 6 different dilutions were prepared considering the following concentrations: 50, 100, 200, 500, 750 and 1000 µg/kg, obtaining a good linearity ($R^2 > 0.99$) for the calibration range.

5.5. Mass Balance Calculation

The mass balance was calculated as described by Camenzuli et al. [20] on the basis of the amount of substrates used for insects' growth, the amount of harvested larvae and of the residual fractions (frass). Furthermore, the accumulated, extracted and potential metabolized mycotoxins were calculated as follow:

$$\% \text{ accumulated mycotoxin} = \frac{\text{amount of harvested insects} \times \text{concentration mycotoxin detected in insects}}{\text{amount of substrates} \times \text{concentration mycotoxin detected in substrates}} \times 100,$$

$$\% \text{ excreted mycotoxin} = \frac{\text{amount of frass} \times \text{concentration mycotoxin detected in frass}}{\text{amount of substrates} \times \text{concentration mycotoxin detected in substrates}} \times 100,$$

$$\% \text{ metabolyzed mycotoxin} = 100 - \% \text{ excreted mycotoxin} - \% \text{ accumulated mycotoxin}.$$

Metabolized mycotoxins were referred to the undetected compounds which could be metabolized in different structures not yet identified. All the measurements of mycotoxin below the LOD were considered as equal to LOD values.

Author Contributions: Conceptualization, S.S.; Data curation, G.L. and M.C.; Formal analysis, G.L. and M.C.; Methodology, M.C., J.J., S.D. and N.G.; Supervision, C.D.; Writing–original draft, G.L., M.C., S.S. and C.D.

Funding: This project received funding from the Bio Based Industries Joint Undertaking under the European Union's Horizon 2020 research and innovation programme under grant agreement No. 720715 (InDIRECT project).

Conflicts of Interest: The authors declare no conflict of interest.

References

1. Food Wastage Footprint: Impacts on Natural Resources (Summary Report). Available online: http://www.fao.org/3/i3347e/i3347e.pdf (accessed on 18 August 2019).
2. Veldkamp, T.; Van Duinkerken, G.; Van Huis, A.; Lakemond, C.M.M.; Ottevanger, E.; Bosch, G.; Van Boekel, M.A.J.S. *Insects as a Sustainable Feed Ingredient in Pig and Poultry Diets—A Feasibility Study*; Wageningen University Livestock Research: Wageningen, The Netherlands, 2012.
3. Van Huis, A.; Oonincx, D.G.A.B. The environmental sustainability of insects as food and feed. A review. *Agron. Sustain. Dev.* **2017**, *37*, 43. [CrossRef]

4. Charlton, A.J.; Dickinson, M.; Wakefield, M.E.; Fitches, E.; Kenis, M.; Han, R.; Zhu, F.; Kone, N.; Grant, M.; Devic, E.; et al. Exploring the chemical safety of fly larvae as a source of protein for animal feed. *J. Insects Food Feed* **2015**, *1*, 7–16. [CrossRef]
5. Rumpold, B.A.; Schlüter, O.K. Potential and challenges of insects as an innovative source for food and feed production. *Innov. Food Sci. Emerg. Technol.* **2013**, *17*, 1–11. [CrossRef]
6. REGULATION (EU) 2015/2283 OF THE EUROPEAN PARLIAMENT AND OF THE COUNCIL of 25 November 2015 on Novel Foods, Amending Regulation (EU) No. 1169/2011 of the European Parliament and of the Council and Repealing Regulation (EC) No. 258/97 of the European Parliament and of the Council and Commission Regulation (EC) No. 1852/2001. Available online: www.eur-lex.europa.eu/legal-content/en/TXT/?uri=CELEX%3A32015R2283 (accessed on 10 June 2019).
7. Van Raamsdonk, L.W.D.; van der Fels-Klerx, H.J.; de Jong, J. New feed ingredients: the insect opportunity. *Food Addit. Contam. Part A* **2017**, *34*, 1384–1397. [CrossRef] [PubMed]
8. COMMISSION REGULATION (EU) 2017/893 of 24 May 2017 Amending Annexes I and IV to Regulation (EC) No. 999/2001 of the European Parliament and of the Council and Annexes X, XIV and XV to Commission Regulation (EU) No. 142/2011 as Regards the Provisions on Processed Animal Protein. Available online: https://eur-lex.europa.eu/legal-content/EN/TXT/?uri=CELEX%3A32017R0893 (accessed on 10 June 2019).
9. REGULATION (EC) No. 999/2001 OF THE EUROPEAN PARLIAMENT AND OF THE COUNCIL of 22 May 2001 Laying down Rules for the Prevention, Control and Eradication of Certain Transmissible Spongiform Encephalopathies. Available online: www.eur-lex.europa.eu/legal-content/EN/ALL/?uri=CELEX%3A32001R0999 (accessed on 10 June 2019).
10. EFSA Scientific Committee. Scientific Opinion on a Risk Profile Related to Production and Consumption of Insects as Food and Feed. Available online: www.efsa.europa.eu/it/efsajournal/pub/4257 (accessed on 10 June 2019).
11. European Commission (EC). Council Directive (EC) 2002/32/ EC of 7 May 2002 on Undesirable Substances in Animal Feed. *Off. J. Eur. Union* **2002**, *L140*, 10–21. Available online: www.eur-lex.europa.eu/legal-content/en/ALL/?uri=CELEX:32002L0032 (accessed on 10 June 2019).
12. COMMISSION RECOMMENDATION 2006/576/EC of 17 August 2006 on the Presence of Deoxynivalenol, Zearalenone, Ochratoxin A, T-2 and HT-2 and Fumonisins in Products Intended for Animal Feeding. *Off. J. Eur. Union* **2019**, *L229*, 7–9. Available online: www.eur-lex.europa.eu/LexUriServ/LexUriServ.do?uri=OJ:L:2006:229:0007:0009:EN:PDF (accessed on 10 June 2019).
13. Hussein, H.S.; Brasel, J.M. Toxicity, metabolism, and impact of mycotoxins on humans and animals. *Toxicology* **2001**, *167*, 101–134. [CrossRef]
14. Steinkellner, H.; Binaglia, M.; Dall'Asta, C.; Gutleb, A.C.; Metzler, M.; Oswald, I.P.; Parent-Massin, D.; Alexander, J. Combined hazard assessment of mycotoxins and their modified forms applying relative potency factors: Zearalenone and T2/HT2 toxin. *Food Chem. Toxicol.* **2019**, *131*, 110599. [CrossRef]
15. Binder, E.M.; Tan, L.M.; Chin, L.J.; Handl, J.; Richard, J. Worldwide occurrence of mycotoxins in commodities, feeds and feed ingredients. *Anim. Feed Sci. Tech.* **2007**, *137*, 265–282. [CrossRef]
16. Berthiller, F.; Krska, R.; Domig, K.J.; Kneifel, W.; Juge, N.; Schuhmacher, R.; Adam, G. Hydrolytic fate of deoxynivalenol-3-glucoside during digestion. *Toxicol. Lett.* **2011**, *206*, 264–267. [CrossRef]
17. De Zutter, N.; Audenaert, K.; Arroyo-Manzanares, N.; De Boevre, M.; Van Poucke, C.; De Saeger, S.; Haesaert, G.; Smagghe, G. Aphids transform and detoxify the mycotoxin deoxynivalenol via a type II biotransformation mechanism yet unknown in animals. *Sci. Rep.* **2016**, *6*, 38640. [CrossRef]
18. Van Broekhoven, S.; Gutierrez, J.M.; De Rijk, T.C.; De Nijs, W.C.M.; Van Loon, J.J.A. Degradation and excretion of the Fusarium toxin deoxynivalenol by an edible insect, the Yellow mealworm (*Tenebrio molitor* L.). *World Mycotoxin J.* **2017**, *10*, 163–169. [CrossRef]
19. Niermans, K.; Woyzichovski, J.; Kröncke, N.; Benning, R.; Maul, R. Feeding study for the mycotoxin zearalenone in yellow mealworm (*Tenebrio molitor*) larvae—Investigation of biological impact and metabolic conversion. *Mycotoxin Res.* **2019**, *35*, 231–242. [CrossRef]
20. Camenzuli, L.; Van Dam, R.; de Rijk, T.; Andriessen, R.; Van Schelt, J.; Van der Fels-Klerx, H.J. Tolerance and Excretion of the Mycotoxins Aflatoxin B1, Zearalenone, Deoxynivalenol, and Ochratoxin A by *Alphitobius diaperinus* and *Hermetia illucens* from contaminated substrates. *Toxins* **2018**, *10*, 91. [CrossRef]

21. Purschke, B.; Scheibelberger, R.; Axmann, S.; Adler, A.; Jäger, H. Impact of substrate contamination with mycotoxins, heavy metals and pesticides on the growth performance and composition of black soldier fly larvae (*Hermetia illucens*) for use in the feed and food value chain. *Food Addit. Contam. Part A.* **2017**, *34*, 1410–1420. [CrossRef]
22. Sanabria, C.O.; Hogan, N.; Madder, K.; Gillott, C.; Blakley, B.; Reaney, M.; Beattie, A.; Buchanan, F. Yellow Mealworm Larvae (*Tenebrio molitor*) Fed Mycotoxin-Contaminated Wheat—A Possible Safe, Sustainable Protein Source for Animal Feed? *Toxins* **2019**, *11*, 282. [CrossRef]
23. Dall'Erta, A.; Cirlini, M.; Dall'Asta, M.; Del Rio, D.; Galaverna, G.; Dall'Asta, G. Masked Mycotoxins Are Efficiently Hydrolyzed by Human Colonic Microbiota Releasing Their Aglycones. *Chem. Res. Toxicol.* **2013**, *26*, 305–312. [CrossRef]
24. Gratz, S.W.; Dinesh, R.; Yoshinari, T.; Holtrop, G.; Richardson, A.J.; Duncan, G.; MacDonald, G.; Lloyd, A.; Tarbin, J. Masked trichothecene and zearalenone mycotoxins withstand digestion and absorption in the upper GI tract but are efficiently hydrolyzed by human gut microbiota in vitro. *Mol. Nutr. Food Res.* **2017**, *61*, 1600680. [CrossRef]
25. Rychlik, M.; Humpf, H.U.; Marko, D.; Dänicke, S.; Mally, A.; Berthiller, F.; Klaffke, H.; Lorenz, N. Proposal of a comprehensive definition of modified and other forms of mycotoxins including "masked" mycotoxins. *Mycotoxin Res.* **2014**, *30*, 197–205. [CrossRef]
26. Damiani, T.; Righetti, L.; Suman, M.; Galaverna, G.; Dall'Asta, C. Analytical issue related to fumonisins: A matter of sample comminution? *Food Control.* **2019**, *95*, 1–5. [CrossRef]
27. Leni, G.; Soetemans, L.; Jacobs, J.; Depraetere, S.; Gianotten, N.; Bastiaens, L.; Caligiani, A.; Sforza, S. Protein hydrolysates from *Alphitobius diaperinus* and *Hermetia illucens* larvae treated with commercial proteases. *Food Res. Int.* **2019**, under review.
28. Sulyok, M.; Berthiller, F.; Krska, R.; Schuhmacher, R. Development and validation of a liquid chromatography/tandem mass spectrometric method for the determination of 39 mycotoxins in wheat and maize. *Rapid Commun. Mass Spectrom.* **2006**, *20*, 2649–2659. [CrossRef]
29. Dall'Asta, C.; Galaverna, G.; Aureli, G.; Dossena, A.; Marchelli, R. LC/MS/MS method for the simultaneous quantification of free and masked fumonisins in maize and maize-based products. *World Mycotoxin J.* **2008**, *1*, 237–246. [CrossRef]

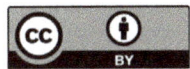

© 2019 by the authors. Licensee MDPI, Basel, Switzerland. This article is an open access article distributed under the terms and conditions of the Creative Commons Attribution (CC BY) license (http://creativecommons.org/licenses/by/4.0/).

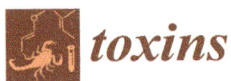

Article

Target Analysis and Retrospective Screening of Multiple Mycotoxins in Pet Food Using UHPLC-Q-Orbitrap HRMS

Luigi Castaldo [1,2], Giulia Graziani [1], Anna Gaspari [1], Luana Izzo [1], Josefa Tolosa [3], Yelko Rodríguez-Carrasco [3,*] and Alberto Ritieni [1]

1. Department of Pharmacy, Faculty of Pharmacy, University of Naples "Federico II", Via Domenico Montesano 49, 80131 Naples, Italy
2. Department of Clinical Medicine and Surgery, University of Naples "Federico II", Via S. Pansini 5, 80131 Naples, Italy
3. Laboratory of Food Chemistry and Toxicology, Faculty of Pharmacy, University of Valencia, Av. Vicent Andrés Estellés s/n, Burjassot, València 46100, Spain
* Correspondence: yelko.rodriguez@uv.es; Tel.: +34-96-354-4117; Fax: +34-96-354-4954

Received: 18 June 2019; Accepted: 22 July 2019; Published: 24 July 2019

Abstract: A comprehensive strategy combining a quantitative method for 28 mycotoxins and a post-target screening for other 245 fungal and bacterial metabolites in dry pet food samples were developed using an acetonitrile-based extraction and an ultrahigh-performance liquid chromatography coupled to high-resolution mass spectrometry (UHPLC-Q-Orbitrap HRMS) method. The proposed method showed satisfactory validation results according to Commission Decision 2002/657/EC. Average recoveries from 72 to 108% were obtained for all studied mycotoxins, and the intra-/inter-day precision were below 9 and 14%, respectively. Results showed mycotoxin contamination in 99% of pet food samples (n = 89) at concentrations of up to hundreds µg/kg, with emerging *Fusarium* mycotoxins being the most commonly detected mycotoxins. All positive samples showed co-occurrence of mycotoxins with the simultaneous presence of up to 16 analytes per sample. In the retrospective screening, up to 54 fungal metabolites were tentatively identified being cyclopiazonic acid, paspalitrem A, fusaric acid, and macrosporin, the most commonly detected analytes.

Keywords: mycotoxins; monitoring; pet food; HRMS-orbitrap; co-occurrence; retrospective screening

Key Contribution: The manuscript contributes to the understanding of a wide range of mycotoxins including emerging *Fusarium* toxins in pet food samples from Italy by using the capability provided by the UHPLC-Q-Orbitrap HRMS technology.

---

1. Introduction

Mycotoxins are a group of toxic secondary metabolites produced by fungi mainly belonging to *Aspergillus, Penicillium, Fusarium,* and *Alternaria* genera [1]. Due to the great structural diversity of these toxic compounds, they display a wide range of deleterious effects, including carcinogenic, hepatotoxic, nephrotoxic, teratogenic, heamatotoxic, immunotoxic, and hormonal or reproductive effects [2,3]. Mycotoxins pose a challenge to food safety as they are unavoidable and unpredictable contaminants in crops. In fact, the Food and Agriculture Organization (FAO) estimated that over one-quarter of the world's food crop are contaminated with mycotoxins [4]. The mycotoxins with greatest agro-economic and health impact are aflatoxins (AFs), ochratoxin A (OTA), zearalenone (ZEN), fumonisins (FBs), and trichothecenes [5]. In the last decade, attention to the risk posed to human and animal health has also been extended to the so-called emerging *Fusarium* mycotoxins (including enniatins (ENNs) and beauvericin (BEA)) as well as the *Alternaria* toxins [6]. The factors affecting molds growth and/or mycotoxin production, and thus contamination of raw materials and feed, are associated with yield conditions (i.e., temperature, humidity, insect damage). Moreover, in post harvesting, other factors, such as moisture and storage conditions, could contribute to increasing risk of mycotoxin production [7].

Food crops susceptible to mycotoxin contamination include corn, wheat, barley, rye, rice, nuts, dried fruit, vegetables, and their derivatives [8]. It is remarkable that cereals and cereal by-products that are often unfit for human consumption are frequently used in feed formulations and act as excellent substrates for the fungal proliferation and production of mycotoxins. Recent surveys indicate that 70% of raw materials are contaminated with these toxins [9,10]. On the other hand, cereal processing, including dry milling, affects mycotoxin occurrence, especially for the fractions commonly designed for animal feeding [11,12]. Consequently, animal exposure to mycotoxins via plant-derived foods is of important consideration [13–16].

To limit the exposure to mycotoxins, the European Commission (EC) has set maximum limits of undesirable substances in both foodstuffs (EC/1881/2006 and amendments) and feedstuffs (2003/100/EC). As far as mycotoxins in feedstuffs are concerned, the Commission Directive 2003/100/EC has only established maximum admissible content of AFB1 in complete feedstuffs at 20 µg/kg. As regards the other mycotoxins, the European Union established in the Commission Decision 2006/576/EC guidance values regarding presence of deoxynivalenol (DON), ZEN, FBs, and OTA in products used as animal feeding (Table 1).

In the last decades, improvement of analytical methods for the detection of mycotoxins at low ng/g range in a wide variety of foodstuffs has been performed [17]. Mass spectrometry-based techniques, such as MS and MS/MS, in combination with gas chromatography (GC) or liquid chromatography (LC) allowed the development of multi-mycotoxins methodologies [18]. Over recent years, there have been improvements in the LC-technique with the development of ultra-high-performance liquid chromatography (UHPLC), leading to higher peak efficiency and shorter chromatography run time [19]. In addition, the use of high-resolution mass spectrometry (HRMS), such as Orbitrap mass analyzers, is growing up in the ambit of food toxicology. HRMS analyzers have good specificity and high resolution due to mass accuracy provided by the resolution of Q-Orbitrap detectors combined with structural information obtained in MS/MS mode [20]. This technique enable the identification of untarget compounds and retrospective data analysis without the need to re-run samples.

Even though investigations on mycotoxin distribution in feedstuffs are regularly conducted by competent authorities, the information on mycotoxin distribution of feedstuffs is limited [21]. Among the available studies focused on mycotoxins occurrence in feedstuffs, most of them have been performed in feed aimed to livestock production, whereas scarce literature have reported the occurrence of these toxic compounds in pet foods [22–25]. Therefore, the development and validation of analytical strategies to evaluate the occurrence of traditional and emerging mycotoxins in pet food to guarantee their quality, as well as to comply with trade requirements, are needed. Hence, the aim of this work was to develop an analytical tool based on a UHPLC-Q-Orbitrap HRMS method that combines quantitative target analysis for detection, quantification, and reliable identification of 28 mycotoxins from different fungi genera in pet food, with post-target screening (identification) of other 245 fungal and bacterial metabolites based on a comprehensive spectral library. In addition, the proposed methodology was applied to 89 dry commercially available pet food samples acquired from pet shops located in Campania region, Southern Italy.

Table 1. Regulated and recommended maximum levels of mycotoxins in feed materials set by the European Commission.

Mycotoxin	Products	[a] Regulated Maximum Level (mg/kg) Relative to a Feedingstuff	[b] Guidance Value (mg/kg) Relative to a Feedingstuff	[c] Guidance Value in mg/kg (ppm) Relative to a Feedingstuff with a Moisture Content of 12 %
AFB1	All feed materials; complete feedingstuffs for pigs and poultry (except young animals); complementary feedingstuffs for cattle, sheep and goats (except complementary feedingstuffs for dairy animals, calves and lambs); complementary feedingstuffs for pigs and poultry (except young animals); complete feedingstuffs for cattle, sheep and goats with the exception of:	0.02		
	complete feedingstuffs for dairy animals	0.005		
	complete feedingstuffs for calves and lambs	0.01		
DON	Maize by-products		12	
	Other cereals and cereal products		8	
	Complementary and complete feedingstuffs with the exception of:		5	
	complementary and complete feedingstuffs for pigs		0.9	
	complementary and complete feedingstuffs for calves (<4 months), lambs and kids		2	
ZEN	Maize by-products		2	
	Other cereals and cereal products		3	
	Complementary and complete feedingstuffs for piglets and young sows		0.1	
	Complementary and complete feedingstuffs for sows and fattening pigs		0.25	
	Complementary and complete feedingstuffs for calves, dairy cattle, sheep and goats		0.50	
OTA	Cereals and cereal products		0.25	
	Complementary and complete feedingstuffs for pigs		0.05	
	Complementary and complete feedingstuffs for poultry		0.1	
FBs	Maize and maize products		60	
	Complementary and complete feedingstuffs for pigs, horses, rabbits and pet animals		5	
	Complementary and complete feedingstuffs for fish		10	
	Complementary and complete feedingstuffs for poultry, calves (<4 months), lambs and kids		20	
	Complementary and complete feedingstuffs for adult ruminants (>4 months) and mink		50	
T-2 + HT-2 toxin	Compound feed for cats			0.05

[a] Directive Commission 2003/100/EC; [b] Recommendation Commission 2006/576/EC; [c] Commission Recommendation 2013/637/EU; Abbreviations: AFB1: aflatoxin B1; DON: deoxynivalenol; ZEN: zearalenone; OTA: ochratoxin A; FBs: fumonisins (FB1 and FB2).

2. Results and Discussion

2.1. Optimization of the Ultrahigh-Performance Liquid Chromatography Coupled to High-Resolution Mass-Spectrometry (UHPLC-Q-Orbitrap HRMS) Analysis

The optimization of the Q-Orbitrap HRMS parameters was performed via direct infusion of each mycotoxin standard ($n = 28$) diluted at 1 µg/mL into the Q-Orbitrap system using a flow rate of 8 µL/min. According to the literature, the addition of formic acid-ammonium formate shows better ionization efficiency of the studied analytes than acetic acid-ammonium acetate, and thus these additives were added to the mobile phases [26]. The most intense and signal stable adducts were selected for each analyte. Precursor ions were subjected to different values of collision energies (between 10 and 60 eV) to perform their fragmentation. Table 2 shows the UHPLC-HRMS parameters for the determination of mycotoxins included in this study.

On the other hand, three gradient programs were tested to achieve a good separation of the 28 mycotoxins:

(i) Gradient 1: started with 20% B, kept up to 1 min, and then increased to 95% B in 1 min, followed by a hold-time of 0.5 min at 95% B. Afterward, the gradient switched back to 75% in 2.5 min, and decreased again reaching 60% B in 1 min. The gradient returned in 0.5 min at 20%, and 1.5 min column re-equilibration at 20%;

(ii) Gradient 2: started with 10% B, kept up to 1 min, and then increased to 95% B in 1 min, followed by a hold-time of 0.5 min at 95% B. Afterward, the gradient switched back to 75% in 2.5 min, and decreased again reaching 60% B in 1 min. The gradient returned in 0.5 min at 10%, and 1.5 min column re-equilibration at 10%;

(iii) Gradient 3: started with 0% B, kept up to 1 min, and then increased to 95% B in 1 min, followed by a hold-time of 0.5 min at 95% B. Afterward, the gradient switched back to 75% in 2.5 min, and decreased again reaching 60% B in 1 min. The gradient returned in 0.5 min at 0%, and 1.5 min column re-equilibration at 0%.

The results showed that several peaks eluted within the column dead time when starting the gradient program with high organic phase (20%, gradient 1) and the peak response was irregular. The second tested gradient (initial phase B set at 10%) decreased the number of analytes non-retained in the chromatographic column but still DON and its acetylated forms eluted within the first 1.0 min. The chromatographic separation of analytes was performed with a Luna Omega Polar C18 column. Optimal results in terms of retention time and good peak shape were achieved when the initial phase B was at 0%, obtaining good separation of the 28 mycotoxins in a total run time of 8 min (Table 2).

2.2. Optimization of Sample Preparation Procedure

Sample preparation has been recognized as a critical step in the chemical analysis workflow [27]. Few multi-mycotoxin methods have been reported in literature regarding pet food samples and most of them were performed with immunoaffinity column assays, increasing the cost of the method significantly [23,25,28]. Recently, a relatively cheap acetonitrile-based extraction was proposed in literature to determine seven *Fusarium* toxins in laboratory rat feed [11]. In this work, the sample preparation protocol reported by those authors was adopted as a starting point and slightly modified to extend it for the simultaneous determination of up to 28 target mycotoxins from different genera, including *Aspergillus, Penicillium, Fusarium,* and *Alternaria*. Critical extraction parameters were evaluated namely stirring time, sonication treatment, clean-up, and sample amount (Supplementary Table S1). All experiments were performed in triplicate using spiked samples at 20 µg/kg.

Table 2. Ultrahigh-performance liquid chromatography coupled to high-resolution mass-spectrometry (UHPLC-HRMS) parameters for the determination of mycotoxins included in this study.

Mycotoxins	Retention Time (min)	Elemental Composition	Adduct Ion	Theoretical Mass (m/z)	Product Ion	Collision Energy (eV)
AFB1	4.64	$C_{17}H_{12}O_6$	$[M+H]^+$	313.07066	285.07489; 269.04373	36
AFB2	4.98	$C_{17}H_{14}O_6$	$[M+H]^+$	315.08631	287.09064; 259.05945	36
AFG1	4.79	$C_{17}H_{12}O_7$	$[M+H]^+$	329.06558	243.06467; 200.04640	40
AFG2	4.61	$C_{17}H_{14}O_7$	$[M+H]^+$	331.08123	313.07010; 245.08032	37
OTA	6.50	$C_{20}H_{18}NO_6Cl$	$[M+H]^+$	404.08954	358.08304; 341.05658	16
FB1	6.03	$C_{34}H_{59}NO_{15}$	$[M+H]^+$	722.39575	352.32010; 334.30963	48
FB2	6.78	$C_{34}H_{59}NO_{14}$	$[M+H]^+$	706.40083	336.32547; 318.31488	58
DON	4.18	$C_{15}H_{20}O_6$	$[M+HCOOH]^-$	341.12451	295.1189; 265.10822	−12
3-ADON	3.83	$C_{17}H_{22}O_7$	$[M+H]^+$	339.14383	231.10118; 203.10638	20
15-ADON	4.02	$C_{17}H_{22}O_7$	$[M+H]^+$	339.14383	261.11154; 137.05957	20
HT-2	5.63	$C_{22}H_{32}O_8$	$[M+NH_4]^+$	442.24354	263.12744; 215.10641	27
T-2	6.13	$C_{24}H_{34}O_9$	$[M+NH_4]^+$	484.25411	215.10603; 185.09561	23
NEO	4.32	$C_{19}H_{26}O_8$	$[M+NH_4]^+$	400.19659	305.13803; 141.0053	10
DAS	5.11	$C_{19}H_{26}O_7$	$[M+NH_4]^+$	384.20168	307.15329; 105.06977	15
FUS-X	4.28	$C_{17}H_{22}O_8$	$[M+Na]^+$	377.12073	228.16002; 175.07550	20
ZEN	6.55	$C_{18}H_{22}O_5$	$[M-H]^-$	317.13945	175.03989; 131.05008	−32
α-ZEL	4.87	$C_{18}H_{24}O_5$	$[M-H]^-$	319.15510	174.95630; 129.01947	36
β-ZEL	4.98	$C_{18}H_{24}O_5$	$[M-H]^-$	319.15510	174.95604; 160.97665	36
α-ZAL	4.81	$C_{18}H_{26}O_5$	$[M-H]^-$	321.17044	259.09497; 91.00272	29
β-ZAL	4.94	$C_{18}H_{26}O_5$	$[M-H]^-$	321.17044	259.09497; 91.00272	40
ZAN	5.00	$C_{18}H_{24}O_5$	$[M-H]^-$	319.15510	273.01187; 131.05020	35
BEA	5.77	$C_{45}H_{57}N_3O_9$	$[M+NH_4]^+$	801.44331	262.76715; 244.18239	70
ENN A	8.17	$C_{36}H_{63}N_3O_9$	$[M+NH_4]^+$	699.49026	228.15900; 210.14847	43
ENN A1	8.16	$C_{35}H_{61}N_3O_9$	$[M+NH_4]^+$	685.47461	228.15900; 210.14847	48
ENN B	7.87	$C_{33}H_{57}N_3O_9$	$[M+NH_4]^+$	657.44331	214.14320; 196.13280	50
ENN B1	8.06	$C_{34}H_{59}N_3O_9$	$[M+NH_4]^+$	671.45986	214.14343; 196.13295	48
AOH	5.88	$C_{14}H_{10}O_5$	$[M-H]^-$	257.04555	215.03490; 213.05569	−32
AME	6.82	$C_{15}H_{12}O_5$	$[M-H]^-$	271.06120	256.03751; 228.04276	−36

Abbreviations: Aflatoxins (AFB1, AFB2, AFG1 and AFG2), ochratoxin A (OTA), fumonisins (FB1 and FB2), deoxynivalenol (DON), 3-acetyl-deoxynivalenol (3-AcDON), 15-acetyl-deoxynivalenol (15-AcDON), HT-2 toxin, T-2 toxin, neosolaniol (NEO), diacetoxyscirpenol (DAS) fusarenon-X (FUS-X), zearalenone (ZEN), α-zearalenol (α-ZEL), β-zearalenol (β-ZEL), α-zearalanol (α-ZAL), β-zearalanol (β-ZAL), zearalanone (ZAN), beauvericin (BEA), enniatins (ENNA, ENNA1, ENNB and ENNB1), alternariol (AOH) and alternariol monomethyl ether (AME).

2.2.1. Stirring Time

Three stirring times (15, 30, and 60 min) were tested to evaluate the effect of agitation in the extraction of mycotoxins. Results showed that 15 min of stirring time was not enough to reach acceptable recoveries (recovery range obtained for all mycotoxins: ≤40%) and RSD values (<23%). By increasing the stirring time up to 30 min, the recoveries for the wide majority of compounds increased (from 65 to 78%) except for AFs, for which recovery values lower than 55% were obtained. On the other hand, optimal results (recovery range: 72–105%, RSD < 16%) were achieved with 60 min of stirring for all studied compounds fulfilling the requirements set at Commission Decision EC 2002/657.

2.2.2. Sonication Treatment

A sonication time of 15 min (with manual shaking every 5 min) was assayed and compared with samples in which the sonication step was not conducted. Results showed that when the sonication step was not performed, the accuracy and precision of the studied mycotoxins (recoveries ranging from 58 to 89%, RSD < 21%) were not as good as those obtained with sonicated samples (recoveries ranging from 72 to 114%, RSD < 14%); and therefore sonication treatment was included in the sample preparation procedure.

2.2.3. Clean-Up Step

In the original method, a freeze-out step was carried out (minimum 2 h) to promote the precipitation of compounds that may interfere in the analysis based on the complexity of the samples [11]. Nonetheless, it significantly increases the time of the analysis. To overcome that, a clean-up step to reduce both matrix interferences and contamination of the instrument was evaluated. The efficiency of this strategy was evaluated by comparing the accuracy and precision data of the results obtained with samples stored in a freezer (2 h) and those submitted with a clean-up. According to literature, the mixture of 300 mg $MgSO_4$ and 100 mg C18 (ratio 3:1, w/w) was selected as appropriate dispersive clean-up [16]. The results showed an improvement in accuracy and precision data due to the efficacy of the clean-up in removing interferences. Furthermore, the matrix effect was significantly minimized (range from 71 to 86%) with the addition of the clean-up, leading to an improved selectivity and robustness. In the samples in which the freezing out was conducted, impurities appeared. The usage of the clean-up step instead of freezing out made the extraction procedure faster and the extract obtained was much cleaner, as evidenced by the chromatographic response.

2.2.4. Sample Amount

Despite the significant reduction of interferences observed by the addition of a clean-up step, moderate signal suppression was obtained for most of the analyzed compounds, as specified in Section 2.2.3. To overcome that, the effect of reducing the sample amount was evaluated. Results showed that no matrix effect or slight signal suppression (≥85%) was obtained for all studied compounds when using 2 g of sample instead of 5 g, and therefore it allowed the quantification of the studied mycotoxins in pet food samples based on external calibration curves.

2.3. Method Validation

Calibration curves were prepared in triplicate at 8 concentration levels. Correlation coefficients (r^2) greater than 0.9990 were obtained for all studied analytes within the linear range from limits of quantification (LOQs) to 1000 µg/kg. No matrix effect or slight signal suppression was observed for all mycotoxins ranging from 75 to 98%. Limits of detection (LODs) obtained were between 0.06 and 0.62 µg/kg; LOQs were calculated from 0.013 and 1.25 µg/kg, being lower than those reported in recent literature (Table 3). Average recoveries were in the range 75–112% for all studied mycotoxins at the fortification levels assayed (10, 20, and 100 µg/kg). Those results highlighted that the proposed methodology is accurate enough for the quantitative determination of the target mycotoxins. Intra-day and inter-day relative standard deviations (RSDs) showed reliable repeatability (RSD < 12%) and within-laboratory repeatability (RSD < 17%) of the developed method (Supplementary Table S2). The carry-over was evaluated by injecting a blank sample after the highest calibration point. No carry-over was present since no peaks were detected in retention time zone of all studied mycotoxins. In the Quality Assurance/Quality Control (QA/QC) procedure, the spiked sample was used in each sample batch in order to assess the accuracy and precision of the proposed method. To guarantee the quality of the results, every one of QA/QC criteria had to be achieved. To provide method reliability, satisfactory recoveries (between 70% and 120%, RSD < 20%) for all samples were required. When the results did not fit the expected criteria, the extractions were repeated in order to achieve this range. After the optimization and validation procedure and during the sample analysis, none of the QA/QC samples were outside of the expected criteria in any batch of samples.

Table 3. Recent surveys reporting the occurrence of mycotoxins in pet foods samples.

Analyzed Samples (n)	Analytes Investigated	Mycotoxins	Positive Samples (%)	[a] Range or Average (µg/kg)	Detection Methods	LOQ (µg/kg)	Reference
89	28	AFB1	25.8	3.3–7.9	UHPLC-Q-Orbitrap	0.013	This work
		AFB2	5.6	1.8–16.6		0.013	
		AFG1	1.1	11.1			
		AFG2	5.6	1.7–31.6		0.125	
		OTA	2.2	1.4–1.5		1.25	
		ZEN	91.0	0.9–60.6		0.013	
		Σ α + β-ZEL	87.6	0.9–58.9		α-ZEL = 1.25; β-ZEL = 0.125	
		Σ α + β -ZAL	79.8	<LOQ		α-ZAL = 1.25; β-ZAL = 0.125	
		ZAN	n.f.	n.f.		0.125	
		DON	30.3	7.6–297.3		1.25	
		Σ 3 + 15 AcDON	5.6	10.9–63.2		3-AcDON = 1.25; 15-AcDON = 1.25	
		NEO	n.f.	n.f.		0.188	
		HT2	32.6	3.3–110.1		1.25	
		T2	47.2	0.7–9.0		0.125	
		BEA	86.5	0.8–176.1		0.013	
		ENNA	10.1	0.3–9.6		0.125	
		ENNA1	22.5	0.4–28.1		0.125	
		ENNB	93.3	0.4–212.4		0.125	
		ENNB1	58.4	0.3–71.8		0.013	
		AOH	82.0	0.2–12.8		0.125	
		AME	84.3	0.1–15.6		0.125	
		FB1	66.3	11.8–990.1		0.125	
		FB2	52.8	10.5–556.3		0.250	
		DAS	n.f.	n.f.			
		FUS-X	n.f.	n.f.			
48	5	ENNA	n.a.	n.a.	LC-MS/MS	5	Tolosa et al., 2019 [16]
		ENNA1	41.5	8.1–11.9		1	
		ENNB	89	2.0–89.5		1	
		ENNB1	64	7.4–28.5		1	
		BEA	62	4.6–129.6		5	

Table 3. Cont.

Analyzed Samples (n)	Analytes Investigated	Mycotoxins	Positive Samples (%)	[a] Range or Average (µg/kg)	Detection Methods	LOQ (µg/kg)	Reference
32	8	AFB1	47.7	30.3–242.7	LC-MS/MS	1.7	Shao et al., 2018 [29]
		AFG1	13.9	13.9		0.7	
		OTA	16.2	15.1–17.3		10.7	
		ZEN	54.5	14.5–389.2		2.5	
		DON	66.3	22.8–421.3		16.5	
		T-2	15.4	15.4		3.3	
		BEA	19.1	0.2–153.4		2.5	
		FB1	87.2	6.6–191.9		10.0	
12	6	AFB1	n.a.	83.3	HPLC-FLD	41.57	Singh et al., 2017a [24]
		AFB2	n.a.	9.0		11.77	
		OTA	n.a.	1.0		-	
		ZEN	n.a.	5.7		-	
		FB1	n.a.	106.3		202.53	
		FB2	n.a.	61.9		118.37	
49	3	AFs	100	0.16–5.39	HPLC-FLD	AFB1 = 0.13; AFB2 = 0.59; AFG1 = 0.03; AFG2 = 0.22	Teixeira et al., 2017 [25]
		ZEN	95.9	4.07–98.3		3.95	
		FBs	77.6	37.4–1015		FB1 = 27.5; FB2 = 35.3	
100	4	AFLs	68	0.34–3.88	HPLC-FLD	B1=0.13; G1 = 0.03; B2 = 0.59; G2 = 0.22	Bissoqui et al., 2016 [23]
		ZEN	95	5.45–442.2		3.95	
		FB1	68	20.0–220		27.5	
		FB2	35	40.0–160		35.3	
20	3	AFs	n.a.	n.a.	ELISA-UV	5	Yasmina et al., 2016 [21]
		AFB1	15	2.6–18.4		1	
		OTA	70	2.62–6.65		2.5	
		ZEN	20	148–1170		1.75	
49	2	AFB1	8.2	<0.05–0.21	HPLC-FLD	0.15	Błajet-Kosicka et al., 2014 [22]
		OTA	46.9	<0.13–3		0.40	
	5	DON	100	22.7–436	LC-MS/MS	20.0	
		T-2	87.7	<0.5–13.3		1.50	
		HT-2	83.7	<1.60–19.6		5.00	
		ZEN	100	1.81–123		0.30	
7		FBs	28.6	<5–108		FB1 = 1.60; FB2 = 1.60; FB3 = 1.60	
76	4	DON	97	>250	ELISA-UV	-	Böhm et al., 2010 [30]
		OTA	5	3.5		-	
		ZEN	47	80		-	
		FBs	42	178		-	
29	3	DON	83	409	HPLC-FLD	25	
22		ZEN	68	185		20	
3		FBs	67	69		15	
180	1	AFB1	70.5	0.3–9.43	HPLC-FLD	0.1	Campos et al., 2008 [31]

Abbreviations: Aflatoxins (AFB1, AFB2, AFG1 and AFG2), ochratoxin A (OTA), fumonisins (FB1 and FB2), deoxynivalenol (DON), 3-acetyl-deoxynivalenol (3-AcDON), 15-acetyl-deoxynivalenol (15-AcDON), HT-2 toxin, T-2 toxin, neosolaniol (NEO), diacetoxyscirpenol (DAS) fusarenon-X (FUS-X), zearalenone (ZEN), α-zearalenol (α-ZEL), β-zearalenol (β-ZEL), α-zearalanol (α-ZAL), β-zearalanol (β-ZAL), zearalanone (ZAN), beauvericin (BEA), enniatins (ENNA, ENNA1, ENNB and ENNB1), alternariol (AOH) and alternariol monomethyl ether (AME). [a] Range or arithmetic mean of all positive samples. n.f. (not found) is shown if there was no readable value below LOD. n.a. not available.

2.4. Occurrence of Mycotoxins in Pet Food Samples

The optimized and validated multi-mycotoxin method was applied to 89 dry pet food samples (55 for dogs and 34 for cats) acquired from different pet shops located in Campania region, Southern Italy. Table 3 shows the results here obtained, as well as reviewing the available studies published in the last decade regarding the occurrence of mycotoxins in pet food samples.

In these analyzed samples, 99% of pet foods showed mycotoxin contamination. Despite the significantly high incidence, the concentration levels found were below the maximum level and/or maximum permissible levels set for mycotoxins in feedstuffs (2003/100/EC; 2006/576/EC). Nonetheless, special attention must be considered for the aflatoxins group. 25.8% of analyzed samples showed AFB1 contamination in a concentration range from 3.3 to 7.9 µg/kg (average content: 4.3 µg/kg). Similar AFB1 findings were reported in petfoods from Poland ($n = 49$) in a concentration range from <LOQ to 0.2 µg/kg [22], and from Brazil ($n = 180$) with AFB1 contamination levels ranging from 0.3 to 9.4 µg/kg [31]. In another survey, 4 out of 70 Brazilian pet food samples showed AFB1 contamination in a range from 15 to 37 µg/kg. This high contamination level reported by these authors was related to the presence of contaminated peanuts present in all positive samples. Despite some samples exceeded the maximum limit set by the EU for complete feedstuffs (20 µg/kg), those levels were below the permitted limits adopted in Brazil (50 µg/kg).

On the other hand, OTA was quantified in 2.2% of the here analyzed pet food samples at average content of 1.5 µg/kg. These levels are in agreement with previous studies as reviewed in Table 3. However, a wide range of OTA incidence reported by the different surveys was observed. Concerning the occurrence of fumonisins in pet food samples, the available studies reported both high incidence (>50%) and concentrations up to hundreds/thousands µg/kg (Table 3). Recently, Teixeira et al. [25] reported FBs contamination in 70% ($n = 87$) of Brazilian pet food samples at a concentration range from 30 to 1015 µg/kg. These findings are also in line with the data here obtained in which 67% of analyzed samples showed FBs contamination ranging from 10.5 to 990.1 µg/kg, being FB1 the most commonly detected fumonisin. The particularly high levels and incidence of FBs in feed could be related to the quality of corn (grain) and corn-based ingredients used in the formulations of these feedstuffs.

As far as trichothecenes are concerned, DON (and its acetylated forms) were the most commonly reported type B trichothecene in pet food samples reported in literature at concentration levels of hundreds µg/kg (Table 3). Similar results were here found; in fact, 30% of samples were DON-contaminated at concentration range from 7.6 to 297.3 µg/kg. On the other hand, type A trichothecenes mainly represented by HT-2 and T-2 toxins, has been barely investigated in pet food samples despite the fact that these toxins have been proven to have a higher toxicity than DON. In these analyzed samples, HT-2 (32.6% positive samples) and T-2 (47.2% positive samples) were detected at levels from 3.3 to 110.1 µg/kg, and from 0.7 to 9.0 µg/kg, respectively. Higher HT-2 and T-2 incidences (of up to 87.7%) than those here obtained were reported by Błajet-Kosicka et al. [22], in the 49 Polish pet food samples, but the concentration levels in that study were below 20 µg/kg in all positive samples. In line with that, ZEN (and its derivative forms) were found in 91% of the here analyzed samples at levels ranging from < LOQ to 60.6 µg/kg. These results are in agreement with recent surveys carried out in Brazilian [23,25], Egyptian [21], Polish [22], and Austrian [30] pet food samples (Table 3).

Emerging *Fusarium* mycotoxins (ENs and BEA) and *Alternaria* mycotoxins (AOH and AME), have been barely investigated in feed samples. The results showed a high incidence (>80%) of enniatins with concentration up to hundreds µg/kg (Table 3). Among enniatins, ENNB was the most commonly detected mycotoxin in the assayed samples (83 out of 89). The results obtained in this work are according to contents reported in different feedstuffs samples. Tolosa et al. [32] reported a high incidence of ENs (100% positive samples) and BEA (95% positive samples) in 20 Spanish fish feed at levels ranging from 0.1 to 10.0 µg/kg and from 0.1 to 6.6 µg/kg respectively. These results are also according to those reported by Warth et al. [33] in which ENs and BEA were present in 70% and 100% ($n = 10$) of animal feed samples from Burkina Faso and Mozambique, with concentration levels ranging from 0.1 to 114.0 µg/kg and from 3.3 to 418 µg/kg, respectively. On the other hand, Warth et al. [33]

reported also AOH and AME contamination in 75% and 25% in a low number of samples analyzed ($n = 4$) at average content of 15.1 and 11.1 µg/kg, respectively. Similar high incidence was reported by Streit et al. [34], in which AOH and AME were found in 80% and 82% of feed and feed raw materials ($n = 83$) from Europe at concentration levels of hundreds µg/kg.

2.5. Co-occurrence of Mycotoxins in Analyzed Samples

All contaminated pet food samples here analyzed showed co-occurrence from three to sixteen mycotoxins in a sum concentration range from 1.6 to 1700.0 µg/kg (Figure 1). Three multicontaminated samples showed sum concentrations above 1000 µg/kg, with several *Fusarium, Aspergillus* and *Alternaria* toxins. A significant number of pet food samples (77.3%) were co-contaminated from 8 to 12 mycotoxins. Similarly, Böhm et al. [30] reported the co-occurrence of mycotoxins in 33% Austrian pet food samples ($n = 76$), and *Fusarium* toxins such as DON, ZEA, and FBs were the most predominant. The simultaneous occurrence complicates the evaluation of toxicological potential of feed. Additive and synergistic effects on overall toxicity are frequently observed when mycotoxin mixtures are evaluated [9,35,36].

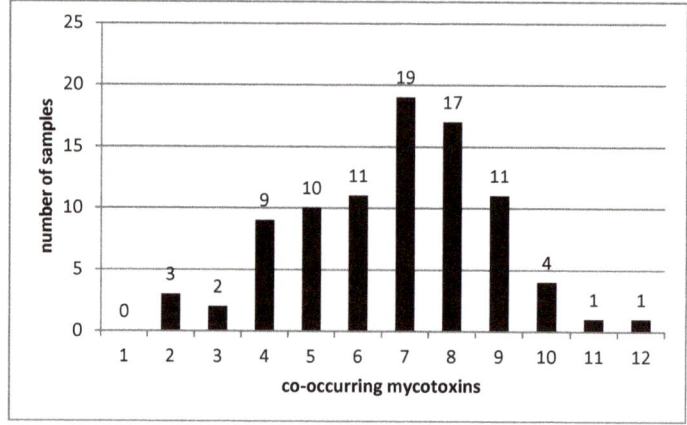

Figure 1. Number of samples co-contaminated with a given number of mycotoxins (total samples analyzed; $n = 89$).

2.6. Identification of Non Target Coumpounds Based on A Retrospective Screening Analysis

The developed strategy based on Q-Orbitrap HRMS combines the quantitative target determination with the post-target screening approach. The possibilities of the Q-Orbitrap HRMS were further explored by subjecting the full scan data of the pet food samples to untargeted screening with the major data processing parameters set as follows: ionization patterns $[M + H]^+$ and $[M - H]^-$, a minimum peak area of 1×10^5 a.u., a maximum mass window of 5 ppm, and a retention time width of 1 min. The confirmation of the structural characterization of unknown compounds and untargeted analytes was based on the accurate mass measurement, elemental composition assignment, and MS/MS spectrum interpretation. Untargeted data processing was carried out using structural formula finder tool and the online high-quality mass spectral database. The advantage of using a full-scan acquisition mode is to allow the retrospective analysis of samples for the identification of up to 245 fungal and bacterial metabolites included in spectral library database by processing the raw data of the analyzed pet food samples. Fifty-four fungal metabolites were tentatively identified in the here analyzed samples (Figure 2). Cyclopiazonic acid, paspalitrem A, fusaric acid, and macrosporin were the most commonly detected mycotoxins in the assayed samples (98.9%). Cyclopiazonic acid and paspalitrem A are produced by *Aspergillus* and *Penicillium* spp. Fusaric acid is produced by some *Fusarium* spp. Macrosporin is mainly produced by *Stemphylium* spp. These metabolites have been already found in contaminated cereal crops such as oats, barley, millet, corn, and rice [37–39].

In these analyzed samples, emodin was also identified in 97.8% of feed samples. This compound was already reported in Spanish feed and feed raw material but lower incidence (57.1%; n = 62) [40].

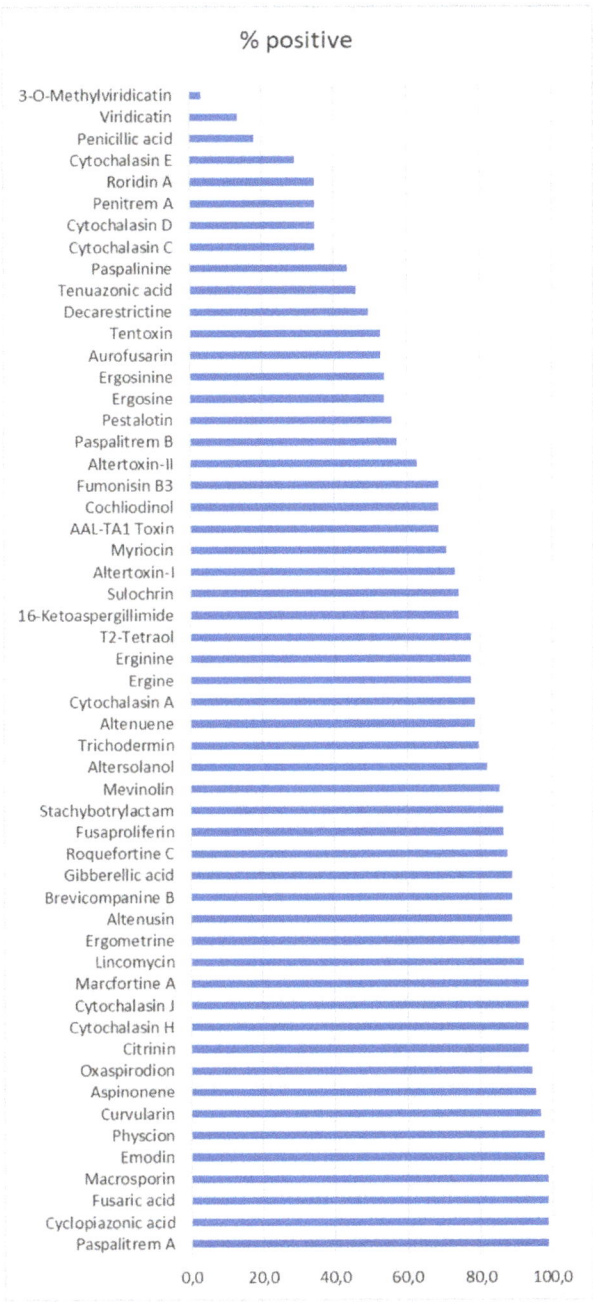

Figure 2. Non-target mycotoxins identified in samples based on ultrahigh-performance liquid chromatography coupled to high-resolution mass-spectrometry (UHPLC-Q-Orbitrap HRMS) library.

3. Conclusions

A UHPLC-Q-Orbitrap HRMS method for simultaneous determination of mycotoxins from different fungal species in pet food samples was in-house optimized and validated according to the criteria set by Commission Decision 2002/657/EC. In addition, mycotoxin spectral library of 245 analytes was used for post-run retrospective screening. The developed method was successfully applied to eighty-nine petfood samples and twenty-six different mycotoxins were found at high incidence (98.9%) but at concentrations below the maximum permissible limits. Co-occurrence of mycotoxins was found in all contaminated samples with up to sixteen analytes per sample. The established method was rapid and efficient, and capable of covering more analytes compared to the previous methods for the detection and quantitation of mycotoxins in pet food products. Moreover, this is the first work describing the simultaneous detection, quantification, and retrospective screening of a wide range of mycotoxins from different genera in pet food samples by using the capability provided by the UHPLC-Q-Orbitrap HRMS technology.

4. Materials and Methods

4.1. Chemical and Reagents

Mycotoxin standards and metabolites namely aflatoxins (AFB1, AFB2, AFG1, and AFG2), ochratoxin A (OTA), fumonisins (FB1 and FB2), deoxynivalenol (DON), 3-acetyl-deoxynivalenol (3-AcDON), 15-acetyl-deoxynivalenol (15-AcDON), HT-2 toxin, T-2 toxin, neosolaniol (NEO), diacetoxyscirpenol (DAS), fusarenon-X (FUS-X), zearalenone (ZEN), α-zearalenol (α-ZEL), β-zearalenol (β-ZEL), α-zearalanol (α-ZAL), β-zearalanol (β-ZAL), zearalanone (ZAN), beauvericin (BEA), enniatins (ENNA, ENNA1, ENNB, and ENNB1), alternariol (AOH), and alternariol monomethyl ether (AME) were purchased from Sigma Aldrich (Milan, Italy). Individual stock solutions of all analytes were prepared by diluting 1 mg of each mycotoxin in 1 mL of methanol and further diluted for preparing working standard solutions. All these solutions were kept in safe conditions at −20 °C.

All solvents, acetonitrile (AcN), methanol (MeOH) and water (LC-MS grade) were purchased from Merck (Darmstadt, Germany) whereas formic acid (mass spectrometry grade) and ammonium formate (analytical grade) were obtained from Fluka (Milan, Italy). Magnesium sulphate was obtained from VWR Chemicals BDH Prolabo, (Leuven, Belgium) and C18 (analytical grade) was purchased from Supelco (Bellafonte, Pennsylvania, PA, USA).

Syringe filters with polytetrafluoroethylene membrane (PTFE, 15 mm, diameter 0.2 μm) were provided by Phenomenex (Castel Maggiore, Italy); conical centrifuge polypropylene tubes of 50 mL and 15 mL were obtained from BD Falcon (Milan, Italy).

4.2. Sampling

A total of eighty-nine standard dry pet food samples was randomly purchased from different pet shops located in Campania region, Southern Italy. The acquired pet food samples were classified as follows: dogs ($n = 55$) and cats ($n = 34$). The nutritional composition of the analyzed samples is shown in Table 4. The main ingredients declared in labels from samples were rice, corn, corn flour, wheat, tapioca, wheat flour, oat, and barley. All samples were homogenized using a laboratory mill (particle size 200 μm) and then stored in a dark and dry place until analysis. The analysis was performed within 3 days after sample registration [40].

Table 4. Nutritional composition of standard dry pet food samples.

Composition (%)	Dog ($n = 55$)	Cat ($n = 34$)
Proteins	25.8 ± 5.2	33.8 ± 3.8
Fats	14.9 ± 3.4	15.2 ± 4.4
Fibers	6.8 ± 1.2	7.5 ± 1.1
Total minerals	3.0 ± 2.1	3.9 ± 2.9

4.3. Sample Preparation

In this work, a sample preparation procedure for extraction of mycotoxins from laboratory rat feed reported in literature was selected as starting point and slightly modified [11]. In brief, homogenous representative samples (2 g) were weighted into 50 mL falcon tube and 10 mL of AcN:H$_2$O mixture (80:20, v/v with 0.1% of formic acid) were added. The mixture was placed in a horizontal shaker for 60 min at 245× g and then placed into an ultrasonic bath for 15 min. Samples were centrifuged for 3 min at 3435× g at 4 °C, and 2 mL of the upper layer were submitted to a dispersive-SPE with a mixture of 300 mg of anhydrous MgSO$_4$ and 100 mg of C18, and vortexed for 1 min. The mixture was centrifuged for 1 min at 1472× g at 4 °C. Finally, the extract was evaporated to dryness under gentle nitrogen flow at 45 °C, reconstituted with 0.5 mL of MeOH/H$_2$O (70:30, v/v), and filtered (0.22 µm filter) prior to the UHPLC-Q Orbitrap HRMS analysis.

4.4. Method Validation

The method validation was performed in-house with respect to linearity, matrix effect, sensitivity, accuracy, and precision, as expected with compliance to Commission Decision 2002/657/EC. For the spiking and recovery studies, there were employed a pool of blank pet food samples ($n = 10$) (dog, $n = 5$; and cat, $n = 5$) of previous studies. Linearity was evaluated throughout standard solutions and matrix-matched calibrations. A graphic scatter plot test was used to assess the linearity, and lack-of-fit test was performed in linear regression model. Linear range of the method was assessed from limit of quantification to 1000 µg/kg for all mycotoxins. Matrix effect was evaluated by comparing the slopes of standard solutions built in neat solvent and the matrix-matched calibration curve. Values around 100% mean that there are no matrix effects, signal suppression, or enhancement if the value obtained was lower or higher than 100%, respectively. The sensitivity was evaluated by LODs and LOQs. LOD was defined as the minimum concentration where the molecular ion can be identified with a mass error below 5 ppm, and LOQ was set as the lowest concentration of the analyte that produce a chromatographic peak with precision and accuracy <20%. The accuracy of the method was evaluated with recovery studies. Blank samples were spiked and left to equilibrate overnight and then extracted as previously described. Method recovery was performed at three spiking levels (10, 20, and 100 µg/kg). Precision was expressed as relative standard deviation (% RSD) and calculated by triplicate measurements carried out on a single day (repeatability) and on three non-consecutive days (within-laboratory repeatability) [41].

4.5. Quality Assurance/Quality Control

For the confirmation criteria, the peaks for the studied compounds in the samples were confirmed by comparing the retention times of the peak with those of standard solutions at a tolerance of ± 2.5%. To ensure a higher level of confidence in the identification, the precursors and product ions were recognized with a mass error below 5 ppm. In the QA/QC procedure, a sample blank, a reagent blank, a replicate sample, and a matrix-matched external calibration were added at the beginning and end of each sample batch in order to assess the effectiveness of the developed method. Spiked pet food samples at three concentration levels (10, 20, and 100 µg/kg) were used for analytical quality control.

4.6. Ultrahigh-Performance Liquid Chromatography Coupled to High-Resolution Mass-Spectrometry (UHPLC-Q-Orbitrap HRMS) Analysis

Detection and quantitation were performed with a UHPLC instrument (Dionex Ultimate 3000, Thermo Fisher Scientific, Waltham, Ma, USA) equipped with a degassing system, a Quaternary UHPLC pump working at 1250 bar, and an autosampler device. Chromatographic separation of analytes was performed with a thermostated Luna Omega Polar C18 column (50 × 2.1 mm, 1.6 µm, Phenomenex) kept at 30 °C. Both mobile phases contained 0.1% formic acid and 5 mM ammonium formate and were H$_2$O (phase A) and MeOH (phase B). The LC gradient started with 0% B, kept up to 1 min, and then increased to 95% B in 1 min, followed by a hold-time of 0.5 min at 95% B. Afterward, the gradient switched back to 75% in 2.5 min, and decreased again reaching 60% B in 1 min. The gradient returned in 0.5 min at 0%, and 1.5 min column re-equilibration at 0%. The injection volume was 5 µL with flow rate of 0.4 mL/min. The UHPLC system was coupled to a Q-Exactive Orbitrap mass spectrometer (UHPLC, Thermo Fischer Scientific, Waltham, Ma, USA). The mass spectrometer was operated in both positive and negative ion mode using fast polarity switching by setting two scan events (Full ion MS and All ion fragmentation, AIF). Full scan data were acquired at a resolving power of 35,000 FWHM at *m/z* 200. The conditions in positive ionization mode (ESI$^+$) were: spray voltage 4 kV; capillary temperature 290 °C; S-lens RF level 50; sheath gas pressure (N_2 > 95%) 35, auxiliary gas (N_2 > 95%) 10, and auxiliary gas heater temperature 305 °C. Ion source parameters in negative (ESI$^-$) mode were: spray voltage −4 kV; capillary temperature 290 °C; S-lens RF level 50; sheath gas pressure (N_2 > 95%) 35, auxiliary gas (N_2 > 95%) 10, and auxiliary gas heater temperature 305 °C. Value for automatic gain control (AGC) target was set at 1×10^6, a scan range of *m/z* 100–1000 was selected and the injection time was set to 200 ms. Scan-rate was set at 2 scans/s. For the scan event of AIF, the parameters in the positive and negative ion mode were: mass resolving power = 17,500 FWHM; maximum injection time = 200 ms; scan time = 0.10 s; ACG target = 1×10^5; scan range = 100–1000 *m/z*, isolation window to 5.0 *m/z*, and retention time window to 30 *s*. The collision energy was optimized individually for each compound. Different collision energies were tested while the infusion of the compound was performed into the HRMS. The optimal energy was chosen when at least the parent compound remained at 10% intensity and it produced characteristic product ions from 80–100% intensity. Data processing were performed by the Quan/Qual Browser Xcalibur software, v. 3.1.66. (Xcalibur, Thermo Fisher Scientific). Retrospective screening was carried out on spectral data collected using a mycotoxin spectral library (Mycotoxin Spectral Library v1.1 for LibraryView™ Software, AB SCIEX, Framingham, USA). The identification was based on accurate mass measurement with a mass error below 5 ppm for the molecular ion; while regarding the fragments on the intensity threshold of 1000 and a mass tolerance of 5 ppm. Quantitative results were obtained working in scan mode with HRMS exploiting the high selectivity achieved in full-scan mode, whereas MS/HRMS information was used for confirmatory purposes.

4.7. Statistics and Data Analysis

All validation experiments were performed in triplicate, and the results were expressed as the average values ± relative standard deviation (RSD, %). Student's *t*-test statistical analysis was performed for data evaluation; *p* values < 0.05 were considered significant.

Supplementary Materials: The following are available online at http://www.mdpi.com/2072-6651/11/8/434/s1, Table S1: Optimization of sample preparation procedure, Table S2: Accuracy and precision of the developed method.

Author Contributions: A.R and Y.R.-C conceived and designed the experiments; L.I. and J.T. performed the experiments, G.G. and A.G. analyzed the data, L.C. and Y.R.-C. wrote the paper.

Funding: Authors thanks the financial support given by Spanish Ministry of Economy and Competitiveness (AGL-2016-77610-R).

Conflicts of Interest: The authors declare no conflict of interest.

References

1. Jedidi, I.; Soldevilla, C.; Lahouar, A.; Marin, P.; Gonzalez-Jaen, M.T.; Said, S. Mycoflora isolation and molecular characterization of Aspergillus and Fusarium species in Tunisian cereals. *Saudi J. Biol. Sci.* **2018**, *25*, 868–874. [CrossRef] [PubMed]
2. Iqbal, S.Z.; Selamat, J.; Ariño, A. Mycotoxins in food and food products: Current status. In *Food Safety*; Springer: Berlin, Germany, 2016; pp. 113–123.
3. Chhonker, S.; Rawat, D.; Naik, R.; Koiri, R. An Overview of Mycotoxins in Human Health with Emphasis on Development and Progression of Liver Cancer. *Clin. Oncol.* **2018**, *3*, 1408.

4. Meeting, J.F.W.E.C.o.F.A. *Safety Evaluation of Certain Mycotoxins in Food*; Food & Agriculture Org.: Rome, Italy, 2001.
5. Pascari, X.; Ramos, A.J.; Marin, S.; Sanchis, V. Mycotoxins and beer. Impact of beer production process on mycotoxin contamination. A review. *Food Res. Int.* **2018**, *103*, 121–129. [CrossRef] [PubMed]
6. Gruber-Dorninger, C.; Novak, B.; Nagl, V.; Berthiller, F. Emerging mycotoxins: Beyond traditionally determined food contaminants. *J. Agric. Food Chem.* **2016**, *65*, 7052–7070. [CrossRef] [PubMed]
7. Suleiman, R.; Rosentrater, K.; Chove, B. Understanding postharvest practices, knowledge, and actual mycotoxin levels in maize in three agro-ecological zones in Tanzania. *J. Stored Prod. Postharvest Res.* **2017**, *8*, 73.
8. Unusan, N. Systematic review of mycotoxins in food and feeds in Turkey. *Food Control* **2018**, *97*, 1–14. [CrossRef]
9. Streit, E.; Schatzmayr, G.; Tassis, P.; Tzika, E.; Marin, D.; Taranu, I.; Tabuc, C.; Nicolau, A.; Aprodu, I.; Puel, O. Current situation of mycotoxin contamination and co-occurrence in animal feed—Focus on Europe. *Toxins* **2012**, *4*, 788–809. [CrossRef]
10. Soler, L.; Oswald, I. The importance of accounting for sex in the search of proteomic signatures of mycotoxin exposure. *J. Proteom.* **2018**, *178*, 114–122. [CrossRef]
11. Escrivá, L.; Font, G.; Berrada, H.; Manyes, L. Mycotoxin contamination in laboratory rat feeds and their implications in animal research. *Toxicol. Mech. Methods* **2016**, *26*, 529–537. [CrossRef]
12. Vila-Donat, P.; Marín, S.; Sanchis, V.; Ramos, A. A review of the mycotoxin adsorbing agents, with an emphasis on their multi-binding capacity, for animal feed decontamination. *Food Chem. Toxicol.* **2018**, *114*, 246–259. [CrossRef]
13. Rodríguez-Carrasco, Y.; Moltó, J.C.; Berrada, H.; Mañes, J. A survey of trichothecenes, zearalenone and patulin in milled grain-based products using GC–MS/MS. *Food Chem.* **2014**, *146*, 212–219. [CrossRef] [PubMed]
14. Adeyeye, S.A. Fungal mycotoxins in foods: A review. *Cogent Food Agric.* **2016**, *2*, 1213127. [CrossRef]
15. Mahmoud, A.F.; Escrivá, L.; Rodríguez-Carrasco, Y.; Moltó, J.C.; Berrada, H. Determination of trichothecenes in chicken liver using gas chromatography coupled with triple-quadrupole mass spectrometry. *LWT* **2018**, *93*, 237–242. [CrossRef]
16. Tolosa, J.; Rodríguez-Carrasco, Y.; Ferrer, E.; Mañes, J. Identification and Quantification of Enniatins and Beauvericin in Animal Feeds and Their Ingredients by LC-QTRAP/MS/MS. *Metabolites* **2019**, *9*, 33. [CrossRef] [PubMed]
17. Rico-Yuste, A.; Walravens, J.; Urraca, J.; Abou-Hany, R.; Descalzo, A.; Orellana, G.; Rychlik, M.; De Saeger, S.; Moreno-Bondi, M. Analysis of alternariol and alternariol monomethyl ether in foodstuffs by molecularly imprinted solid-phase extraction and ultra-high-performance liquid chromatography tandem mass spectrometry. *Food Chem.* **2018**, *243*, 357–364. [CrossRef] [PubMed]
18. Kaczynski, P.; Hrynko, I.; Lozowicka, B. Evolution of novel sorbents for effective clean-up of honeybee matrix in highly toxic insecticide LC/MS/MS analysis. *Ecotoxicol. Environ. Saf.* **2017**, *139*, 124–131. [CrossRef]
19. Rodríguez-Carrasco, Y.; Gaspari, A.; Graziani, G.; Sandini, A.; Ritieni, A. Fast analysis of polyphenols and alkaloids in cocoa-based products by ultra-high performance liquid chromatography and Orbitrap high resolution mass spectrometry (UHPLC-Q-Orbitrap-MS/MS). *Food Res. Int.* **2018**, *111*, 229–236. [CrossRef] [PubMed]
20. Van Wijk, X.M.; Goodnough, R.; Colby, J.M. Mass spectrometry in emergency toxicology: Current state and future applications. *Crit. Rev. Clin. Lab. Sci.* **2019**, *56*, 225–238. [CrossRef]
21. Abd-Elhakim, Y.M.; El Sharkawy, N.I.; Moustafa, G.G. An investigation of selected chemical contaminants in commercial pet foods in Egypt. *J. Vet. Diagn. Investig.* **2016**, *28*, 70–75. [CrossRef]
22. Błajet-Kosicka, A.; Kosicki, R.; Twarużek, M.; Grajewski, J. Determination of moulds and mycotoxins in dry dog and cat food using liquid chromatography with mass spectrometry and fluorescence detection. *Food Addit. Contam. Part B* **2014**, *7*, 302–308. [CrossRef]
23. Bissoqui, L.Y.; Frehse, M.S.; Freire, R.L.; Ono, M.A.; Bordini, J.G.; Hirozawa, M.T.; de Oliveira, A.J.; Ono, E.Y. Exposure assessment of dogs to mycotoxins through consumption of dry feed. *J. Sci. Food Agric.* **2016**, *96*, 4135–4142. [CrossRef] [PubMed]
24. Singh, S.D.; Baijnath, S.; Chuturgoon, A.A. A comparison of mycotoxin contamination of premium and grocery brands of pelleted cat food in South Africa. *J. S. Afr. Vet. Assoc.* **2017**, *88*. [CrossRef] [PubMed]

25. Teixeira, E.; Frehse, M.; Freire, R.; Ono, M.; Bordini, J.; Hirozawa, M.; Ono, E. Safety of low and high cost dry feed intended for dogs in Brazil concerning fumonisins, zearalenone and aflatoxins. *World Mycotoxin J.* **2017**, *10*, 273–283. [CrossRef]
26. Mao, J.; Zheng, N.; Wen, F.; Guo, L.; Fu, C.; Ouyang, H.; Zhong, L.; Wang, J.; Lei, S. Multi-mycotoxins analysis in raw milk by ultra high performance liquid chromatography coupled to quadrupole orbitrap mass spectrometry. *Food Control* **2018**, *84*, 305–311. [CrossRef]
27. Kabir, A.; Locatelli, M.; Ulusoy, H. Recent trends in microextraction techniques employed in analytical and bioanalytical sample preparation. *Separations* **2017**, *4*, 36. [CrossRef]
28. Singh, S.D.; Chuturgoon, A.A. A comparative analysis of mycotoxin contamination of supermarket and premium brand pelleted dog food in Durban, South Africa. *J. S. Afr. Vet. Assoc.* **2017**, *88*, 1–6. [CrossRef] [PubMed]
29. Shao, M.; Li, L.; Gu, Z.; Yao, M.; Xu, D.; Fan, W.; Yan, L.; Song, S. Mycotoxins in commercial dry pet food in China. *Food Addit. Contam. Part B* **2018**, *11*, 237–245. [CrossRef]
30. Böhm, J.; Koinig, L.; Razzazi-Fazeli, E.; Blajet-Kosicka, A.; Twaruzek, M.; Grajewski, J.; Lang, C. Survey and risk assessment of the mycotoxins deoxynivalenol, zearalenone, fumonisins, ochratoxin A, and aflatoxins in commercial dry dog food. *Mycotoxin Res.* **2010**, *26*, 147–153. [CrossRef]
31. Campos, S.; Keller, L.; Cavaglieri, L.; Krüger, C.; Fernández Juri, M.; Dalcero, A.; Magnoli, C.; Rosa, C. Aflatoxigenic fungi and aflatoxin B1 in commercial pet food in Brazil. *World Mycotoxin J.* **2009**, *2*, 85–90. [CrossRef]
32. Tolosa, J.; Font, G.; Mañes, J.; Ferrer, E. Natural occurrence of emerging Fusarium mycotoxins in feed and fish from aquaculture. *J. Agric. Food Chem.* **2014**, *62*, 12462–12470. [CrossRef]
33. Warth, B.; Parich, A.; Atehnkeng, J.; Bandyopadhyay, R.; Schuhmacher, R.; Sulyok, M.; Krska, R. Quantitation of mycotoxins in food and feed from Burkina Faso and Mozambique using a modern LC-MS/MS multitoxin method. *J. Agric. Food Chem.* **2012**, *60*, 9352–9363. [CrossRef] [PubMed]
34. Streit, E.; Schwab, C.; Sulyok, M.; Naehrer, K.; Krska, R.; Schatzmayr, G. Multi-mycotoxin screening reveals the occurrence of 139 different secondary metabolites in feed and feed ingredients. *Toxins* **2013**, *5*, 504–523. [CrossRef] [PubMed]
35. Alassane-Kpembi, I.; Schatzmayr, G.; Taranu, I.; Marin, D.; Puel, O.; Oswald, I.P. Mycotoxins co-contamination: Methodological aspects and biological relevance of combined toxicity studies. *Crit. Rev. Food Sci. Nutr.* **2017**, *57*, 3489–3507. [CrossRef] [PubMed]
36. Smith, M.-C.; Madec, S.; Coton, E.; Hymery, N. Natural co-occurrence of mycotoxins in foods and feeds and their in vitro combined toxicological effects. *Toxins* **2016**, *8*, 94. [CrossRef] [PubMed]
37. Di Marino, D.; D'Annessa, I.; Coletta, A.; Via, A.; Tramontano, A. Characterization of the differences in the cyclopiazonic acid binding mode to mammalian and P. Falciparum Ca^{2+} pumps: A computational study. *Proteins Struct. Funct. Bioinform.* **2015**, *83*, 564–574. [CrossRef] [PubMed]
38. Anjorin, S.T.; Fapohunda, S.; Sulyok, M.; Krska, R. Natural Co-occurrence of Emerging and Minor Mycotoxins on Maize Grains from Abuja, Nigeria. *Ann. Agric. Environ. Sci.* **2016**, *1*, 1.
39. Ogara, I.M.; Zarafi, A.B.; Alabi, O.; Banwo, O.; Ezekiel, C.N.; Warth, B.; Sulyok, M.; Krska, R. Mycotoxin patterns in ear rot infected maize: A comprehensive case study in Nigeria. *Food Control* **2017**, *73*, 1159–1168. [CrossRef]
40. Romera, D.; Mateo, E.M.; Mateo-Castro, R.; Gomez, J.V.; Gimeno-Adelantado, J.V.; Jimenez, M. Determination of multiple mycotoxins in feedstuffs by combined use of UPLC–MS/MS and UPLC–QTOF–MS. *Food Chem.* **2018**, *267*, 140–148. [CrossRef] [PubMed]
41. Antignac, J.-P.; Le Bizec, B.; Monteau, F.; Andre, F. Validation of analytical methods based on mass spectrometric detection according to the "2002/657/EC" European decision: Guideline and application. *Anal. Chim. Acta* **2003**, *483*, 325–334. [CrossRef]

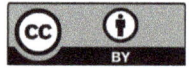

© 2019 by the authors. Licensee MDPI, Basel, Switzerland. This article is an open access article distributed under the terms and conditions of the Creative Commons Attribution (CC BY) license (http://creativecommons.org/licenses/by/4.0/).

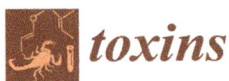

Article

Pig Urinary Concentration of Mycotoxins and Metabolites Reflects Regional Differences, Mycotoxin Intake and Feed Contaminations

Lucia Gambacorta [1], Monica Olsen [2,*] and Michele Solfrizzo [1]

1. Institute of Sciences of Food Production (ISPA), National Research Council (CNR), Via Amendola 122/O, 70126 Bari, Italy
2. National Food Agency, Department of Risk Benefit Assessment, P.O. Box 622, 751 26 Uppsala, Sweden
* Correspondence: monica.olsen@slv.se

Received: 16 June 2019; Accepted: 28 June 2019; Published: 30 June 2019

Abstract: The determination of mycotoxin and metabolite concentrations in human and animal urine is currently used for risk assessment and mycotoxin intake measurement. In this study, pig urine ($n = 195$) was collected at slaughterhouses in 2012 by the Swedish National Food Agency in three counties representing East, South and West regions of Sweden. Urinary concentrations of four mycotoxins, (deoxynivalenol (DON), zearalenone (ZEA), fumonisin B_1 (FB_1), and ochratoxin A (OTA)), and four key metabolites, (deepoxy-deoxynivalenol (DOM-1), aflatoxin M_1 (AFM_1, biomarker of AFB_1), α-zearalenol (α-ZOL), and β-zearalenol (β-ZOL)) were identified and measured by UPLC-MS/MS. Statistically significant regional differences were detected for both total DON (DON + DOM-1) and total ZEA (ZEA + α-ZOL + β-ZOL) concentrations in pig urine from the three regions. These regional differences were in good agreement with the occurrence of *Fusarium graminearum* mycotoxins (DON + ZEA) in cereal grains harvested in 2011 in Sweden. There were no statistically significant differences in FB_1, AFM_1 and OTA urinary concentrations in pigs from the three regions. The overall incidence of positive samples was high for total ZEA (99–100%), total DON (96–100%) and OTA (85–95%), medium for FB_1 (30–61%) and low for AFM_1 (0–13%) in the three regions. Urinary mycotoxin biomarker concentrations were used to estimate mycotoxin intake and the level of mycotoxins in feeds consumed by the monitored pigs. The back-calculated levels of mycotoxins in feeds were low with the exception of seven samples that were higher the European limits.

Keywords: mycotoxins; biomarkers; urine; UPLC-MS/MS; intake; feed; grain

Key Contribution: This is the first manuscript that provides data on the occurrence of the five agriculturally important mycotoxins and metabolites in pig urine collected in three regions of Sweden. A statistically significant difference in total DON and total ZEA concentrations were observed in the three monitored regions, which reflected a similar situation in the grain grown in the respective areas.

1. Introduction

Deoxynivalenol (DON), zearalenone (ZEA), fumonisin B_1 (FB_1), ochratoxin A (OTA) and aflatoxin B_1 (AFB_1) were defined as the five agriculturally important mycotoxins for their impact on the safety of human food and feed [1]. Pigs are quite susceptible to mycotoxin toxicity; therefore, the guidance values for cereals and cereal products and compound feed for animal feeding are lower for those destined for pigs [2]. In developed countries, feeds are constantly monitored for mycotoxins to protect animal health and increase animal productivity and farmer's income. Monitoring mycotoxins in cereal grain is expensive and laborious due to the inhomogeneous distribution of mycotoxins in raw materials, which requires the application of adequate sampling plans that comprise the collection of a high number of samples to be analyzed. Hult et al. (1979) demonstrated the efficacy of biomonitoring of OTA in pig's blood to determine OTA levels in feeds consumed by the monitored pigs [3]. Subsequently, Gilbert et al.; (2001) demonstrated a better correlation between OTA consumption and urinary OTA as compared to blood OTA [4]. More recently, with the availability of better performing LC-MS/MS instrumentation, new and high performing analytical methods, such as those reviewed by Vidal et al.; (2018) [5], were developed for multiple mycotoxins and their phase I and II metabolites determination in biological fluids, especially urine. The introduction of an enzymatic digestion step in the sample preparation of urine was used in several analytical methods in order to hydrolyze conjugated mycotoxins, phase II metabolites and conjugated phase I metabolites of mycotoxins into free analytes. This approach reduces the number of analytes to be monitored, increases the sensitivity of the analytical method and avoids producing/synthesizing commercially unavailable conjugated standards. A good dose response was demonstrated in piglets between the consumption of the five agriculturally important mycotoxins and urinary concentrations of mycotoxins and their metabolites [6]. Urinary concentrations of mycotoxins and their metabolites were also successfully used to demonstrate the efficacy of grape pomace to significantly reduce the bioavailability of AFB_1 and ZEA in pigs [7]. Few studies have been conducted in the past to assess pig exposure to mycotoxins, and most of them considered only one mycotoxin and its metabolites [8–13]. The main aim of the present work was to assess pig exposure to the five agriculturally important mycotoxins through the determination of mycotoxin biomarkers in urine collected at slaughterhouses in three regions of Sweden and to evaluate any regional differences. The main conclusion of this study was that mycotoxin exposure of Swedish pigs was low with a few exceptions. Moreover, our results indicate that pig urine can be used for monitoring both pig exposure to mycotoxins as well as the trends of DON and ZEA in cereal grains.

2. Results and Discussion

2.1. Occurrence, Intake, Feed Contamination and Regional Differences

The UPLC-MS/MS method and MS/MS parameters used in this study to analyze pig urine were previously reported [6,7]. As a minor modification, 5 mL of urine was used instead of 6 mL. The method performance was verified by a recovery experiment conducted with Swedish pig urine. As shown in Table 1, mean recoveries (>70%) and the repeatability of results (1–12%) were all acceptable, with the exception of FB_1 that gave a mean recovery of 64% but a good repeatability of results (7%). In Table 1, we also report the values of the limit of detection (LOD) (0.006–0.36 ng/mL) and the limit of quantification (LOQ) (0.02–1.21 ng/mL) for each analyte. LOD and LOQ were calculated as three times and 10 times the noise, respectively.

Table 1. Results of in-house validation of the LC-MS/MS method for mycotoxin biomarkers in pig urine. DON = deoxynivalenol; ZEA = zearalenone; FB_1 = fumonisin B_1; OTA = ochratoxin A; DOM-1 = deepoxy-deoxynivalenol; AFM_1 = aflatoxin M_1; α-ZOL = α-zearalenol; β-ZOL = β-zearalenol.

Mycotoxin	Spike levels (ng/mL)	Recovery (%)	RSD [a] (%)	LOD [b] (ng/mL)	LOQ [c] (ng/mL)
DON	90	93	6.8	0.18	0.61
DOM-1	45	82	3.6	0.36	1.21
ZEA	45	98	1.1	0.02	0.07
α-ZOL	45	100	0.9	0.04	0.13
β-ZOL	45	96	12.3	0.04	0.15
OTA	0.9	71	5.0	0.006	0.02
FB_1	18	64	6.7	0.02	0.06
AFM_1	9.0	96	0.7	0.01	0.03

[a] RSD: within-day relative standard deviation [b] LOD: limit of detection [c] LOQ: limit of quantification.

In Table 2, we report the incidence of positive samples, and the mean, median and max concentration of each analyte, reported as ng/mL and as ng/mg creatinine (crea). The total concentrations of DON (DON + DOM-1) and ZEA (ZEA + α-ZOL + β-ZOL) are also reported. The high percentages of samples positive for DON, ZEA and their metabolites was not surprising and were comparable to those previously reported by other authors for pig urine [9,11,13].

Table 2. Urinary concentrations of mycotoxins and their metabolites in samples of Swedish pigs collected in 2012 ($n = 195$).

Mycotoxin [a]	% Positives [b] (n)	Mean ± SD [c] (ng/mL)	Median (ng/mL)	Max (ng/mL)	Mean ± SD [c] (ng/mg crea)	Median (ng/mg crea)	Max (ng/mg crea)
DON	93% (181)	19.35 ± 49.53	5.91	510.64	17.25 ± 56.28	3.43	491.25
DOM-1	95% (186)	12.89 ± 20.55	4.95	120.63	10.71 ± 27.14	3.75	318.69
Total DON	98% (192)	32.25 ± 59.92	12.46	538.51	27.95 ± 77.64	7.84	809.94
ZEA	92% (179)	2.44 ± 4.39	0.77	28.32	2.32 ± 7.63	0.58	76.68
α-ZOL	90% (176)	2.72 ± 4.78	1.02	33.86	3.31 ± 13.87	0.69	162.47
β-ZOL	81% (158)	0.75 ± 1.59	0.21	14.69	0.73 ± 1.97	0.13	18.15
Total ZEA	99% (194)	5.91 ± 9.78	2.13	65.66	6.37 ± 22.35	1.41	257.29
OTA	95% (185)	0.31 ± 0.65	0.23	7.94	0.39 ± 2.03	0.11	25.57
FB_1	42% (82)	0.080 ± 0.256	0.01	2.58	0.084 ± 0.256	0.01	2.08
AFM_1	7% (14)	0.015 ± 0.063	0.01	0.74	0.014 ± 0.057	0.003	0.50

[a] DON = deoxynivalenol; DOM-1 = deepoxy-deoxynivalenol; Total DON = DON + DOM-1; ZEA = zearalenone; α-ZOL = α-zearalenol; β-ZOL = β-zearalenol; Total ZEA = ZEA + α-ZOL + β-ZOL; OTA = ochratoxin A; FB_1 = fumonisin B_1, AFM_1 = aflatoxin M_1; crea = creatinine. [b] Positives are considered the samples above the LOD, n = number of samples. [c] To calculate mean concentrations, values below the LOD were assigned a fixed value of LOD/2, values between the LOD and the LOQ were assigned a fixed value of LOQ/2. SD = standard deviation.

The occurrence of multiple mycotoxins and metabolites in pig urine is reported in Figure 1. The most common combinations were total DON + total ZEA + OTA (50.3% of samples) followed by total DON + FB_1 + total ZEA + OTA (34.9% of samples) (Figure 1). Each of the seven other combinations occurred in less than 6% of urine.

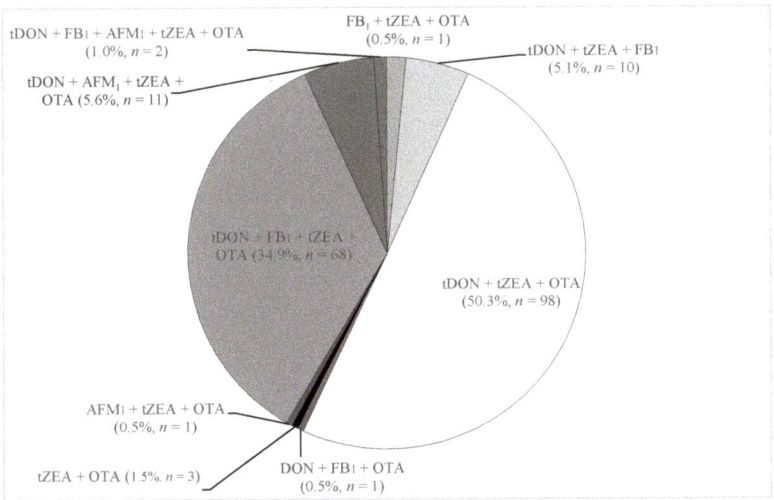

Figure 1. Mycotoxin combinations and their incidence in 195 Swedish pig urine samples collected in 2012. tDON = total DON; tZEA = total ZEA.

In Table 3, we compare the results of the present study (percentage of positives and mean concentrations of positive samples) with those reported in other studies conducted with pigs or piglets bred in six different countries. Mean concentrations of mycotoxin biomarkers in Swedish pigs were within the concentrations reported by other authors for this animal species. In particular, the urinary mean DON concentration of Swedish pigs was lower than that measured in Belgian pigs [12] but higher than those measured in Vietnamese pigs [13] and French piglets [7]. Mean urinary concentrations of ZEA and total ZEA were lower than those reported from Croatia [9,10], Austria [11] and Vietnam [13] but higher than those reported from France for piglets [7]. A high mean concentration of ZEA (206 ng/mL) was reported in Croatia for 30 pigs showing clear symptoms of hyperestrogenism, probably because they were fed with feed highly contaminated by ZEA [9]. Swedish pig urine showed incidences of positive samples and a mean OTA concentration higher than those reported for Belgian pigs and French piglets [7,12]. On the other hand, the incidence of positive samples and mean concentration of FB_1 in Swedish pigs was comparable to those reported for Belgian pigs and French piglets [7,12]. A remarkable difference was observed when comparing the AFM_1 results of Swedish and Vietnamese pigs. As reported in Table 3, the Swedish pig urine showed an incidence of positive samples and mean AFM_1 concentration 8–11 and 4–27 times lower compared to Vietnamese pig urine, respectively [8,13]. These results confirmed that the feeds used to fed Swedish pigs were only sporadically and marginally contaminated by AFB_1 which is mainly excreted in urine as AFM_1. Taken together, the results reported in Table 3 gave a picture about the differing occurrence of the eight biomarkers of the five agriculturally important mycotoxins in the urine of pigs bred in Sweden and France, and for 1–6 biomarkers of 1–3 mycotoxins in five more countries.

The urinary mycotoxin and metabolite concentrations measured in this study and the urinary excretion rate of the five target mycotoxins and their metabolites in pigs [6] were used to calculate the probable daily intake (PDI) of the target mycotoxins in Swedish pigs using Formula (1). The calculated mean and max PDI values of each mycotoxin in exposed pigs is shown in Table 4.

The mean PDI value of DON was higher than those of ZEA, OTA, FB_1 and AFB_1. The calculated PDI values, mean pig weight, mean daily urine volume and mean weight of feed consumed daily by pigs were used to calculate the level of each mycotoxin in the feed consumed by each pig monitored in this study according to Formula (2), reported in the experimental section. The results of this evaluation are reported in Table 5, which also shows the maximum permitted level of AFB_1 [14] and the guidance levels of DON, ZEA, OTA and fumonisins in feeds for pigs [2]. The estimated mean level of DON in feed was 116.8 µg/kg, whereas for ZEA, OTA, FB_1 and AFB_1, they ranged from 16.1–0.6 µg/kg. These values are largely below the limits for DON (900 µg/kg), ZEA (250 µg/kg), OTA (50 µg/kg), AFB_1 (20 µg/kg) and FB_1 (5000 µg/kg). However, the estimated mycotoxin levels of the feeds consumed by seven pigs were higher the limits of DON, OTA or AFB_1. Five out of the seven pigs were bred in the West region and three of them consumed feed with high DON levels, whereas two pigs consumed feeds with high levels of OTA (Table 5). On the other hand, only one pig from the East region and one from the South region consumed feed contaminated with high levels of AFB_1 and OTA, respectively.

Table 3. Occurrence of urinary mycotoxins and their metabolites in pigs from different countries fed with naturally contaminated feeds.

Country	Method	Mean Biomarker Concentrations (ng/mL) in Positive Samples (% Positive Samples)											References
		DON	DOM-1	Total DON	OTA	AFM$_1$	FB$_1$	ZEA	α-ZOL	β-ZOL	Total ZEA		
Sweden (n = 195) [a]	LC-MS/MS	20.8 (93)	13.5 (95)	32.7 (98)	0.33 (95)	0.15 (7)	0.18 (42)	2.7 (92)	3.0 (90)	0.9 (81)	5.9 (99)	Present study
Croatia (n = 11) [a]	ELISA	na[b]	na	na	na	na	na	40.5 (100)	na	na	na	[10]
Croatia (n = 30) [a]	ELISA	na	na	na	na	na	na	206	na	na	na	[9]
Austria (n = 6) [a]	LC-MS/MS	na	na	na	na	na	na	5.9 (100)	3.2 (100)	2.1 (83)	10.0 (100)	[11]
Belgium (n = 19) [c]	LC-MS/MS	54.6 (74)	na	na	0.11 (26)	nd[d]	0.30 (21)	nd	nd	nd	nd	[12]
Vietnam (n = 15) [a]	LC-UV/FLD	10.3 (60)	10.3 (40)	na	na	4.1 (80)	na	6.9 (7)	2.8 (47)	10 (7)	19.7 (93)	[13]
Vietnam (n = 1920) [c]	ELISA	na	na	na	na	0.63 (53.9)	na	na	na	na	na	[8]
France (n = 28) [a,e]	LC-MS/MS	12.6 (93)	0.5 (11)	13.4 (11)	0.2 (43)	nd	0.5 (29)	0.5 (89)	0.3 (18)	nd	0.86 (18)	[7]

[a] using enzymatic hydrolysis prior to analysis. [b] not analyzed. [c] not using enzymatic hydrolysis prior to analysis. [d] not detected. [e] piglet urine was collected before the administration of contaminated feed boluses.

Table 4. Probable daily intake (PDI) (μg/kg bw[a]) of total DON (DON + DOM-1), total ZEA (ZEA + α-ZOL + β-ZOL), OTA, AFB$_1$ and FB$_1$ in 195 Swedish pigs.

Analyte	Mean ± SD	Median	Max
Total DON	2.66 ± 4.93	1.03	44.34
Total ZEA	0.36 ± 0.60	0.13	4.06
OTA	0.27 ± 0.57	0.20	6.94
FB$_1$	0.07 ± 0.22	0.01	2.26
AFB$_1$	0.01 ± 0.06	0.005	0.67

[a] bw = body weight.

Table 5. Comparison of EU limits and mean levels of DON, ZEA, OTA, AFB$_1$, and FB$_1$ in pig feeds calculated from urinary biomarker concentrations.

Mycotoxin	Limits (μg/kg)	Mean ± SD (μg/kg)	Median (μg/kg)	Max (μg/kg)	n > limit East	n > limit South	n > limit West
DON	900 [1]	116.84 ± 217.09	45.14	1951.11	0	0	3
ZEA	250 [1]	16.06 ± 26.57	5.78	178.42	0	0	0
OTA	50 [1]	11.87 ± 25.02	8.85	305.25	1	0	2
FB$_1$	5000 [1]	3.08 ± 9.84	0.38	99.26	0	0	0
AFB$_1$	20 [2]	0.60 ± 2.51	0.20	29.64	0	1	0

[1] Commission Recommendation (EC) n. 2006/576. [2] Commission Regulation (EC) n. 574/2011.

These results prompted us to statistically compare the mycotoxin concentrations in the urine of pigs bred in the West, South and East regions of Sweden (Figure 2). The results of this statistical evaluation were reported in Table 6 as ng/mL and as ng/mg crea. A significant difference ($p < 0.001$) was observed for total DON between West (56.8 ± 88.7 ng/mL) and South (19.3 ± 22.8 ng/mL) and between West and East (12.8 ± 13.6 ng/mL). The statistical analyses of crea adjusted urine concentrations confirmed the significant difference ($p < 0.009$) of total DON between West (45.7 ± 106 ng/mg crea) and South (12.9 ± 15.1 ng/mg crea), but no differences were observed between West and East and between South and East. Total ZEA was significantly higher ($p < 0.009$) in the West (7.8 ± 10.4 ng/mL) compared to South (4.3 ± 9.5 ng/mL) but no significant difference was found to the East. Similar results were obtained for crea adjusted concentrations, although a significant difference ($p < 0.05$) was also observed between East (12.5 ± 42.2 ng/mg crea) and South (3.7 ± 10.5 ng/mg crea).

These regional differences were in good agreement with the differing occurrence of *Fusarium graminearum* mycotoxins (DON and ZEA) in cereal grains harvested in 2011 in different Swedish regions [15,16]. Moreover, data pertaining to DON in oats in 2011 collected by the Swedish grain industry (Thomas Börjesson, personal communication) showed similar differences between West (mean level 4287 ± 4120 μg/kg, $n = 1300$) and South (mean level 572 ± 655 μg/kg, $n = 160$). Despite the fact that pigs are not fed oats, the data reflect the situation of a high infection rate with *F. graminearum* in the fields of the West region, which was particularly troublesome in oats this year.

According to the Kruskal–Wallis equality of population rank test, there was no difference ($p > 0.05$) in FB$_1$, AFM$_1$ and OTA between the three regions. Considering that AFB$_1$ and FB$_1$ were not found in Swedish grains, the positive samples were most likely due to other feed components or the farmer was not producing their own feed and used commercial feed; in that case, we should not expect regional differences. Protein concentrates were found to contain AFB$_1$ from 5–500 μg/kg and the more heavily contaminated samples were destined for pig rations [17].

Table 6. Statistical comparison of urinary mycotoxin biomarker concentrations in pigs bred in three Swedish regions.

Mycotoxin	East Region (n = 38)			South Region (n = 83)			West Region (n = 74)		
	Positives (%) [1]	Mean ± SD (ng/mL)	Mean ± SD (ng/mg crea)	Positives (%) [1]	Mean ± SD (ng/mL)	Mean ± SD (ng/mg crea)	Positives (%) [1]	Mean ± SD (ng/mL)	Mean ± SD (ng/mg crea)
DON	90	7.80 ± 12.0 [a]	19.8 ± 78.3 [AB]	94	9.37 ± 11.9 [a]	6.47 ± 9.29 [A]	93	36.5 ± 76.3 [b]	28.0 ± 70.4 [B]
DOM-1	90	4.95 ± 4.47 [a]	6.60 ± 10.3 [A]	93	9.95 ± 16.2 [a]	6.41 ± 9.18 [A]	86	20.3 ± 26.8 [b]	17.6 ± 41.6 [B]
Total DON	100	12.8 ± 13.6 [a]	26.3 ± 87.5 [AB]	96	19.3 ± 22.8 [a]	12.9 ± 15.1 [B]	99	56.8 ± 88.7 [b]	45.7 ± 106 [A]
ZEA	92	1.93 ± 3.04 [ab]	3.97 ± 12.8 [A]	94	1.76 ± 3.89 [a]	1.33 ± 3.65 [B]	95	3.47 ± 5.27 [b]	2.59 ± 7.39 [A]
α-ZOL	84	2.62 ± 4.46 [a]	6.90 ± 26.5 [A]	96	2.01 ± 5.18 [a]	1.84 ± 5.97 [B]	89	3.57 ± 4.38 [b]	3.12 ± 10.3 [A]
β-ZOL	84	1.25 ± 2.72 [ab]	1.66 ± 3.66 [A]	81	0.50 ± 1.07 [a]	0.51 ± 1.38 [B]	81	0.77 ± 1.22 [b]	0.50 ± 0.89 [AB]
Total ZEA	100	5.80 ± 8.83 [ab]	12.5 ± 42.2 [A]	100	4.27 ± 9.47 [a]	3.67 ± 10.5 [B]	99	7.80 ± 10.35 [b]	6.21 ± 18.2 [A]
OTA	85	0.26 ± 0.37 [a]	0.90 ± 4.13 [A]	98	0.26 ± 0.16 [a]	0.19 ± 0.19 [A]	95	0.39 ± 1.01 [a]	0.36 ± 1.43 [A]
FB$_1$	61	0.11 ± 0.41 [a]	0.11 ± 0.23 [A]	30	0.09 ± 0.26 [a]	0.10 ± 0.33 [A]	50	0.06 ± 0.10 [a]	0.05 ± 0.15 [A]
AFM$_1$	0	0.01 ± 0.00 [a]	0.02 ± 0.08 [A]	13	0.03 ± 0.09 [a]	0.02 ± 0.06 [A]	5	0.01 ± 0.01 [a]	0.01 ± 0.03 [A]

[1] % of samples > nd. [a] or [b] ([A] or [B]): the mean concentration, in ng/mL or ng/mg crea, of a specific mycotoxin is not significantly different ($p > 0.05$, Mann–Whitney test) between the three regions if the letter is the same in the same line.

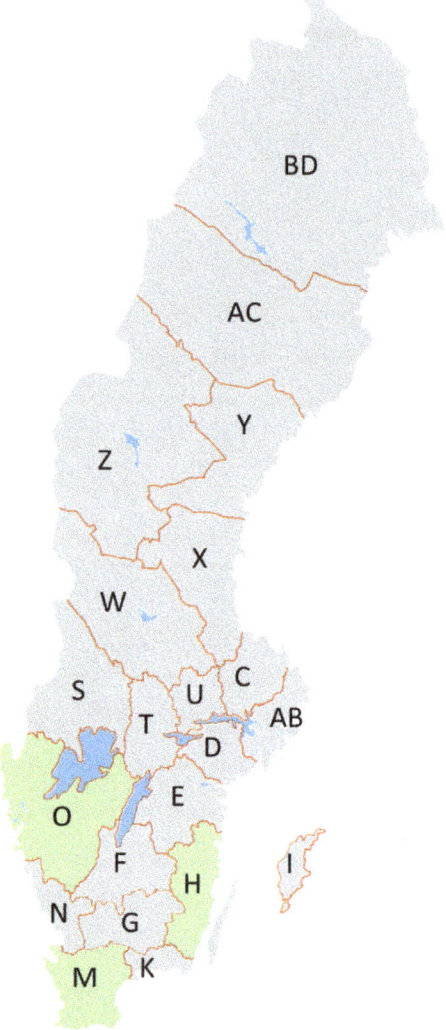

Figure 2. Map of the Sweden showing from which county the pig urine samples were collected. The West region is represented by Västra Götaland county (O), the South region is represented by Skåne county (M) and the East region is represented by Kalmar county (H). The names of other counties are reported here https://www.iso.org/obp/ui/#iso:code:3166:SE.

2.2. Comparison of Urinary Mycotoxin/Metabolite Ratios in Naturally Exposed Pigs and Pigs Fed with Experimental Contaminated Diets

In Figure 3, the ratios of DON/DOM-1, ZEA/α-ZOL, ZEA/β-ZOL and ZEA/α-ZOL + β-ZOL measured in the urine of pigs chronically exposed to naturally contaminated feeds are compared to pigs exposed for a short period (1–29 days) to relatively high DON and/or ZEA doses in experimental *in vivo* studies [6,7,18–22]. All mean ratios measured in the occurrence studies [7,11,13], including the present study, were statistically lower ($p < 0.05$) than those measured in *in vivo* studies where pig diets contained higher levels of DON and/or ZEA (Figure 3). The calculated total mean level of DON in feeds consumed by the monitored pigs of the three occurrence studies [7,13], including the present study, was 60 µg/kg, whereas the calculated total mean level of DON in the various feeds used in the seven *in vivo* studies was 2321 µg/kg [6,7,18–22]. The calculated total mean level of ZEA in feeds consumed by pigs of the four occurrence studies [7,11,13], including the present study, was 21 µg/kg, whereas the total mean level of ZEA in various feeds used in the six *in vivo* studies was 920 µg/kg [6,7,18,19,21,23]. The data shown in Figure 3 suggested that pigs chronically exposed to relatively low levels of DON and/or ZEA (occurrence studies) had an improved capacity to metabolize DON into DOM-1 as compared to pigs exposed for a relatively short period to high levels of these mycotoxins, i.e. DON/DOM-1 ratio was lower in occurrence studies as compared to *in vivo* studies. Moreover, the results shown in Figure 3 confirmed that pigs mainly metabolize ZEA into α-ZOL, and to a lesser extent into β-ZOL, i.e. ZEA/α–ZOL ratios were always lower that ZEA/β-ZOL ratios both in occurrence results and *in vivo* results (Figure 3).

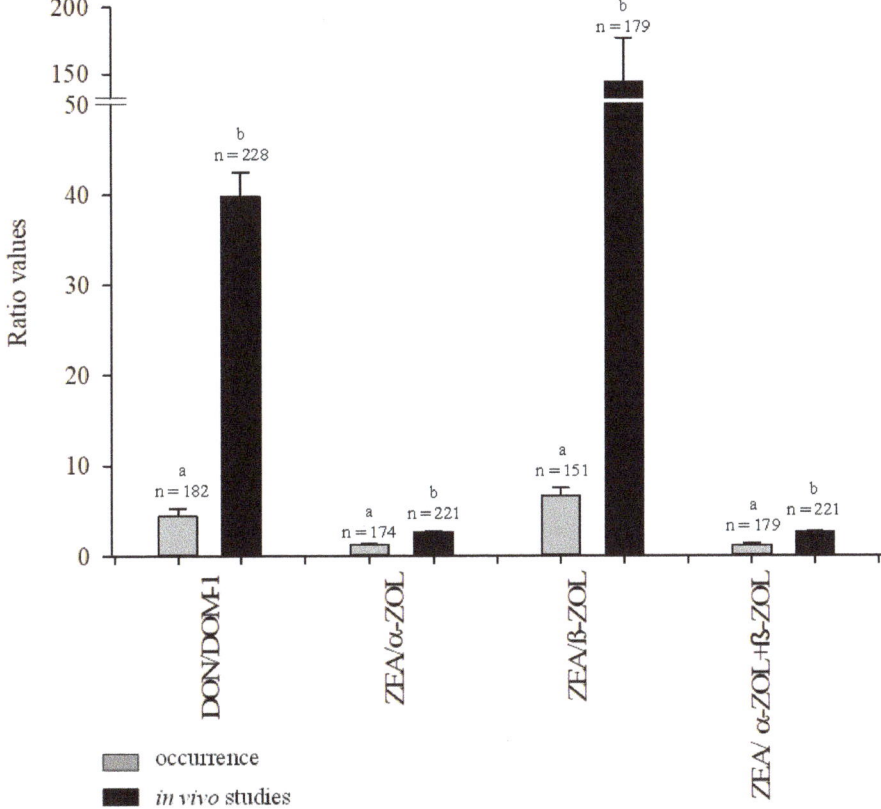

Figure 3. Ratios of DON/DOM-1, ZEA/α-ZOL, ZEA/β-ZOL and ZEA/α-ZOL + β-ZOL in the urine of pigs chronically exposed to naturally contaminated feeds (grey bars) [7,11,13] and pigs exposed for a short period to relatively high doses of DON and/or ZEA (black bars) [6,7,19–23]. [a,b] Different letters within each couple of bars represent statistically significant difference ($p < 0.05$).

3. Conclusions

The UPLC-MS/MS method used herein for the determination of urinary biomarkers of DON, FB_1, OTA, AFB_1 and ZEA was suitable to measure the low concentrations naturally occurring in pig urine from pigs bred in three Swedish regions. A multiple mycotoxin exposure was detected in all samples and the more frequent mycotoxin combinations were total DON + total ZEA + OTA followed by total DON + FB$_1$ + ZEA + OTA. Urinary biomarker concentrations were used to estimate PDI and mycotoxin levels in feeds consumed by pigs. The overall mycotoxin levels in feeds were lower the European limits with the exception of 4% of the samples that were found to be contaminated with levels of either DON, OTA or AFB$_1$ that were higher than the recommended/regulatory limits. Within the three regions monitored in this study, the pigs bred in the West region were more exposed to DON and ZEA compared to pigs in the South and East regions. Monitoring of urinary mycotoxin biomarkers was quite effective to assess pig exposure to mycotoxins, the mycotoxin levels in consumed grains and to identify the regions at higher risk for mycotoxin accumulation in the grains produced.

4. Materials and Methods

4.1. Collection of Samples

The sampling of pig urine, collected from slaughterhouses, was conducted from January–December 2012 by the Swedish National Food Agency. The age of the pigs at slaughter were, on average, 6 months with a range of 5–8 months. The West, South and East regions of Sweden were represented by Västra Götaland county ($n = 74$), Skåne county ($n = 83$) and Kalmar county ($n = 38$), respectively (Figure 2). Soon after collection, urine samples were frozen and sent from the National Food Agency (Uppsala, Sweden) to the Institute of Sciences of Food Production (Bari, Italy) for UPLC-MS/MS analysis of biomarkers of the five agriculturally important mycotoxins, i.e.; DON and DOM-1 for DON, AFM$_1$ for AFB$_1$, FB$_1$ for FB$_1$, ZEA, α-ZOL and β-ZOL for ZEA, and OTA for OTA.

4.2. Chemicals and Reagents

Standard solutions of mycotoxins and their key metabolites were purchased from Romer Labs Diagnostic (Tulln, Austria). In particular, solutions of DON (100 µg/mL), DOM-1 (50 µg/mL), AFM$_1$ (0.5 µg/mL), ZEA (100 µg/mL), α-ZOL (10 µg/mL), β-ZOL (10 µg/mL) and OTA (10 µg/mL) were prepared in acetonitrile (ACN), whereas FB$_1$ solution (50 µg/mL) was prepared in acetonitrile–water (50:50 v/v). The enzymatic solution β-glucuronidase/sulfatase type H-2 from *Helix pomatia* (specific activity 130,200 units/m L β-glucuronidase, 709 units/mL sulfatase) was purchased by Sigma Aldrich (Milan, Italy). Chromatography-grade methanol (MeOH) and glacial acetic acid were obtained from Carlo Erba (Milan, Italy). Ultrapure water was obtained from a Milli-Q system (Millipore, Bedford, MA, USA). Myco6in1+TM immunoaffinity columns were purchased from Vicam L.P (Watertown, MA, USA). OASIS HLB® columns (60 mg, 3 mL) were purchased from Waters (Milford, MA, USA) and regenerated cellulose filters (0.45 µm) were purchased from Sartorius Stedim Biotech (Goettingen, Germany).

4.3. Urine Analysis

The analyses of pig urinary mycotoxin biomarkers (DON, DOM-1, AFM$_1$, FB$_1$, ZEA, α-ZOL, β-ZOL and OTA) were performed using an ultra-performance liquid chromatography tandem mass spectrometry (UPLC-MS/MS) method reported elsewhere [6,7]. Briefly, 5 mL of pig urine was treated with the aqueous solution of β-glucuronidase/sulfatase type H-2 from *Helix pomatia* to hydrolyze glucuronide- and sulfate- conjugates of mycotoxins and their key metabolites. The digested sample was diluted with water (1:1, v/v) and purified on a Myco6in1+TM multi-antibody immunoaffinity column and OASIS HLB® column connected in tandem. The purified urine was dried down and reconstituted in 200 µl of mobile phase (MeOH:H$_2$O, 20:80, v/v) and analyzed by UPLC-MS/MS with a triple quadrupole API 5000 mass spectrometer (Applied Biosystems, Foster City, CA, USA), equipped with an ESI interfaced to an Acquity UPLC system comprising a binary pump and a microautosampler (Waters, Milford, MA, USA). Data acquisition and processing was performed with Analyst version 1.5.1 software (Applied Biosystems 2011, Foster City, CA, USA). Detailed chromatographic and mass spectrometric operating conditions are reported elsewhere [24,25]. Crea concentrations in urine samples were analyzed according to an enzymatic method described by [26].

4.4. Calibration Curves

Quantification of mycotoxin biomarkers in the 195 purified pig urine sample extracts was performed using matrix-matched calibration curves. For each set of samples (one for each day), matrix-matched calibration solutions were prepared for 6 purified urinary extracts: one aliquot was analyzed as a control and 5 aliquots were used to prepare calibration samples. In particular, aliquots of urine from 5 pigs were pooled and mixed, then 6 aliquots (5 mL each) were purified according to the protocol reported above. After purification, adequate and increasing amounts of standard solutions of DON, DOM-1, AFM_1, FB_1, ZEA, α-ZOL, β-ZOL and OTA were added to the 5 purified extracts, dried down, reconstituted in 200 μL of LC–MS/MS mobile phase and filtered. The calibration ranges in the matrix ranged between: 0.1–100 ng/mL for DON, 0.75–24.85 ng/mL for DOM-1, 0.01–7 ng/mL for AFM_1, 0.10–101.6 ng/mL for FB_1, 0.03–20.6 ng/mL for β-ZOL and α-ZOL, 0.01–100 ng/mL for ZEA, 0.01–5.01 ng/mL for OTA.

4.5. Recovery Experiment

A mixture of 3 blank pig urine samples was used for the recovery experiment of DON, DOM-1, AFM_1, FB_1, ZEA, α-ZOL, β-ZOL and OTA. Triplicate experiments were performed. The spiking concentration of each analyte was reported in Table 1. They ranged from 0.9 ng/mL for OTA to 90 ng/mL for DON. Matrix matched calibration curves were used to quantify each analyte. LOD and LOQ were calculated as 3 times and 10 times the noise, respectively.

4.6. Censoring

Left-censored analytical results, i.e.; values below the limit of detection (LOD) and the limit of quantification (LOQ), were evaluated with the substitution method as suggested by the European Food Safety Authority (EFSA 2010) [27]. Within the three scenarios proposed by EFSA (lower, middle and upper bound), we used the middle bound approach, i.e.; results below the LOD (or the LOQ), were given the value LOD/2 (or LOQ/2). To calculate the mean concentration in positive samples (Table 3), the values between the LOD and the LOQ were assigned a fixed value of LOQ/2. LOD and LOQ values for all mycotoxins and metabolites were reported in Table 1.

4.7. Estimation of Mycotoxin Intake

Calculation of intake estimation was performed for DON, ZEA, FB_1, OTA and AFB_1 in pigs using urinary biomarker concentrations measured in this study according Formula (1), reported by [25]:

$$PDI = (C \times V \times 100)/(W \times E) \quad (1)$$

where:

PDI: probable daily intake of each mycotoxin (μg/kg body weight);
C: pig urinary biomarker concentration (μg/L);
V: mean 24 h pig urine volume (2.5 L);
W: mean pig body weight (110 kg);
E: mean urinary excretion rate of each mycotoxin in 24 h post dose in piglets (36.8% for total ZEA, 27.9% for total DON, 2.6% for FB_1, 2.6% for OTA and 2.5% for AFB_1 excreted as AFM_1 [6]).

4.8. Estimation of Feed Contamination

The DON, ZEA, FB_1, OTA and AFB_1 contamination in feeds consumed by the pigs monitored in this study was calculated using the calculated PDI of each mycotoxin and Formula (2).

$$ML = PDI \times W/V \quad (2)$$

where:

ML: mycotoxin level in the feed (µg/kg);
PDI: probable daily intake of the mycotoxin (µg/kg body weight);
W: mean pig body weight (110 kg)
V: mean 24 h pig urine volume (2.5 L)

4.9. Statistical Analyses of Urinary Biomarker Concentrations and Geographical Areas

Mean, median and standard deviation of the results were calculated using Microsoft Excel 2013 software (Microsoft Corporation, Redmond, WA, USA). Statistical analyses were performed using GraphPad Instat software version 3.00 (Instat 1997, San Diego, CA, USA). Data were subjected to the unpaired t-test (one-tail p value). Values were judged to be significantly different if p values were < 0.05.

The Mann–Whitney test and the Kruskal–Wallis equality of population rank test were performed in STATA version 12.1 (STATA Corp. 2017, College Station, TX, USA). A p-value < 0.05 was considered significant.

Author Contributions: Funding acquisition, M.O.; Investigation, L.G. and M.O.; Methodology, L.G. and M.S.; Project administration, M.O.; Resources, M.O.; Validation, M.S.; Writing – original draft, M.S.; Writing – review and editing, M.O.

Funding: This research was funded by the Swedish National Food Agency and the Swedish Civil Contingencies Agency.

Conflicts of Interest: The authors declare no conflict of interest.

References

1. Miller, J.D. Fungi and mycotoxins in grain: Implications for stored product research. *J. Stored Prod. Res.* **1995**, *31*, 1–16. [CrossRef]
2. European Commission (EC). Commission Recommendation 2006/576/EC of 17 August 2006 on the presence of deoxynivalenol, zearalenone, ochratoxin A, T-2 and HT-2 and fumonisins in products intended for animal feeding. *Off. J. Eur. Union* **2006**, *L229*, 7–9.
3. Hult, K.; Hokby, E.; Hagglund, U.; Gatenbeck, S.; Rutqvist, L.; Sellyey, G. Ochratoxin A in pig blood: Method of analysis and use as a tool for feed studies. *Appl. Environ. Microbiol.* **1979**, *38*, 772–776. [PubMed]
4. Gilbert, J.; Brereton, P.; MacDonald, S. Assessment of dietary exposure to ochratoxin A in the UK using a duplicate diet approach and analysis of urine and plasma samples. *Food Addit. Contam.* **2001**, *18*, 1088–1093. [CrossRef] [PubMed]
5. Vidal, A.; Mengelers, M.; Yang, S.; De Saeger, S.; De Boevre, M. Mycotoxin biomarkers of exposure: A comprehensive review. *Compr. Rev. Food Sci. F.* **2018**, *17*, 1127–1155. [CrossRef]
6. Gambacorta, L.; Solfrizzo, M.; Visconti, A.; Powers, S.; Cossalter, A.M.; Pinton, P.; Oswald, I.P. Validation study on urinary biomarkers of exposure for aflatoxin B1, ochratoxin A, fumonisin B1, deoxynivalenol and zearalenone in piglets. *World Mycotoxin J.* **2013**, *6*, 299–308. [CrossRef]
7. Gambacorta, L.; Pinton, P.; Avantaggiato, G.; Oswald, I.P.; Solfrizzo, M. Grape Pomace, an Agricultural Byproduct Reducing Mycotoxin Absorption: In Vivo Assessment in Pig Using Urinary Biomarkers. *J. Agric. Food Chem.* **2016**, *64*, 6762–6771. [CrossRef]
8. Lee, H.S.; Lindahl, J.; Nguyen-Viet, H.; Khong, N.V.; Nghia, V.B.; Xuan, H.N.; Grace, D. An investigation into aflatoxin M_1 in slaughtered fattening pigs and awareness of aflatoxins in Vietnam. *BMC Vet. Res.* **2017**, *13*, 363. [CrossRef]
9. Pleadin, J.; Mihaljević, Z.; Barbir, T.; Vulić, A.; Kmetič, I.; Zadravec, M.; Brumen, V.; Mitak, M. Natural incidence of zearalenone in Croatian pig feed, urine and meat in 2014. *Food Addit. Contam. Part B* **2015**, *8*, 277–283. [CrossRef]
10. Vulić, A.; Pleadin, J.; Perši, N.; Mitak, M. Analysis of naturally occurring zearalenone in feeding stuffs and urine of farm animals in Croatia. *J. Immunoass. Immunochem.* **2012**, *33*, 369–376. [CrossRef]
11. Jodlbauer, J.; Zöllner, P.; Lindner, W. Determination of zeranol, taleranol, zearalenone, α-and β-zearalenol in urine and tissue by high-performance liquid chromatography-tandem mass spectrometry. *Chromatographia* **2000**, *51*, 681–687. [CrossRef]

12. Song, S.; Ediage, E.N.; Wu, A.; De Saeger, S. Development and application of salting-out assisted liquid/liquid extraction for multi-mycotoxin biomarkers analysis in pig urine with high performance liquid chromatography/tandem mass spectrometry. *J. Chromatogr. A* **2013**, *1292*, 111–120. [CrossRef] [PubMed]
13. Thieu, N.Q.; Pettersson, H. Zearalenone, deoxynivalenol and aflatoxin B1 and their metabolites in pig urine as biomarkers for mycotoxin exposure. *Mycotox. Res.* **2009**, *25*, 59–66. [CrossRef] [PubMed]
14. European Commission. European Commission (EC) Commission Regulation 574/2011 of 16 June 2011 amending Annex I to Directive 2002/32/EC of the European Parliament and of the Council as regards maximum levels for nitrite, melamine, *Ambrosia* spp. and carry-over of certain coccidiostats and histomonostats and consolidating Annexes I and II thereto. *Off. J. Eur. Union* **2011**, *7*, L159.
15. Lindblad, M.; Gidlund, A.; Sulyok, M.; Börjesson, T.; Krska, R.; Olsen, M.; Fredlund, E. Deoxynivalenol and other selected Fusarium toxins in Swedish wheat—Occurrence and correlation to specific Fusarium species. *Int. J. Food Microbiol.* **2013**, *167*, 284–291. [CrossRef] [PubMed]
16. Fredlund, E.; Gidlund, A.; Sulyok, M.; Börjesson, T.; Krska, R.; Olsen, M.; Lindblad, M. Deoxynivalenol and other selected Fusarium toxins in Swedish oats—Occurrence and correlation to specific Fusarium species. *Int. J. Food Microbiol.* **2013**, *167*, 276–283. [CrossRef]
17. European Food Safety Authority (EFSA). Opinion of the scientific panel on contaminants in the food chain on a request from the commission related to aflatoxin B_1 as undesirable substance in animal feed. *EFSA J.* **2004**, *39*, 1–27.
18. Brezina, U.; Rempe, I.; Kersten, S.; Valenta, H.; Humpf, H.-U.; Dänicke, S. Diagnosis of intoxications of piglets fed with Fusarium toxin-contaminated maize by the analysis of mycotoxin residues in serum, liquor and urine with LC-MS/MS. *Arch. Anim. Nutr.* **2014**, *6*, 425–447. [CrossRef]
19. Dänicke, S.; Brüssow, K.P.; Valenta, H.; Ueberschär, K.H.; Tiemann, U. and Schollenberger, M. On the effects of graded levels of Fusarium toxin contaminated wheat in diets for gilts on feed intake, growth performance and metabolism of deoxynivalenol and zearalenone. *Mol. Nutr. Food Res.* **2005**, *49*, 932–943. [CrossRef]
20. Dänicke, S.; Goyarts, T.; Valenta, H.; Razzazi, E.; Bohm, J. On the effects of deoxynivalenol (DON) in pig feed on growth performance, nutrients utilization and DON metabolism. *J. Anim. Feed Sci.* **2004**, *13*, 539–556. [CrossRef]
21. Döll, S.; Dänicke, S.; Ueberschär, K.H.; Valenta, H.; Schnurrbusch, U.; Ganter, M.; Klobasa, F.; Flachowsky, G. Effects of graded levels of Fusarium toxin contaminated maize in diets for female weaned piglets. *Arch. Anim. Nutr.* **2003**, *57*, 311–334. [CrossRef]
22. Goyarts, T.; Dänicke, S. Bioavailability of the Fusarium toxin deoxynivalenol (DON) from naturally contaminated wheat for the pig. *Toxicol. Lett.* **2006**, *163*, 171–182. [CrossRef] [PubMed]
23. Lásztity, R.; Bata, Á.; Palyusyk, M. Investigation of the distribution of zearalenone and its metabolites in the pigs fed with feed contaminated by zearalenone. *Period. Polytech. Chem. Eng.* **1989**, *33*, 203–209.
24. Wallin, S.; Gambacorta, L.; Kotova, N.; Lemming, E.W.; Nälsén, C.; Solfrizzo, M.; Olsen, M. Biomonitoring of concurrent mycotoxin exposure among adults in Sweden through urinary multi-biomarker analysis. *Food Chem. Toxicol.* **2015**, *83*, 133–139. [CrossRef] [PubMed]
25. Solfrizzo, M.; Gambacorta, L.; Visconti, A. Assessment of Multi-Mycotoxin Exposure in Southern Italy by Urinary Multi-Biomarker Determination. *Toxins* **2014**, *6*, 523–538. [CrossRef]
26. Mazzachi, B.C.; Peake, M.J.; Ehrhardt, V. Reference range and method comparison studies for enzymatic and Jaffé creatinine assays in plasma and serum and early morning urine. *Clin. Lab.* **2000**, *46*, 53–55. [PubMed]
27. European Food Safety Authority (EFSA). Management of left-censored data in dietary exposure assessment of chemical substances. *EFSA J.* **2010**, *8*, 1557.

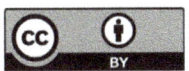

© 2019 by the authors. Licensee MDPI, Basel, Switzerland. This article is an open access article distributed under the terms and conditions of the Creative Commons Attribution (CC BY) license (http://creativecommons.org/licenses/by/4.0/).

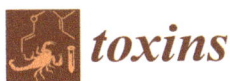

Review

In-Vitro Cell Culture for Efficient Assessment of Mycotoxin Exposure, Toxicity and Risk Mitigation

Ran Xu [1], Niel A. Karrow [1,*], Umesh K. Shandilya [1], Lv-hui Sun [2] and Haruki Kitazawa [3,4]

1. Department of Animal Biosciences, University of Guelph, Guelph, ON N1G 2W1, Canada; rxu02@uoguelph.ca (R.X.); ushand@uoguelph.ca (U.K.S.)
2. Department of Animal Nutrition and Feed Science, College of Animal Science and Technology, Huazhong Agricultural University, Wuhan 430070, China; lvhuisun@mail.hzau.edu.cn
3. Food and Feed Immunology Group, Laboratory of Animal Products Chemistry, Graduate School of Agricultural Science, Tohoku University, Sendai 980-8572, Japan; haruki.kitazawa.c7@tohoku.ac.jp
4. Livestock Immunology Unit, International Education and Research Center for Food and Agricultural Immunology (CFAI), Graduate School of Agricultural Science, Tohoku University, Sendai 980-8572, Japan
* Correspondence: nkarrow@uoguelph.ca; Tel.: +1-519-824-4120 (ext. 53646)

Received: 11 February 2020; Accepted: 25 February 2020; Published: 27 February 2020

Abstract: Mycotoxins are toxic secondary fungal metabolites that commonly contaminate crops and food by-products and thus, animal feed. Ingestion of mycotoxins can lead to mycotoxicosis in both animals and humans, and at subclinical concentrations may affect animal production and adulterate feed and animal by-products. Mycotoxicity mechanisms of action (MOA) are largely unknown, and co-contamination, which is often the case, raises the likelihood of mycotoxin interactions. Mitigation strategies for reducing the risk of mycotoxicity are diverse and may not necessarily provide protection against all mycotoxins. These factors, as well as the species-specific risk of toxicity, collectively make an assessment of exposure, toxicity, and risk mitigation very challenging and costly; thus, in-vitro cell culture models provide a useful tool for their initial assessment. Since ingestion is the most common route of mycotoxin exposure, the intestinal epithelial barrier comprised of epithelial cells (IECs) and immune cells such as macrophages, represents ground zero where mycotoxins are absorbed, biotransformed, and elicit toxicity. This article aims to review different in-vitro IEC or co-culture models that can be used for assessing mycotoxin exposure, toxicity, and risk mitigation, and their suitability and limitations for the safety assessment of animal foods and food by-products.

Keywords: mycotoxins; in-vitro cell culture; toxicity assessment and mitigation

Key Contribution: This article reviews previous studies assessing *Fusarium* and *Penicillium* mycotoxin exposure, toxicity, and risk mitigation using a range of intestinal epithelial cell (IEC) and immune cell models cultured in different systems that can be used as efficient in vitro models of in vivo intestinal barrier microenvironment, considering their suitability and limitations.

1. Introduction

Mycotoxins are toxic secondary metabolites produced by filamentous fungi that predominantly belong to species from the *Aspergillus, Fusarium,* and *Penicillium* genera. Over 500 different classes of mycotoxins have been discovered, many of which have unknown mechanisms of action (MOA) [1]. Ingestion of mycotoxins can lead to mycotoxicosis in both animals and humans, and at subclinical concentrations may affect animal production and adulterate food animal by-products. These toxic compounds of global concern are commonly detected as contaminants in a variety of commodities of plant origin, especially cereal grains, and are therefore often detected in animal feeds. Mycotoxins can also be found in animal-derived products such as meat, eggs, milk, and milk derivatives due to their carry-over from animals that have consumed contaminated feeds [2–4]. Natural co-occurrence of mycotoxins with potential additive, antagonistic, or synergistic effects more commonly occurs in foods and feeds than single mycotoxin contaminants [5]. Mycotoxins inflict high annual economic losses worldwide due to condemned agricultural commodities as well as reduced animal and human health [6]. Weather conditions associated with climate change have been predicted to favor more fungal contamination of foods and feeds as temperature and moisture are major factors influencing fungal growth and mycotoxin production [2,7]. Global trade of food and feed commodities contributes to the worldwide dispersal of mycotoxins [5].

A wealth of toxicity and mechanistic studies have been conducted on mycotoxins at the cellular level using kidney cells and blood lymphocytes [5,8], as well as animal performance studies [9]. However, the effects of mycotoxins on the intestine should be more thoroughly considered and assessed for the following reasons. Firstly, the intestinal epithelium is the initial site of exposure following the ingestion of mycotoxins and the first physical barrier that limits their entry into the animal [10]; damage to this barrier could also facilitate entry of luminal microbes, antigens, and other food contaminants. Secondly, the intestinal mucosa possesses the largest single compartment of the immune system underlying the epithelial lining [11]. Collectively, the gut-associated lymphoid system and intestinal epithelial cells (IECs) forming the intestinal barrier cross-talk with each other to maintain homeostasis of both the intestine and the immune system to elicit an appropriate immune response during microbial infection and to repair damaged tissues [10,12–15]. Mycotoxin exposure could render this important immunological barrier dysfunctional and this, combined with disrupted physical barrier function, could increase host susceptibility to disease. Thirdly, IECs are equipped with metabolizing enzymes and protein pumps that regulate absorption and biotransformation of xenobiotics as well as the possible efflux of metabolites back to the intestinal lumen. Mycotoxins may be able to alter the expression and activity of IEC proteins involved in absorption, efflux, and biotransformation [16], which could compromise their ability to regulate the bioavailability of other xenobiotics and nutrients. A fourth reason is that IECs may be repeatedly exposed to high concentrations of mycotoxins, which could increase the likelihood of impairment to the intestinal barrier function [17,18]. Specifically, after absorption by IECs, mycotoxins such as Ochratoxin A (OTA) and zearalenone (ZEA) could be returned to intestinal lumen either by IECs through efflux proteins, or via bile after undergoing entero-hepatic circulation [10,16,19,20]. This recirculation could result in the reabsorption of mycotoxins and prolonged exposure of IECs at the intestinal barrier, which could increase the risk of mycotoxins interacting with each other and other xenobiotics [5,21]. A fifth reason is that IECs undergo continuous renewal in order to maintain barrier function, and a number of mycotoxins are known to inhibit protein synthesis [22,23], which could impair the renewal process. A sixth reason is a potential interaction between mycotoxins and gut microbiota. Rumen and intestinal microflora are able to metabolically inactivate certain mycotoxins [9,24], however, some mycotoxins that exhibit antimicrobial activity may reduce detoxification efficiency [25–27]. Since the intestinal microbiota also contributes to intestinal barrier function, immune system development, and mediates the production of neurotransmitters associated with brain function [28–30], disrupted intestinal microbial populations could also potentially impair gut–immune and gut–brain communication.

The effects of various mycotoxins on the intestinal mucosal components have been studied both in-vivo and in-vitro. Since in-vitro cell culture models provide a cost-effective and high throughput means for the initial screening and assessment of mycotoxins, and mitigation approaches, this review will provide a summary of in vitro studies that have been carried out on individual and combined mycotoxins acting on the intestinal epithelial and gut immunological barrier using IEC and immune cell models, and explore different in-vitro IEC or co-culture models and their suitability and limitations for assessing mycotoxin exposure. The mycotoxins most commonly addressed in this review include deoxynivalenol (DON), ZEA, aflatoxin B1 (AFB1), citrinin (CIT), OTA, and mycophenolic acid (MPA) in terms of their prevalence, toxicity, and occurrence of pre- and post-harvest in animal feeds. The review also summarizes the in-vitro assessment of mycotoxin detoxifying agents (i.e. mycotoxin binders and modifiers) as feed additives that are widely used in the animal feed industry to mitigate the risk of exposure. Lastly, this review points out the need for co-culture models that are better able to more physiologically and immunologically reflect the intestinal mucosa to better assess the effects of mycotoxins on the intestine.

2. Mycotoxins

Mycotoxins are structurally diverse low-molecular-weight metabolites that are chemically and thermally stable [10,31]. The three most predominant mycotoxin-producing fungi species *Aspergillus*, *Fusarium*, and *Penicillium* can be classified as either field (*Fusarium* spp.) or storage fungi (*Aspergillus* spp. and *Penicillium* spp.) [32]; field fungi produce mycotoxins (DON and ZEA) prior to harvest [33,34], while storage fungi initially colonize plants prior to harvest and continue to grow and produce mycotoxins (AFB1, CIT, OTA, and MPA) under improper grain and silage storage conditions that favor fungal development and mycotoxin production [33,35–37].

DON is one of the most commonly detected mycotoxins in cereal crops such as wheat, corn, barley, and rye [38]. Various organ systems can be the targets of DON. Ingestion, for example, causes nausea and vomiting through interactions with the neural dopaminergic system; because of this, DON is also referred to as vomitoxin [39–41]. The immune system is another target for DON; at high concentrations, DON is an immunosuppressant, whereas, at lower concentrations, DON may stimulate the immune system [39,42]. DON also induces caspase-mediated apoptosis via activation of MAPK signaling pathways [39]. One MOA of DON includes disruption of protein translation via binding to the 60S ribosomal subunit of peptidyl transferase [43].

ZEA is another major mycotoxin produced by various *Fusarium* species. ZEA is classified as an estrogenic mycotoxin because it resembles human 17β-estradiol and binds to and activates estrogen receptors expressed mainly within the reproductive system. ZEA has been shown to also be immunotoxic, hepatotoxic, hematotoxic, and genotoxic, which may be partially attributed to ZEA contributing to oxidative DNA damage and cellular apoptosis induced by the production of reactive oxygen species [44–49].

Aflatoxins are produced mainly by species of *Aspergillus flavus* and *Aspergillus parasiticus* [50]. AFB1 is the most potent member of the aflatoxin family based on its well-characterized carcinogenicity leading to hepatocellular carcinoma in both humans and animals [51]. It also causes malnutrition, suppresses growth, and modulates immune function [52]. The formation of DNA adducts and the ability to cause oxidative damage might contribute to AFB1 cytotoxicity and carcinogenicity [53].

CIT is produced predominantly by *Penicillium* spp. [38]. Several species of *Aspergillus* and *Monascus* are also producers of CIT [36,38]. CIT naturally contaminates a variety of foods and feeds such as nuts, grains, barley, wheat, and corn, mainly during storage [6], and has been shown to be nephrotoxic in all tested animal species [38]. CIT genotoxicity is controversial, showing both positive and negative results using various in-vitro systems [54–56].

OTA is produced by *Penicillium* spp. and various *Aspergillus* spp., and it is the most prominent among the family of ochratoxins [57]. OTA has been found to contaminate cereals and cereal by-products such as wheat, rye and barley [10,38], and has been detected in animal products including pork and milk [58]. OTA is a nephrotoxin to all animal species including humans [3,59–61]. OTA has also been shown to be a teratogen, hepatotoxin, immunosuppressant, and carcinogen in various animal species including humans [62,63]. The number of MOAs by which OTA interferes with cellular functions has been determined. OTA inhibits protein synthesis through inhibiting phenylalanyl-tRNA synthetase, thus phenylalanine metabolism. Mitochondria are also targeted by OTA through inhibiting ATP production and inducing the production of reactive oxygen and nitrogen species. OTA also disrupts cell-cycle progression by targeting the cyclin–CDK system, disrupting mitosis, and causing chromosomal instability [64–70]. Lastly, OTA can also induce DNA adducts, particularly deoxyguanosine (dG) adducts [67,71,72].

The mycotoxin MPA is produced by *Penicillium roqueforti* fungi, which is a main silage spoiler and the most prevalent post-harvest fungi found in forage silages due to its capacity to grow in low-oxygen and high carbon dioxide as well as acidic and cold environmental conditions [37,73–78]. MPA is one of the "emerging" mycotoxins that are being detected in feedstuffs. It is frequently detected in forages, particularly silage [79]. MPA is able to inhibit B and T lymphocyte proliferation and inhibit the production of cytotoxic T cells [80,81]. MPA also exhibits antibacterial, antifungal, antitumor, and antiviral properties [80,82]. However, MPA's immunosuppressive properties may increase the susceptibility of exposed animals to infectious diseases and sensitivity to other mycotoxins [83], and MPA's antimicrobial properties could disrupt the normal function of the microflora in ruminants, including the detoxication of other *Penicillium* mycotoxins [84,85]

3. The Intestinal Barrier

3.1. Physical Barrier

The intestine forms a physical barrier between the microbial-rich luminal environment and sterile internal host tissues [86]. This selectively permeable barrier allows for the exchange of nutrients and antigens, while preventing the penetration of opportunistic commensal and pathogenic microorganisms and their toxins into host tissues [87,88]. The intestinal barrier consists of an external "physical" barrier mainly formed by mucous-coated IECs, and an underlying functional "immunological" barrier [13,89]. Collectively, these barriers communicate and interact with each other to maintain intestinal barrier function and optimize the outcome of the host defense against microbial infection [13,89].

The intestinal physical barrier is made up of a variety of polarized IECs. Five major specialized mucosal IEC lineages have been found to differentiate from multipotential stem cells located at the base of the intestinal crypts of Lieberkühn; these include enterocytes, which are the most abundant IECs [13,90], goblet cells, enteroendocrine cells, Paneth cells, and microfold (M) cells. These specialized IECs reside in different proportions at different locations along the epithelium and carry out different functions. Goblet cells contribute to intestinal physical barrier function by secreting mucus containing mucin proteins; these mucins help prevent attachment of commensal and pathogenic bacteria to the intestinal epithelium [91]. Intercellular junctions, including tight junctions (TJs) and adhesion molecules, connect adjacent IECs to maintain physical barrier function. The TJs are the major functional elements that seal the paracellular spaces; thus, they play a key role in regulating the flow of ions and small molecules and in preventing fluid leaking between the lumen and underlying tissues [92,93]. TJs are composed of transmembrane proteins and cytoplasmic scaffold proteins. The transmembrane proteins, whose extracellular domains horizontally cross the plasma membrane of adjacent cells, including occludin (OCLN), the claudin protein family (CLDNs), and the junctional adhesion molecules marvel D3, and tricellulin [92]. The cytoplasmic scaffold proteins are intracellular TJs that link the actin cytoskeleton to transmembrane TJs, and the zonula occludin proteins (ZOs) are an important group [92].

Commensal microbiota residing within the intestine can also contribute to the intestinal barrier function by competitively excluding attachment sites and nutrients from pathogenic microorganisms [13]. The commensal barrier is beyond the scope of this review; however, it is worth noting that commensal microorganisms can become opportunistic pathogens when the intestinal barrier function is compromised [94,95].

3.2. Immunological Barrier

3.2.1. IECs and Intraepithelial Lymphocytes (IELs)

The intestine also possesses a functional innate and acquired immunological barrier that provides localized defense when potentially harmful luminal microorganisms, or their toxins, penetrate the host epithelial barrier. In addition to their physical barrier function discussed above, differentially specialized IECs are an important component of the host innate immune system and are considered the first line of defense provided by the immunological barrier [96]. Paneth cells, for example, are specialized secretory cells that produce large amounts of antimicrobial peptides and proteins such as β-defensins and cathelicidin, and antimicrobial enzymes such as lysozyme [96,97]. Enterocytes, in addition to their specialized role in digestion and nutrient absorption, can also serve as luminal sensors for the immune system since they possess large numbers of pattern-recognition receptors (PRRs) that are expressed both on the cell surface and within the cell. These PRRs recognize conserved structure molecules displayed on the surface of bacteria, fungi, parasites, and viruses that are referred to as pathogen-associated molecular patterns [13,15,98]. Membrane PRRs include the Toll-like receptors (TLRs), and cytoplasmic PRRs include the NOD-like receptors such as NOD1 and NOD2 [99,100]. In addition to producing mucus, goblet cells also have the capacity to take up luminal material and present antigens to dendritic cells in the lamina propria [91,101,102].

Interspersed amongst the IECs lining the epithelium are highly abundant long-living intraepithelial lymphocytes (IELs); the estimated IEL to IEC ratio in the human small intestine is 1:10 [103]. These motile cells have diverse lineages, but the majority can be broadly classified as either "unconventional" IELs that contribute to the innate immunological barrier, or "conventional" IELs that contribute to the acquired immunological barrier. Regardless of the lineage, IELs possess cytotoxic and immunoregulatory properties that are key to regulating homeostatic crosstalk between the innate and acquired immunological barriers and commensal microbiota, and their dysfunction has been implicated in gastrointestinal disease [104].

3.2.2. Lamina Propria

The subepithelial lamina propria is the site were effector immune cells of the intestinal immune system can be found [105], these include numerous innate immune cells such as macrophages ($M_\emptyset$) and innate lymphoid cells (ILCs) and the acquired immune lymphoid B and T cells [105]. The intestine is known to represent the largest pool of tissue $M_\emptyset$ in the body [106,107]. These $M_\emptyset$ are innate immune effectors with potent phagocytic and bactericidal activities [11,96,108], but unlike other macrophage populations, they inflict minimal inflammatory collateral tissue damage [13,96]. This distinct property could be ascribed to high expression of phagocytosis-promoting genes such as Mertk, Cd206, Gas6, Axl, Cd36, Itgav, and Itgb5 [109,110], as well as low or lack of expression of receptors associated with innate immune activation, such as receptors for LPS (CD14), Fcα (CD89), Fcγ (CD64, CD32, and CD16), CR3 (CD11b/CD18), and CR4 (CD11c/CD18) [108]. This special functional adaption of resident intestinal $M_\emptyset$ allows them to maintain local tissue homeostasis in part by preventing excessive immune reactions to commensal microbiota and food antigens that might otherwise elicit chronic inflammation and tissue damage [111]. Resident intestinal $M_\emptyset$ also efficiently remove apoptotic cells and foreign debris and contribute to the repair and remodeling of damaged tissues [112,113]. Collectively, these unique properties ascribe intestinal $M_\emptyset$ to the maintenance of intestinal homeostasis [112,113].

In addition to $M_\emptyset$, a large population of ILCs is also located within lamina propria [114]. This mixed population of ILCs can be classified based on their cytokines and transcription factors, including natural killer cells, ILC1, ILC2, or ILC3 [115–118]; respectively, these ILCs are phenotypically and functionally similar to the T helper (T_H) cell subpopulations T_H1, T_H2, and T_H17 [114]. These ILCs have cytotoxic and immunoregulatory properties that allow them to rapidly respond to and orchestrate the host response against gastrointestinal threats and also maintain epithelial integrity and tissue homeostasis [119].

A number of acquired lymphoid cell populations are also found within the subepithelial lamina propria. Both conventional $CD4^+$ and $CD8^+$ T cells are found and they perform immunoregulatory and cytotoxic activities, respectively [105,120,121]. Immunoglobulin (IgA)-producing B1 cells are also present [105]; the IgA antibodies produced by their differentiated plasma cells are selectively transported across the epithelium into the intestinal lumen where it helps to prevent microbial invasion by decreasing their motility and adhesion to the surface of the epithelium [122,123].

3.2.3. Gut-Associated Lymphoid Tissue (GALT) and Mesenteric Lymph Nodes (MLNs)

A series of events must occur in order for the above-mentioned acquired lymphoid cells to become activated and drive an acquired immune response. M cells must sample and transfer luminal antigens and intact microorganisms to underlying $M_\emptyset$ and dendritic cells, which then migrate the Peyer's patches (PP) of the gut-associated lymphoid tissues (GALT) and/or draining mesenteric lymph nodes (MLN) where they convene with T_H cells to carry out antigen presentation. Although the events are less well characterized in the PP than MLN, it is believed they are analogous [124]; in short, antigen-specific T_H cells become activated during antigen presentation, and then can assist with the activation of antigen-specific B cells, which clonally expand within germinal centers and differentiate into IgA secreting plasma cells.

3.3. Cross-Talk between IECs and Immune Cells

Bidirectional communication between IECs and immune cells facilitates protection from microbial invasion, tissue homeostasis, and repair. This cross-talk is mediated in part by secreted cytokines [12–15], many of which are commonly produced by immune cells and IECs [10,14]. Some of these cytokines include TGF-α, IL-1, IL-10, IL-15, IL-8, IL-1α, and β, IL-6, TNF-α, MCP-1, CCL20, and GM-CSF [14,125]. IECs also possess receptors for various cytokines, which allows them to respond to immune cell signals. For example, it has been reported that goblet cell mucus production and properties can be directly affected by IL-10 produced by $M_\emptyset$ and T-cells within the lamina propria [126]. The expression of IEC TJ proteins can also be inhibited by TNF-α, IFN-γ, and the interleukins IL-2, IL-4, and IL-8, which results in increased gut paracellular permeability [127]. Also, the binding of IL-1 to its receptor on IECs amplifies the secretion of IEC pro-inflammatory cytokines [128].

4. In-vitro Intestinal Epithelial Barrier Models

Although primary cells are most biologically and physiologically similar to the gastrointestinal epithelial barrier, their short-life span and rapid loss of differentiated characteristics limit their use for in vitro studies [129,130]. Instead, immortalized cell lines of animal and human origin including Caco-2, IPEC-1, and IPEC-J2 IECs have been extensively utilized as in vitro models of the intestinal epithelium to study the effects of mycotoxins on intestinal barrier function. These cell lines have been used at various differentiation states, proliferative versus differentiated, for example, to simulate different intestinal microenvironments [131,132]. Undifferentiated IECs present as a tumorigenic phenotype and do not display cell polarity [131,133]; they also appear similar to dividing cells in tissue undergoing regeneration or repair after damage [132,134]. In contrast, differentiated cells mimic the mature small intestinal barrier in that they have defined epithelial characteristics such as TJs and microvilli, which are lacking in undifferentiated cells [135].

4.1. Caco-2

Human Caco-2 cells have been the most widely used IEC line in recent decades [136]; Caco-2 is a cancer-derived cell line originally isolated from a human colon adenocarcinoma [137]. However, once differentiated after 18–21 days of culture post-confluence, they become a homogenously polarized monolayer of enterocyte-like cells with apical and basolateral membranes, a brush border with microvilli and TJs [138–141]. Caco-2 cells have also been shown to express TLRs and produce various cytokines [140,142].

4.2. IPEC-1 and IPEC-J2

IPEC-1 and IPEC-J2 are two other IEC lines that have been used as in vitro models of the intestinal barrier. Both IPEC lines were derived from the porcine small intestine. IPECs are spontaneously immortalized non-transformed and non-carcinoma cell lines, established from normal IECs [143,144]. IPEC-1 was derived from the jejunum and ileum of piglets less than 12 hours old. The IPEC-J2 cell line was originally isolated from the jejunum of neonatal unsuckled pigs [139,143,145]. Both IPECs are able to spontaneously differentiate into multiple IEC types [139], and a continuous polarized monolayer and TJ structure can be formed after differentiation [144]. Compared to Caco-2, the IPEC-1 and IPEC-J2 IECs attain a homogenous appearance and express various differentiation markers within a shorter period of time; within 10 days and 1–2 weeks of culturing post-confluence, respectively [143,146], and the IPEC-J2 line is more morphologically and functionally differentiated than the IPEC-1 line [144]. Since the pig intestine closely resembles the human intestine genetically and physiologically, IPECs have been used to model the human intestinal barrier [129,144].

4.3. In-vitro Cell Culture Systems

In vitro models of the intestinal epithelial barrier have traditionally consisted of one-dimensional (1D) monolayers grown on the surface of culture vessels. With this 1D culture system, functional IEC characteristics, such as cell polarity, are not well defined [147], and misleading results can possibly be obtained. Alternatively, a two-dimensional (2D) monoculture system can be achieved by growing IECs on microporous permeable membrane supports [148,149]; this system structurally mimics the apical and basolateral sides of the intestine and leads to the development of polarized IECs. Most reviewed cytotoxicity studies (Table 1) have been conducted using a 1D monoculture system and the 2D monoculture system has been extensively applied to study the effects of mycotoxins on intestinal barrier function parameters such as transepithelial electrical resistance (TEER) and TJ protein expression.

More complex 1D and 2D co-culture systems that are more physically and functionally similar to the intestinal barrier have also been established. These co-culture systems involve cultivating more than one cell type together within one culture system [129,150,151]. The IEC + immune cell co-culture system involving permeable membrane supports is one such established 2D co-culture model [140].

Table 1. Summary of effects of individual mycotoxins on intestinal epithelial cell (IEC) viability.

Mycotoxin	IEC model	Exposure Duration	Tested Exposure Concentration	Cytotoxicity Assay	LC50/Effective Concentration (ECs)	References
DON	Caco-2 (differentiated)	24 h	0, 1.39, 4.17, 12.5, 37.5 µM	LDH release	EC: 37.5 µM	[152]
	Caco-2	48 h	0, 0.05, 0.1, 0.3, 0.5, 1, 3, 5, 10 µM	Luminescent Cell Viability Assay	LC50 =1.3 uM; EC: 0.5–10µM	[153]
	Caco-2	24 h	0, 0.25, 1, 2.5, 5, 10 µM	MTS Assay	LC50 = 10 µM	[154]
				Neutral Red	LC50 = 3.7 µM	
		72 h	0, 0.25, 1, 2.5, 5, 10 µM	MTS Assay	LC50 = 4.3 µM	
				Neutral Red	LC50 = 3.7 µM	
	Caco-2 (differentiated)	24 h	0, 0.25, 1, 2.5, 5, 10 µM	MTS Assay	LC50 > 10 µM	[154]
				Neutral Red	LC50 > 10 µM	
		72 h	0, 0.25, 1, 2.5, 5, 10 µM	MTS Assay	LC50 > 10 µM	
				Neutral Red	LC50 > 10 µM	
	Caco-2	72 h	1–150 µM	Neutral Red	LC50 = 21.5 µM; EC: 10 µM	[155]
				MTT Assay	LC50 = 25 µM; EC: 10 µM	
	Caco-2	24 h	0, 0.001, 0.01, 0.1, 1, 10, 25, 50, 100 µM	CCK-8	LC50 = 21.94 µM	[156]
		48 h			LC50 = 9.39 µM	
		72 h			LC50 = 6.18 µM	
	IPEC-1	24 h	0, 0.34, 0.67, 1.7, 3.4, 6.7 10.2, 13.4 µM	MTT Assay	EC: 1.7, 3.4, 10.2, 13.4 µM	
		48 h			EC: 0.34 µM; 1.7–13.4 µM	
		72 h			EC: 0.34 µM; 1.7- 13.4 µM	
	IPEC-1 (in serum-free media)	24 h	0, 0.67, 6.7 µM	LDH release	NA	[143]
		48 h			EC: 6.7 µM	
		72 h			EC: 6.7 µM	
	IPEC-1 (in complete media)	24 h	0, 0.67, 6.7 µM	Neutral Red	EC: 0.67, 6.7 µM	
		48 h			EC: 6.7 µM	
		72 h			EC: 6.7 µM	

Table 1. Cont.

Mycotoxin	IEC model	Exposure Duration	Tested Exposure Concentration	Cytotoxicity Assay	LC50/Effective Concentration (ECs)	References
	IPEC-1 (in serum-free media)	24 h	0, 0.67, 6.7 µM	Neutral Red	EC: 0.67, 6.7 µM	
		48 h			EC: 6.7 µM	
		72 h			EC: 6.7 µM	
	IPEC-J2	24 h	0, 0.34, 0.67, 1.7, 3.4, 6.7 10.2, 13.4 µM	MTT Assay	EC: 0.34, 3.4, 6.7, 13.4 µM	[143]
		48 h			EC: 1.7–13.4 µM	
		72 h			EC: 1.7–13.4 µM	
		14 d	0, 0.17, 0.34, 0.67, 1.02, 1.34, 1.7 µM		0.67, 1.02, 1.34, 1.7 µM	
	IPEC-J2	24 h	0, 0.67, 6.7 µM	LDH release	NA	[143]
		48 h			EC: 6.7 µM	
		72 h			NA	
	IPEC-J2	24 h	0, 0.67, 6.7 µM	Neutral Red	EC: 0.67, 6.7 µM	[143]
		48 h			EC: 6.7 µM	
		72 h			EC: 6.7 µM	
	IPEC-J2 (in serum-free media)	24 h	0, 0.67, 6.7 µM	Neutral Red	EC: 0.67, 6.7 µM	[143]
		48 h			EC: 6.7 µM	
		72 h			EC: 6.7 µM	
	IPEC-J2 (basolateral)	24 h	0, 0.67, 1.7, 6.7, 13.4 µM	DAPI staining	NA	[157]
		48 h			EC: 6.7, 13.4 µM	
		72 h			EC: 6.7, 13.4 µM	
	IPEC-J2	24 h	0, 0.034, 0.085, 0.17, 0.34, 0.85, 1.7, 3.4, 17, 34 µM	Neutral Red	EC: 0.85–34 µM	[132]
	IPEC-J2	72 h	0, 3.4, 8.5, 17, 25.5, 34 µM	Annexin-V-FITC/ PI	EC: 8.5–34 µM	[158]
	IPEC-J2	72 h	0, 3.4, 17, 34, 51, 67 µM	Annexin-V-FITC/ PI	LC50 = 10.47 µM	[159]
	IPEC-J2 (differentiated)	72 h	0, 3.4, 17, 34, 51, 67 µM	Annexin-V-FITC/ PI	LC50 = 46.9 µM	[159]
	IPEC-J2	6 h	0, 0.67, 6.7 µM	CCK-8 Assay	EC: 0.67, 6.7 µM	[160]
		12 h				
		24 h				
		48 h				
		72 h				
	IPEC-J2	48 h	0, 0.25, 0.5, 1, 2 µM	MTT Assay	LC50 = 1.83 µM; EC: 1–2 µM	[161]
	IPEC-J2	24 h	0, 0.43, 0.85, 1.7, 3.4, 6.7 µM	CCK-8 Assay	EC: 0.85–6.7 µM	[162]
ZEA	Caco-2	72 h	1–150 µM	Neutral Red	LC50 = 15 µM	[155]
				MTT Assay	LC50 = 25 µM	
	Caco-2	24 h	0, 0.001, 0.01, 0.1, 1, 10, 25, 50, 100 µM	CCK-8	LC50 = 62.67 µM	[156]
		48 h			LC50 = 56.96 µM	
		72 h			LC50 = 34.36 µM	
	IPEC-1	24 h	0, 0.1, 1, 10, 100 µM	XTT Assay	EC: 100 µM	[163]
	IPEC-1	24 h	0, 0.1, 1, 10, 100 µM	XTT Assay	EC: 100 µM	[164]
			0, 0.1, 1, 10, 100 µM	Neutral Red	EC: 100 µM	
	IPEC-J2	48 h	0, 5, 10, 20, 40 µM	MTT Assay	EC: 10, 40 µM	[161]
	IPEC-J2	48 h	0, 15.5, 31, 62, 124, 248 µM	MTT Assay	LC50 = 62.1 µM; EC: 62–248 µM	[46]
	IPEC-J2	72 h	0, 19.9, 39.8, 44.73, 59.7, 79.6, 99.5 µM	Annexin-V-FITC/PI	EC: 44.73–99.5 µM	[158]
AFB1	Caco-2	24 h	0, 0.032, 0.16, 0.32, 1.6, 3.2 µM	MTT Assay	EC: 3.2 µM	[165]
		48 h			EC: 0.32—3.2 µM	
		72 h			EC: 1.6–3.2 µM	
	Caco-2 (differentiated)	24 h	0, 0.032, 0.16, 0.32, 1.6, 3.2 µM	MTT Assay	EC: 1.6 µM	[165]
		48 h			EC: 1.6–3.2 µM	
		72 h			EC: 0.16–3.2 µM	
	Caco-2	24 h	0, 0.032, 0.16, 0.32, 1.6, 3.2 µM	LDH release	EC: 1.6–3.2 µM	[165]
		48 h			EC: 0.32–3.2 µM	
		72 h			EC: 0.32–3.2 µM	

Table 1. Cont.

Mycotoxin	IEC model	Exposure Duration	Tested Exposure Concentration	Cytotoxicity Assay	LC50/Effective Concentration (ECs)	References
	Caco-2 (differentiated)	24 h	0, 0.032, 0.16, 0.32, 1.6, 3.2 µM	LDH release	EC: 3.2 µM	[165]
		48 h			EC: 0.032–3.2 µM	
		72 h			EC: 0.032–3.2 µM	
	Caco-2	24 h	0, 1, 3, 10, 30, 100 µM	MTT Assay	LC50 = 5.39 µM; EC: 1–100 µM	[166]
				LDH release	LC50 = 10 µM; EC: 3–100 µM	
	Caco-2	24 h	0–100 µM	Neutral Red	LC50 = 10 µM	[167]
		48 h			LC50 = 2 µM	
		72 h			LC50 = 0.75 µM	
CIT	Caco-2	48 h	0, 399.6, 999 µM	Crystal Violet staining (CVS)	EC: 399.6, 999 µM	[168]
	HCT116	36 h	0, 75, 150, 300 µM	Fluorescein diacetate (FDA) staining	LC50 = 300 µM; EC: 150–300 µM	[169]
MPA	Caco-2	48 h	0, 0.0078, 0.078, 0.78, 7.8, 78, 780 µM	MTS Assay	LC50 > 780 uM	[75]
	Caco-2 (differentiated)					
OTA	Caco-2	24 h	0, 1, 3, 10, 30, 100 µM	MTT Assay	LC50 = 21.25 µM; EC: 1–100 µM	[166]
				LDH release	LC50 = 16.85 µM; EC: 1–100 µM	
	Caco-2	24 h	1–200 µM	MTT Assay	LC50 = 145.36 µM	[170]

5. Effects of Selected Mycotoxins on Intestinal Barrier Function

5.1. Cytotoxic Effects of Individual or Combined Mycotoxins on IECs

5.1.1. Individual Mycotoxins

The cytotoxicity of selected mycotoxins has been evaluated using various IEC models on the basis of cell viability (Table 1) as well as proliferation at different concentrations and exposure durations. Mycotoxin cytotoxicity is usually the first parameter to be measured, not only to evaluate the cytotoxicity, but also to identify appropriate mycotoxin concentrations that can be used in follow-up experiments of intestinal barrier function.

The cytotoxicity of DON on different IEC models has been the most studied among the five reviewed mycotoxins. Results using various IEC models including Caco-2, IPEC-1, and IPEC-J2 have shown that DON induces cell death at various concentrations and under different durations of exposure (Table 1). A wide range of DON exposure concentrations have been used, ranging from as low as 0.0001 up to 100 µM [156].

A variety of cytotoxicity assays have been applied to assess the cell viability (Table 1) and tetrazolium salt MTT (3-[4,5-dimethylthiazol-2-yl]-2,5-diphenyltetrazolium bromide) was most widely used in the reviewed studies, which was shown to be a quick and suitable assay to detect a wide range of mycotoxins for different cell types [171]. In order to avoid false results, more than one cytotoxicity assay has been applied in parallel in some studies, and both similar and discrepant results have been reported [143,154,164]. The 3-(4,5-dimethylthiazol-2-yl)-5-(3-carboxymethoxyphenyl)-2-(4-sulfophenyl)-2H-tetrazolium, inner salt (MTS), and Neutral Red (NR) assays have been reported to yield similar cell viability results based on Caco-2 cell viability after 24 h DON exposure [154]. The authors in [164] observed similar cell viability results from the 2,3-Bis-(2-Methoxy-4-Nitro-5-Sulfophenyl)-2HTetrazolium-5-Carboxanilide (XTT) and NR assays in IPEC-1 cells. However, [143] reported that the lactate dehydrogenase (LDH) leakage assay was less sensitive to DON toxicity compared to the NR assay using both IPEC cell lines. Interestingly, the route of application, apical versus the basolateral side of IECs, appears to influence DON-mediate changes in cell viability, as IPEC-J2 cell viability was more significantly affected when DON is applied to the basolateral side [157]. This differential susceptibility of apical and basolateral surfaces of IECs to DON exposure could be attributed to their biological and functional distinctions such as different protein and lipid compositions [172]. It could also result from the addition of the mucus produced by IPEC-J2 cells covering the apical side of epithelial monolayer [139] as an extra defense line against DON exposure.

The differentiation status of cells may also influence sensitivity to DON exposure. It has been reported that dividing IPEC-J2 and Caco-2 cells, for example, are both more susceptible to DON than their differentiated counterparts [132,154,159]. Differentiation status is typically defined by cell culture duration in some of the reviewed cytotoxicity studies. For example, Caco-2 cells and IPEC-J2 grown on microplates without membrane inserts less than 4 days after seeding were considered undifferentiated, whereas, cells cultured at least 17 days post-seeding were considered differentiated [153,154].

Cell death has been reported to be induced by DON via both apoptosis and necrosis. Caspase 3, a marker for induction of apoptosis, was activated only at a high concentration of DON (6.7 µM) in both IPEC-1 and IPEC-J2 cell lines indicating DON-induced apoptosis [143]. However, necrosis-induced cell death was observed in both differentiated and undifferentiated IPEC-J2 cells after 72 h exposure to DON (0–67 µM) and it was found that the proportion of necrotic cells was concentration-dependent [158,159].

ZEA has also been reported to have adverse effects on IPEC-1, IPEC-J2, and Caco-2 cell viability at various concentrations after different exposure durations (Table 1). ZEA is less toxic than DON based on viability studies performed by [156,161]. ZEA appears to induce apoptosis via mitochondrial damage by reducing antioxidant enzyme activities; this may lead to an accumulation of ROS and decreased mitochondrial membrane potential [46]. Necrosis-induced cell death in undifferentiated and differentiated IPEC-J2 cells was also observed after 72 h of exposure to ZEA at 19.9–99.5 µM [158].

AFB1 induced a concentration-dependent decrease in the viability of both undifferentiated and differentiated Caco-2 cells between 24 h and 72 h of exposure [165]. In contrast to DON, the differentiated Caco-2 cells were found to be more susceptible to AFB1 than undifferentiated cells after 72 h of exposure, which could be due to more metabolic and transport enzymes being expressed by the differentiated mature enterocytes [165]. A similar concentration-dependent decrease in Caco-2 cell viability was also observed by [166] after 24 h exposure to a range of AFB1 concentrations (0–100 µM) with LC50s reported to be 5.39 and 6.02 µM obtained from MTT and LDH assays, respectively. AFB1 LC50s obtained from NR assay have also been reported by [167] after Caco-2 cells were exposed to AFB1 (0–100 µM) for 24, 48, and 72 h, which were 10, 2, and 0.5 µM, respectively.

Limited results have been reported on the effects of CIT, MPA, and OTA on cell viability compared to DON and ZEA. CIT has been reported to reduce human HCT116 colon cancer cell viability after 36 h exposure at concentrations of 150 and 300 µM, with the identified LC50 being 300 µM [169]. Authors in [168] reported that CIT exposure also resulted in a decrease in Caco-2 cell viability at 399.6 and 999 µM after 48 h exposure. Cell apoptosis was induced by CIT via endoplasmic reticulum stress [169]. Concerning MPA, [75] reported a concentration-dependent cytotoxic effect of MPA after 48 h exposure in both undifferentiated and differentiated Caco-2 cells, however, LC50 was not obtained with the tested concentration range. However, based on the LC20 calculated in the study, undifferentiated Caco-2 cells appeared to be more susceptible to MPA than differentiated cells [75]. Lastly, the cytotoxic effect of OTA was concentration-dependent, and two LC50s have been reported for the Caco-2 cell line after 24 h of OTA exposure using MTT and LDH assays; these were 21.25 and 16.85 µM, respectively [166]. However, a significantly different OTA LC50 of 145.36 µM was recently reported after 24 h of exposure using Caco-2 cells [170].

Mycotoxins have also been reported to affect cell cycle progression and proliferation. The proliferation of IPEC-1 and IPEC-2 cells have been reported to be stimulated at lower DON concentrations or inhibited at higher concentrations [143]. For example, 0.67 µM of DON stimulated IPEC-1 cell proliferation after 48 h exposure and stimulated the proliferation of both IPEC-1 and IPEC-J2 cells after 72 h of exposure [143]. However, it is inconclusive whether the stimulated proliferation of IPEC cells resulted from a primary effect of DON or a secondary effect from DON-induced cell death [157] as almost all types of epithelial cells forming monolayers are capable of undergoing self-repair after injury by inducing cell proliferation and migration to the injured site [173].

DON started to inhibit the proliferation of IPEC-1 cells at higher concentrations ranging from 3.4 to 6.7 µM after 48 and 72 h of exposure [143]. The same pattern of effect was also observed for IPEC-J2 cells after 72 h of exposure [143]. The route of application of DON, the apical versus the basolateral side of IECs for example, has also been reported to influence IPEC-J2 cell proliferation. The authors in [157] reported IPEC-J2 proliferation was more significantly stimulated when DON is applied to the basolateral side. Selected mycotoxins other than DON, only OTA has been investigated and it inhibited the proliferation of Caco-2–14 and HT-29-D4 cells by 50% (IC50) at 30 and 20 µM, respectively [174].

At a higher concentration of 6.7 µM, DON decreased the percentage of IPEC-J2 cells in the G0/G1 phase after 24 [160], 48, and 72 h of exposure [143,157]. The authors in [160] also observed a decrease in the percentage of IPEC-J2 cells in the G0/G1 phase at a lower DON concentration of 0.67 µM after 6, 12, and 24 h of exposure. A prolonged IPEC-J2 cell G2/M phase was also induced by DON after 12 and 24 h [160] and 48 h of exposure at 6.7 µM [143]. However, a decrease in cell percentage in the G2/M phase was observed by [160] after 12 h exposure of DON at a lower concentration of 0.67 µM. A prolonged S phase in IPEC-J2 cells was also reported after 6, 12, and 24 h exposure to DON at 0.67 µM, but S phase was reduced at 6.7 µM after 12 h exposure [160].

DON also induced a reduction in the percentage of cells in the G0/G1 phase and G2/M arrest in IPEC-1 cells after 48 and 72 h of exposure at 6.7 µM [143]. A prolonged S phase was also observed in IPEC-1 cells by [143] after 48 h exposure of DON at 6.7 µM. The results on cell proliferation and cell cycle distribution should be considered integrated with the interpretation of the effect of DON on cell growth. The cell cycle shift from G0/G1 to S and G2/M phases and increase in cell proliferation [173] induced by DON at lower concentration might indicate intestinal epithelial cells were undergoing self-repair after DON-induced injury; whereas exposure to higher concentration of DON could have negative impact on intestinal epithelial cell growth by inducing G2/M arrest [175] that allows the cell to repair the DNA damage or misaligned chromosomes at the mitotic spindle [176].

5.1.2. Mycotoxin Combinations

Mycotoxin mixtures have also been explored for their effects on IEC cytotoxicity. Concerning DON + ZEA, one of the most prevalent mycotoxin combinations, [161] observed antagonism of DON + ZEA mixtures on IPEC-J2 cell viability after 48 h exposure at both tested exposure combinations (2 µM DON + 40 µM ZEA and 0.5 µM DON + 10 µM ZEA). The authors in [177] also observed an antagonistic effect of DON + ZEA (100 µM/ 40 µM) on HTC116 human cell viability after 24 h exposure, whereas [155], reported that all three combinations of DON + ZEA (10/10, 10/20, and 20/10 µM) resulted in a significant reduction in Caco-2 cell viability compared to individual mycotoxins. With the combination of 10 µM DON + 10 µM ZEA, [164] also observed that the mixtures of ZEA and DON elicited synergistic effects on Caco-2 cell lipid peroxidation and antagonistic effects on DNA synthesis. Lastly, the viability of THP-1 immune cells in a Caco-2 + THP-1 co-culture model was decreased after 48 h exposure to DON + ZEA mixture (LC30/LC30, which was not specified in the article) [151].

5.2. Mycotoxins and Intestinal Permeability

Intestinal permeability is one of the key features reflecting the ability of the intestine to function as the barrier [178]. TEER is commonly used to assess IEC permeability in vitro, and a reduction in TEER has been used as an indicator of mycotoxin-induced epithelial damage [152]. Non-cytotoxic concentrations of tested mycotoxins were usually chosen for TEER studies in the reviewed studies to eliminate the effect of uncontrolled cell death on a reduction in TEER [179].

Paracellular tracer flux assays are often applied following the measurement of TEER to investigate if the potential cause of the observed decrease in TEER is increased intestinal epithelial paracellular permeability. The most commonly applied in vitro paracellular markers include fluorescence compounds (e.g., lucifer yellow, LY), or fluorescent-labeled compounds such as fluorescein isothiocyanate (FITC)-dextran and FITC-insulin [180]. As TJs are the major functional components to regulate the paracellular pathway [181], the assessment of TJs at both gene and protein levels can also be performed to further investigate the mechanism by which compromised intestinal barrier function is induced by mycotoxins.

5.2.1. Measurement of Transepithelial Electrical Resistance (TEER)

The impact of DON on TEER has been extensively studied using various in vitro intestinal models. DON decreases TEER values in both concentration- and time-dependent manners regardless of in vitro models used [152,157,182]. The lowest DON concentration that reduced Caco-2 cell TEER values was 0.17 µM after 24 h exposure [183]. A decrease in Caco-2 TEER measurements has also been observed in a Caco-2+ THP-1 co-culture model after 48 h exposure to DON at LC10 and LC30 [151]. In addition to concentration and exposure duration, DON-mediated changes in TEER also depend on cell type. It has been reported that DON reduced IPEC-1 cell TEER measurements more significantly than Caco-2 cells, indicating that IPEC-1 cells are more susceptible to DON exposure [184]. The route of DON application can also affect TEER readings, as it has been reported that the decrease in Caco-2 and IPEC-J2 cell TEER measurements was more pronounced when DON was applied to the basolateral side compared to the apical exposure of DON [143,152]. The authors in [151] reported a decrease in Caco-2 cell TEER readings in a Caco-2 + THP-1 co-culture model after 48 h exposure to both ZEA at LC10 and LC30 (LC10 and LC30 not specified in the article). In a monoculture system, [164] observed that ZEA reduced TEER readings at a concentration of 50 µM over 10 days of exposure duration.

The impact of other mycotoxins on IEC TEER measurements has been less well studied than DON. A decrease in TEER was induced by OTA in Caco-2 and HT-29-D2 cell models [166,174,185,186]. The route of application of OTA can affect TEER readings, as it has been reported that the decrease in HT-29-D2 TEER measurements was more significant and rapid when OTA was applied to the basolateral side compared to the apical exposure of OTA [174]. However, [185] observed the equal toxic effect of OTA on Caco-2 cell TEER measurement on both apical and basolateral exposure. The authors in [186] reported that TEER decrease in Cacao-2/TC7, a clonal derivative of parental Caco-2 cells induced by 48 h exposure to OTA at a concentration up to 200 µM was reversible and the TEER value was fully recovered within 24 h after mycotoxin exposure cessation. AFB1 at 100 µM also decreased the TEER values in Caco-2 cells after 7 days of exposure [166]. Lastly, MPA has also been reported to induce decreased TEER in the Caco-2 cell model after 21 days of continuous exposure at the highest concentration of 190 µM [75].

There are limited data on the effects of mycotoxin mixtures on IEC TEER measurements. Caco-2 cell TEER measurements in the co-culture model were reported to decrease after 48 h exposure to DON + ZEA mixture of two different ratios (LC10/LC10 and LC30/LC30), respectively (LC10 and LC30 were not specified in the article) [151].

Although TEER values that have been reported in the literature have been corrected for the surface area of the membrane inserts used and is typically reported in units of Ω *cm^2 [187], other factors that may have impact on TEER measurements should also be considered for purpose of interlaboratory comparisons, including temperature, cell passage number, the composition of cell culture medium, and duration of cell culture [188].

5.2.2. Assessment of the Expression of TJ Proteins

DON exposure has been reported to induce alterations in the expression of TJs at both gene and protein levels in various in vitro IEC models and contradictory effects have been reported (Table 2). Up-regulation of gene expression has been often observed, whereas a decrease in protein expression has been reported (Table 2). The reduction in protein levels associated with the rise in mRNA levels could indicate a compensatory mechanism in place for repair [183,189]. The inconsistent findings emphasize that analyses of mRNA and protein expression should be performed in parallel since the mRNA level does not necessarily predict the amount of protein [190,191].

Table 2. Summary of effects of selected mycotoxins on tight junction gene and protein expression.

Mycotoxins	IEC model	Exposure Duration	Exposure Concentration	Effects of Selected Mycotoxins on Gene and Protein Expression of TJs		References
				Gene Expression	Protein Expression	
DON	Caco-2	24 h	0, 1.39, 4.17, 12.5 µM	Increase in CLDN1, CLDN3, CLDN4, OCLN, ZO-1	Decrease in CLDN1, CLDN3, CLDN4	[152]
	Caco-2	24 h	0, 0.17, 1.7, 17 µM	Increase in CLDN4, OCLN	Decrease in CLDN4	[183]
	Caco-2	48 h	0, 5, 10, 20, 50, 100 µM	N/A	Decrease in CLDN4	[184]
	IPEC-1	48 h	0, 5, 10, 20, 50 µM	N/A	Decrease CLDN3, CLDN4	[184]
	IPEC-1	48 h	0.67, 6.7 µM	N/A	Decrease in ZO-1	[143]
	IPEC-J2	48 h	0.67, 6.7 µM	N/A	Decrease in ZO-1	[143]
	IPEC-J2	12 h	0, 4 µM	Decrease in CLDN3; increase CLDN4, OCLN, ZO-1	Decrease CLDN3, CLDN4	[189]
AFB1	Caco-2	7 days	0, 1, 3, 10, 30 µM	Decrease in CLDN3, OCLN	N/A	[166]
OTA	Caco-2	24 h	0, 100 µM	N/A	Decrease in CLDN3 and CLDN4	[185]
	Caco-2	24 h	0, 100 µM	N/A	Decrease in CLDN3 and CLDN4	[192]
	Caco-2	7 days	1, 3, 10, 30 µM	Decrease in CLDN3, CLDN4 and OCLN	N/A	[166]

In contrast to DON exposure, [166] observed a decrease in mRNA expression of CLDN3 and OCLN in Caco-2 cells after AFB1 exposure (0–30 µM), but no changes in CLDN4 mRNA expression was observed. OTA exposure decreased in Caco-2 cell mRNA expression of CLDN3, CLDN4, and OCLN [166]. This inhibitory effect at the transcription level could be explained by its ability to form DNA adducts [67,71,72]. A decrease in protein expression of CLDN3 and CLDN4 has also been reported [185,192].

5.2.3. Measurement of Flux of Paracellular Markers

DON induced a dose-dependent increase in the apical to basolateral transport of fluorescence compounds LY and 4 kDa FITC-dextran in Caco-2, IPEC-1 and IPEC-J2 cell lines [152,189,193]. The results on the paracellular passage of 4 kDa FITC–dextran also indicated that IPEC-1 exhibited more sensitivity to DON than Caco-2 cells [184].

It has also been reported that OTA did not affect IEC permeability to 20 and 40 kDa FITC-dextran [194], indicating that the intestinal epithelial cells still partially retain their barrier function during OTA exposure, and that larger molecules are selectively excluded, which is also in agreement with DON exposure.

5.3. Effects of Mycotoxins on Translocation of Intestinal Microorganisms

In addition to increased intestinal permeability and dysfunctional mucosal immune system, impaired intestinal barrier function is also associated with translocation of luminal antigens [92,178,195,196], which is another endpoint that has been used to investigate the effects of mycotoxins on the intestinal barrier. In vitro studies have shown that DON promoted transepithelial passage and invasion of *Salmonella typhimurium* in both differentiated and undifferentiated IPEC-J2 cells; the increased transepithelial passage of *S. typhimurium* was concentration-dependent [132]. DON also increased the transepithelial passage of *Escherichia coli* in IPEC-1 and IPEC-J2 cells [184,189]. MPA did not promote non-invasive *E. coli* to cross the intestinal epithelium in an in vitro study with Caco-2 cells [75].

6. Effect of Selected Mycotoxins on the Intestinal Immune System

Selected mycotoxins also have cytotoxic effects on immune cells. A 0.85 µM DON induced apoptosis in the RAW264.7 macrophage cell line [197]. The apoptosis of Jurkat human T cell line was induced by DON in the concentration range tested (0.85–3.4 µM) [198]. Concerning *Penicillium* mycotoxins, CIT, OTA, and MPA induced cell death and inhibited proliferation of bovine macrophage cell line (BoMacs) in a concentration-dependent manner [199]. A decrease in cell viability of THP-1 cells, human leukemia monocytic cell line, was observed in a Caco-2+THP-1 co-culture system after 48 h exposure to ZEA LC30 (LC30 not specified in the article) [151].

Host mucosal immune response to the invasion of luminal antigens/pathogens requires coordination between IECs and immune cells. Being part of the intestinal innate immune system, IECs serve as dynamic sensors for luminal microbes by expressing PRRs such as TLRs. IECs can also direct the mucosal immune response by producing important chemokines and cytokines that are responsible for the recruitment of immune cells and the induction of the inflammatory response [10,93].

Measuring the expression of cytokine and PRR at gene or protein level has been an endpoint that is commonly used to evaluate the effects of selected mycotoxins on the intestinal immune system using in vitro IEC models. At 2 μM of DON exposure, DON has been reported to up-regulate the expression of IPEC-J2 cell IL1-α, IL1-β, IL-6, IL-8, TNF-α, and MCP1 genes after 48 h of exposure, whereas, 0.5 μM exposure simulated expression of IL1-β, IL-6, and IL-8 genes, and down-regulated expression of IL1-α and MCP1 genes [200]. The up-regulatory effect of DON on IL-6, TNF-α, and IL1-β through the NF-κB pathway was also observed in IPEC-J2 cells after 24 h of DON exposure within the concentration range of 0.34 μM to 6.7 μM [162]. DON also reportedly induced a concentration-dependent increase in the secretion of IL-8 protein by Caco-2 cells through NF-κB after 48 h exposure [201], and [194] reported an increase in IL-8 protein secretion by Caco-2 cells after 12 h, which was associated with NF-κB, PKR, and p38 pathways.

The effect of ZEA on the modulation of cytokine gene expression was carried out using the IPEC-1 and IPEC-J2 cell lines. At a higher concentration of 40 μM, ZEA up-regulated IL1-α, IL1-β, IL-6, IL-8, TNF-α, and MCP1 after 48 h exposure by IPEC-J2 cells, whereas ZEA at 10 μM only stimulated the gene expression of IL1-α, IL1-β, and IL-8 [200]. A stimulatory effect on IFN-λ and IL-4 gene expression was observed in IPEC-1 after 1 h of exposure to 25 μM of ZEA [23]. However, contradictory results have also been reported in other studies. The authors in [163] observed no significant effects on the expression of assessed cytokine genes after IPEC-1 cells were exposed to 10 μM of ZEA for 24 h, including TNF-α, IL1-β, IL-6, IL-8, IL-12p40, IFN-λ, MCP1, IL-10, IL-18, and CCL20, and 10 μM and 25 μM of ZEA exhibited no effect on the expression of IPEC-1 cell IL-8 and IL-10 genes after 24 h of exposure [164].

As for the effect of other mycotoxins, in Caco-2 cells, the protein expression of IL-8 was stimulated in a concentration-dependent manner by MPA at concentrations ranging from 78 μM to 780 μM after 48 h of exposure [75]. Whereas, [194] reported OTA did not have a significant impact on protein secretion of IL-8 in Caco-2 cells. Lastly, [23,163] observed an increase in the expression of TLR2, TLR3, TLR4, and TLR8 genes in IPEC-1 cells after 10 h exposure to 10 μM of ZEA and 1 h exposure to 25 μM of ZEA, respectively.

Exposure of porcine pulmonary alveolar macrophages (PAM) to 0.025 ug/ml DON enhanced the phagocytosis of *S. typhimurium* by macrophages by modulating the macrophage cytoskeleton [202]. The phagocytosis of *Mycobacterium avium ssp. Paratuberculosis* (MAP) by BoMacs was also enhanced by OTA [203]; the other *Penicillium* mycotoxins (CIT and MPA) that this group investigated did not show this stimulatory effect on macrophage phagocytosis [203].

7. In-Vitro Assessment of Efficacy of Risk Mitigation

7.1. Strategies to Counteract Mycotoxin Contamination

In an attempt to mitigate the risk of mycotoxin contamination in food and feed, different pre-and post-harvest physical (e.g., crop rotation, thermal treatment, and irradiation), chemical (e.g., acids/bases and absorbents), and biological (e.g., microbial and enzymatic degradation) strategies have been deployed [27,204–207]. Besides these conventional mitigation methods, nanotechnology may be an innovative solution to mycotoxin contamination [208]. It is not possible in this review to discuss all the approaches; instead, the discussion will focus on remediation strategies that are most widely used in the animal feed industry, especially the use of mycotoxin adsorbents as feed additives.

Among all approaches, the addition of mycotoxin adsorbents to animal feeds, also referred to as "mycotoxin binders", one of the two classes of mycotoxin detoxifying agents [204], is one of the most widely applied and promising remediation approaches to reduce risk of mycotoxicosis in farm animals [209–212]. Mycotoxin adsorbents bind mycotoxins in the gastrointestinal tract after the contaminated feed is ingested [207], and the bioavailability of the mycotoxins is reduced by the formation of toxin-adsorbent complexes, which are later excreted in the feces [204]. Mycotoxin absorbents can be classified as either silica-based inorganic compounds, or carbon-based organic polymers [213]. The inorganic absorbents are further sub-grouped into aluminosilicate minerals (clays, including bentonites, montmorillonites, hydrated sodium calcium aluminosilicate, and zeolites), activated charcoal (AC), and synthetic polymers (e.g., cholestyramine). The aluminosilicate minerals are the most widely studied of the silica-based inorganic mycotoxin absorbents [211,213]. The efficacy of inorganic absorbents depends on the physio-chemical structure of both adsorbent and mycotoxin [206,211,214]; this includes the total charge and charge distribution of adsorbents and mycotoxins, adsorbent pore size, and accessible surface area, as well as mycotoxin polarity, solubility, and three-dimensional structure [204,206,211,212]. The efficacy of aluminosilicate adsorbents for reducing aflatoxin B_1 (AFB_1) bioavailability is fairly efficient [206], but their binding capacity to other mycotoxins is limited [206,214,215]. In contrast, AC has been reported to effectively bind to DON, ZEA, AFB1, fumonisin B1, and OTA, but it can reduce the absorption of some micronutrients which jeopardize the nutritional value of the feed [204,211,214,216]. Cholestyramine is the most well-known of the synthetic polymers and has been shown to be an effective adsorbent for FB_1, OTA, and ZEA [210,212,214,217]. Its high cost limits its practical use as a mycotoxin adsorbent [218], and inorganic binders are typically added to feeds at high concentrations to account for their low efficiency [216]. Lastly, since the degradation of bound mycotoxins after they have been excreted is relatively slow, this is another ecological disadvantage of using inorganic adsorbents [207].

A commonly used organic adsorbent is yeast cell wall (YCW) from *Saccharomyces cerevisiae* yeast strains [204]. The major functional fractions of YCW responsible for mycotoxin binding include β-D-glucan and α-D-mannan (glucomannan), which bind to mycotoxins via hydrogen bonding and van-der-Waal forces [219–224]. The YCW has been shown effective at binding a wide-spectrum of mycotoxins including DON, T-2 toxins, AFB_1, ZEA, and OTA [207,219,222–233]. Heat or acid treatment can further increase the mycotoxin-binding capacity of YCW [229]. Another advantage of YCW products is that they are biodegradable, and therefore the toxin-binder complexes do not accumulate in the environment after being excreted in the feces [219]. The use of lactic acid bacteria (LAB) as an organic dietary mycotoxin-adsorbing agent has recently gained interest [204]. LAB are a group of Gram-positive and non-sporulating bacteria [233], and the strain of LAB that is used to bind to mycotoxins is *Lactobacillus rhamnosus* [204,213]. With glucomannan as the functional component affecting mycotoxin binding capability, the mechanism of LAB is thought to be similar to that of YCW [204].

The second class of mycotoxin detoxifying agents is referred to as mycotoxin modifiers. These agents, which include microorganisms and their enzymes, can be applied to reduce the risk of mycotoxicity by biotransforming mycotoxins to less toxic metabolites [204]. Many commercially available mycotoxin detoxifying agents contain a combination of these two classes, capable of both degradation and adsorption. The authors in [234] conducted a study assessing the efficacy of 20 commercial products incubated under aerobic and anaerobic conditions to detoxify DON and ZEA. Their study revealed that only one out of 20 products under anaerobic incubation was effective at completely degrading DON after 24 h and only one tested product completely degraded ZEA under both incubation conditions after 24 h. All the other products incubated under both aerobic and anaerobic conditions showed maximum DON detoxification of only 17%, and only the other four products showed a reduction of ZEN ≥60% [234].

7.2. In-Vitro Assessment of Mycotoxin Absorbents

The efficacy of mycotoxin adsorbents has been assessed using both in vitro chemical and cell-based bioassays [231,235,236]. With in-vitro chemical assay, the method involves simulating pH conditions in the gastrointestinal tract of different species during adsorbent-mycotoxin co-incubation, and this is followed by chemical chromatographic analysis such as high-performance liquid chromatography with fluorometric detection [205,230–232,234], ultraviolet light detection [237], liquid chromatography-tandem mass spectrometry [238], or gas chromatography [235]. Several adsorption isotherm models have been used following the chromatographic analyses to quantify the adsorption performance of tested adsorbents including the Hill, Langmuir, Freundlich, Brunauer–Emmett–Teller (BET), and non-ideal competitive adsorption (NICA) models [228,230,232]. In a study assessing the binding capacity of various yeast-based products to ZEA, AFB_1, and OTA, the most suitable models were the Hill model for ZEA, the Langmuir model for AFB_1, and the Freundlich model for OTA [232]. When assessing the binding capacity of YCW products and hydrated sodium calcium aluminosilicate to ZEA, [228] reported that the Hill model was or more suitable than the Freundlich model for evaluating YCW adsorption efficacy, but less suitable for HSCAS (hydrated sodium calcium aluminosilicate) adsorbents.

In vitro cell-based bioassays have been less utilized for the assessment of mycotoxin adsorbent efficacy. The endpoints of assessment have included cell viability, proliferation, and TEER measurement [231,235,236]. Different cell lines derived from various species and tissues have been used in assessment studies including Caco-2, NIH/3T3-LNCX murine fibroblasts, and MCF-7 human breast cells [231,235]. A study using the differentiated Caco-2 cell line demonstrated that adsorbents such as AC, aluminosilicate minerals, cholestyramine, mannans, and β-glucans exhibited no significant cytotoxicity; however, cholestyramine induced a decrease in cell viability [235]. In the same study, all tested adsorbents except for cholestyramine mitigated the cytotoxic effects of DON, maintaining higher cell viability than even the control [235]. A study using NIH/3T3-LNCX murine fibroblasts also indicated AC showed the highest binding affinity to DON based on cell viability assessment [231]. The study using the MCF-7 cell line has shown that AC and aluminosilicate minerals adsorbents were effective in binding ZEA [231]. Lastly, [236] assessed the binding capacity of a YCW product to *Penicillium* mycotoxins (i.e., CIT, OTA, MPA, patulin and penicillic acid) using a bovine macrophage (BoMacs) cell line, with cell proliferation as a bioassay endpoint. Their results showed that YCW was the most effective in protecting BoMacs cells against OTA, followed by CIT among all five mycotoxins. A study has also shown that illite mineral clay was for protecting AFB1- and OTA-mediated reductions in Caco-2 cell TEER measurements [166].

8. Suitability and Limitations of Reviewed Intestinal in Vitro Models

In vitro cell culture models have been extensively used in toxicology, mostly for assessing organ-specific effects of xenobiotics. However, they hardly represent the complexity of the human and animal body [239,240]. The simplicity of in vitro models compared to in vivo however makes it possible to study toxic MOAs in a reproducible manner that may be difficult to be achieved in vivo [140]. In vitro experiments also allow for dose–response analysis of individual mycotoxin exposure as well as their mixtures [8]. The Caco-2, IPEC-1, and IPEC-J2 cell lines reported in the reviewed studies were able to exhibit adequate differentiated intestinal epithelial characteristics, such as proper formation of TJs and polarization in certain culture conditions, immune response-related molecular markers, as well as responsiveness of these characters to mycotoxin exposure with or without risk mitigation methods such as mycotoxin adsorbents; they could represent physiological models of the intestinal epithelial barrier. While these IEC models are used at their undifferentiation status where polarization is not displayed and proper TJs are not formed, they could also be a representation of pathological models of the intestinal epithelial barrier, such as inflammatory bowel diseases (IBD) [241]; they also appear similar to dividing cells in tissue undergoing regeneration or repair after damage [132,134]. Moreover, in terms of assessing the efficacy of mycotoxin adsorbents, with the presence of cells, the in-vitro cell culture could also detect unpredictable tenside-like activities of adsorbents that could affect cell membrane permeability and result in an increase in cellular uptake and toxicity of mycotoxins [242].

Although in vitro models are useful tools and provide valuable information, results should be interpreted with care as there are some limitations with these in vitro models. First, cell lines lack cellular diversity in the single-cell type system. For example, the Caco-2 cell line is not able to differentiate into goblet cells that are present in vivo, thus, mucins and mucus, which are present under normal physiological conditions, are lacking in vitro [140,243]. Second, in vitro cell models may lack certain phenotypes and characteristics that are exhibited in vivo [140,243–248]. For example, the HT-29 human colon cancer cell line cannot form proper TJs under certain growth conditions, whereas the T84 human colon cancer cell line is an excellent model to examine epithelial barrier function due to its high TEER properties [139]. Also, the TEER of Caco-2 cells was reported to be smaller than in vivo [249], and neither Caco-2, T84 nor IPEC-J2 cells express claudin-2 [250]. Third, cell culture conditions, such as passage number, media formulation, and culture time, can also affect the conditions of cell lines [139,251]. Other limitations include a lack of relevant factors occurring in vivo, immortalization, limited survival, and metabolic imbalance [231,252].

To date, limited studies have investigated the effects of mycotoxins on the intestinal barrier functions using 2D co-culture models. However, an IEC + immune cell co-culture system may be more appropriate than monocultures to study the effects of mycotoxins on the intestinal barrier function because 2D co-culture models better represent the epithelial structure and function in vivo. This 2D system enables the study of cell–cell interactions by both direct cell contact and soluble factors that are secreted between IECs and immune cells, depending on the co-culture set-up [129,253]. However, 2D co-culture models do have some limitations. Compared to 3D co-culture models, 2D co-culture models have reduced cell–cell interactions, lack cell–matrix interactions, and may be lacking in complete tissue architecture [254]. When compared to monoculture models, a limitation of 2D co-culture is that a wider range of variables could affect the outcomes of co-culture models including cell culture conditions, the size and ratio of different cultured cell populations, and time scale of the experiments with the interactions between populations considered [255].

9. Conclusion and Discussion

Mycotoxins present an issue worldwide due to their ability to contaminate agricultural commodities and to pose a health risk to both humans and animals that have ingested the contaminated food and feed. Climate change will likely favor more mycotoxin contamination [2,7]. Since mycotoxins are commonly present as co-contaminants, it is not only important to understand their MOAs, many of which are unknown, but also to understand how they interact with each other to affect exposed humans and animals.

Since the intestine is the major site of mycotoxin interaction following oral exposure, understanding these interactions at the intestinal level is critical for risk assessment and mitigation. The intestine functions as a semi-permeable physical and immunological barrier and is the major site of nutrient absorption. Therefore, any adverse effects mycotoxins pose to the intestine, such as changes in intestinal permeability, cytokine production, and cell viability may be a constraint to animal health and production.

In vitro cell culture models of the intestinal barrier have been used to mimic oral exposure to mycotoxins. These intestinal models are usually based on a monolayer epithelial cell culture system, sometimes grown on membrane inserts to better mimic the intestinal barrier for assessing the intestinal transport of mycotoxins, the impact of different routes of exposure, and how mycotoxin exposure impacts the translocation of pathogens [143,148,152,256].

A number of different mitigation approaches, including the use of mycotoxin adsorbents, have been developed and applied to help reduce the adverse effects of mycotoxins on animals, but their efficacy varies depending on physio-chemical properties of both adsorbents and mycotoxins. Given this, there is an ongoing need for the development of novel more effective mycotoxin adsorbents and for their efficacy assessment. Given that in-vitro cell culture can help to better understand what actually happens at the intestinal level [235], the possible cytotoxic effects of mycotoxin adsorbents on the gut epithelium and their mycotoxin binding efficacy can be assessed using in-vitro cell-based bioassays based on functional parameters such as cell viability and TEER values [231,235].

Most of the cell culture studies collated in this review are based on the in vitro monoculture system. However, it may be more appropriate and efficient to co-culture various cell types, such as the IEC + macrophage co-culture model, to simulate a more complex in-vitro system that better reflects the intestinal mucosa physiologically and morphologically. Although there are limitations associated with cell culture models, in vitro monoculture, or even better a co-culture system, is an efficient approach for initial toxicity assessment of mycotoxins and their mixtures and assessment of adsorbent efficacy. It is also an efficient approach for determining the MOAs for both individual and combined mycotoxins that exhibit species- and organ-specific toxicity at the cellular and molecular level.

10. Suggestions for Future Research

Although in vitro and in vivo toxicity data for DON is abundant, toxicity data for other mycotoxins is limited, especially with regards to *Penicillium* mycotoxins, which are commonly detected in forage, particularly silage [257,258]. There is also a lack of in vitro and in vivo toxicity data concerning the combined toxic effects of mycotoxins. Moreover, exposure guidelines throughout the world are all based on individual mycotoxins, and multi-exposure has raised a question about the health risk of co-occurring mycotoxins. As in most cases, feed and food can be contaminated with multiple mycotoxins and the combined toxicity of mycotoxin mixtures cannot always be predicted based on their individual toxicity [5]. Thus, more studies should investigate the effects of multi-mycotoxin exposure to provide guidance for toxicological evaluation and reflect on the suitability of current mycotoxin exposure guidelines.

In vitro and in vivo mycotoxin toxicity studies have focused more on monogastric animals over ruminants, as ruminants are considered more resistant to mycotoxins due to the ability of rumen microbes to detoxify mycotoxins into non-toxic compounds [259]. However, the safety of ruminant species should be more thoroughly considered. Certain mycotoxins with antimicrobial properties, for example, can impair the function of the rumen and intestinal microflora, thus, decreasing their capacity to degrade mycotoxin [25,27]. Moreover, ruminant animals in certain production stages are more susceptible to mycotoxins. For example, ruminants in the transition period have a negative energy balance and are particularly sensitive to mycotoxin contamination in feed [25]. Also, newly-weaned ruminants can be prone to mycotoxin exposure because the rumen microbiota is not fully established or functional to protect young ruminants from mycotoxins [260]. Some mycotoxins may by-pass the rumen intact instead of being detoxified in the rumen [79].

In vitro cell culture systems (monoculture or co-culture systems) could be a useful and effective approach to start with for studying organ- and species-specific complicated issues of mycotoxin toxicity at the cellular and molecular levels such as interactions between different mycotoxins [151], comparative toxicity of mycotoxins, and their metabolites [155]. Moreover, cell culture systems could be appropriate methods to study biotransformation of mycotoxins in animal cells, for example, the cell models could express certain enzymes such as Cytochromes P450 (CYPs) that might interact with tested mycotoxins by biotransforming them to the resulting metabolites [16,261].

Author Contributions: Writing—original draft preparation, R.X.; writing—review and editing, N.A.K., R.X., U.K.S., L.-h.S., and H.K; supervision, N.A.K.; project administration, U.K.S.; funding acquisition, N.A.K.; H.K. All authors have read and agreed to the published version of the manuscript.

Funding: This work has been funded by Natural Sciences and Engineering Research Council of Canada and Alltech Inc, KY, US [532378-18] to N.A.K and Grant-in-Aid for Scientific Research (A) [19H00965] from the Japan Society for the Promotion of Science (JSPS) to H.K., and by JSPS Core-to-Core Program, A. Advanced Research Networks entitled Establishment of international agricultural immunology research-core for a quantum improvement in food safety.

Acknowledgments: We appreciate the work of all colleagues on this topic.

Conflicts of Interest: The authors declare no conflict of interest.

References

1. Mohammadi, H. A Review of Aflatoxin M1, Milk, and Milk Products. In *Aflatoxins–Biochemistry and Molecular Biology*; IntechOpen: London, UK, 2011; pp. 397–414.
2. Bryden, W.L. Mycotoxin contamination of the feed supply chain: Implications for animal productivity and feed security. *Anim. Feed Sci. Technol.* **2012**, *173*, 134–158. [CrossRef]
3. Marin, S.; Ramos, A.J.; Cano-Sancho, G.; Sanchis, V. Mycotoxins: Occurrence, toxicology, and exposure assessment. *Food Chem. Toxicol.* **2013**, *60*, 218–237. [CrossRef] [PubMed]
4. Völkel, I.; Schröer-Merker, E.; Czerny, C.-P. The Carry-Over of Mycotoxins in Products of Animal Origin with Special Regard to Its Implications for the European Food Safety Legislation. *Food Nutr. Sci.* **2011**, *2*, 852–867. [CrossRef]
5. Smith, M.-C.; Madec, S.; Coton, E.; Hymery, N. Natural Co-Occurrence of Mycotoxins in Foods and Feeds and Their in vitro Combined Toxicological Effects. *Toxins* **2016**, *8*, 94. [CrossRef] [PubMed]
6. Council for Agricultural Science and Technology. *Mycotoxins: Risks in Plant, Animal, and Human Systems*; Council for Agricultural Science and Technology: Ames, IA, USA, 2003; ISBN 978-1-887383-22-6.
7. Lee, H.-S.; Kwon, N.J.; Kim, Y.; Lee, H. Prediction of mycotoxin risks due to climate change in Korea. *Appl. Biol. Chem.* **2018**, *61*, 389–396. [CrossRef]
8. Alassane-Kpembi, I.; Puel, O.; Oswald, I.P. Toxicological interactions between the mycotoxins deoxynivalenol, nivalenol and their acetylated derivatives in intestinal epithelial cells. *Arch. Toxicol.* **2015**, *89*, 1337–1346. [CrossRef] [PubMed]
9. Grenier, B.; Applegate, T. Modulation of Intestinal Functions Following Mycotoxin Ingestion: Meta-Analysis of Published Experiments in Animals. *Toxins* **2013**, *5*, 396–430. [CrossRef]
10. Bouhet, S.; Oswald, I.P. The effects of mycotoxins, fungal food contaminants, on the intestinal epithelial cell-derived innate immune response. *Vet. Immunol. Immunopathol.* **2005**, *108*, 199–209. [CrossRef]
11. Bain, C.C.; Mowat, A.M. Macrophages in intestinal homeostasis and inflammation. *Immunol. Rev.* **2014**, *260*, 102–117. [CrossRef]
12. Bain, C.C.; Scott, C.L.; Uronen-Hansson, H.; Gudjonsson, S.; Jansson, O.; Grip, O.; Guilliams, M.; Malissen, B.; Agace, W.W.; Mowat, A.M. Resident and pro-inflammatory macrophages in the colon represent alternative context-dependent fates of the same Ly6C hi monocyte precursors. *Mucosal Immunol.* **2013**, *6*, 498–510. [CrossRef] [PubMed]
13. Pelaseyed, T.; Bergström, J.H.; Gustafsson, J.K.; Ermund, A.; Birchenough, G.M.H.; Schütte, A.; Van der Post, S.; Svensson, F.; Rodríguez-Piñeiro, A.M.; Nyström, E.E.L.; et al. The mucus and mucins of the goblet cells and enterocytes provide the first defense line of the gastrointestinal tract and interact with the immune system. *Immunol. Rev.* **2014**, *260*, 8–20. [CrossRef] [PubMed]
14. Stadnyk, A.W. Intestinal Epithelial Cells as a Source of Inflammatory Cytokines and Chemokines. *Can. J. Gastroenterol.* **2002**, *16*, 241–246. [CrossRef] [PubMed]
15. Swamy, M.; Jamora, C.; Havran, W.; Hayday, A. Epithelial decision makers: In search of the "epimmunome". *Nat. Immunol.* **2010**, *11*, 656–665. [CrossRef] [PubMed]
16. Sergent, T.; Ribonnet, L.; Kolosova, A.; Garsou, S.; Schaut, A.; De Saeger, S.; Van Peteghem, C.; Larondelle, Y.; Pussemier, L.; Schneider, Y.-J. Molecular and cellular effects of food contaminants and secondary plant components and their plausible interactions at the intestinal level. *Food Chem. Toxicol.* **2008**, *46*, 813–841. [CrossRef] [PubMed]
17. Prelusky, D.B.; Trenholm, H.L.; Rotter, B.A.; Miller, J.D.; Savard, M.E.; Yeung, J.M.; Scott, P.M. Biological Fate of Fumonisin B1 in Food-Producing Animals. In *Fumonisins in Food*; Jackson, L.S., DeVries, J.W., Bullerman, L.B., Eds.; Springer: Boston, MA, USA, 1996; pp. 265–278. ISBN 978-1-4899-1379-1.
18. Shephard, G.S.; Thiel, P.G.; Sydenham, E.W.; Savard, M.E. Fate of a single dose of 14C-labelled fumonisin B1 in vervet monkeys. *Nat. Toxins* **1995**, *3*, 145–150. [CrossRef] [PubMed]
19. Biehl, M.L.; Prelusky, D.B.; Koritz, G.D.; Hartin, K.E.; Buck, W.B.; Trenholm, H.L. Biliary Excretion and Enterohepatic Cycling of Zearalenone in Immature Pigs. *Toxicol. Appl. Pharmacol.* **1993**, *121*, 152–159. [CrossRef]

20. Roth, A.; Chakor, K.; EkuéCreepy, E.; Kane, A.; Roschenthaler, R.; Dirheimer, G. Evidence for an enterohepatic circulation of ochratoxin A in mice. *Toxicology* **1988**, *48*, 293–308. [CrossRef]
21. De Angelis, I.; Friggè, G.; Raimondi, F.; Stammati, A.; Zucco, F.; Caloni, F. Absorption of Fumonisin B1 and aminopentol on an in vitro model of intestinal epithelium; the role of P-glycoprotein. *Toxicon* **2005**, *45*, 285–291. [CrossRef]
22. Creppy, E.E. Update of survey, regulation and toxic effects of mycotoxins in Europe. *Toxicol. Lett.* **2002**, *127*, 19–28. [CrossRef]
23. Taranu, I.; Marin, D.E.; Pistol, G.C.; Motiu, M.; Pelinescu, D. Induction of pro-inflammatory gene expression by Escherichia coli and mycotoxin zearalenone contamination and protection by a Lactobacillus mixture in porcine IPEC-1 cells. *Toxicon* **2015**, *97*, 53–63. [CrossRef] [PubMed]
24. Liew, W.-P.-P.; Mohd-Redzwan, S. Mycotoxin: Its Impact on Gut Health and Microbiota. *Front. Cell. Infect. Microbiol.* **2018**, *8*. [CrossRef] [PubMed]
25. Fink-Gremmels, J. The role of mycotoxins in the health and performance of dairy cows. *Vet. J.* **2008**, *176*, 84–92. [CrossRef] [PubMed]
26. Maresca, M.; Fantini, J. Some food-associated mycotoxins as potential risk factors in humans predisposed to chronic intestinal inflammatory diseases. *Toxicon* **2010**, *56*, 282–294. [CrossRef] [PubMed]
27. Wambacq, E.; Vanhoutte, I.; Audenaert, K.; Gelder, L.D.; Haesaert, G. Occurrence, prevention and remediation of toxigenic fungi and mycotoxins in silage: A review. *J. Sci. Food Agric.* **2016**, *96*, 2284–2302. [CrossRef]
28. Kashyap, P.C.; Marcobal, A.; Ursell, L.K.; Larauche, M.; Duboc, H.; Earle, K.A.; Sonnenburg, E.D.; Ferreyra, J.A.; Higginbottom, S.K.; Million, M.; et al. Complex Interactions Among Diet, Gastrointestinal Transit, and Gut Microbiota in Humanized Mice. *Gastroenterology* **2013**, *144*, 967–977. [CrossRef]
29. Patel, R.M.; Lin, P.W. Developmental biology of gut-probiotic interaction. *Gut Microbes* **2010**, *1*, 186–195. [CrossRef]
30. Yano, J.M.; Yu, K.; Donaldson, G.P.; Shastri, G.G.; Ann, P.; Ma, L.; Nagler, C.R.; Ismagilov, R.F.; Mazmanian, S.K.; Hsiao, E.Y. Indigenous Bacteria from the Gut Microbiota Regulate Host Serotonin Biosynthesis. *Cell* **2015**, *161*, 264–276. [CrossRef]
31. Karlovsky, P.; Suman, M.; Berthiller, F.; De Meester, J.; Eisenbrand, G.; Perrin, I.; Oswald, I.P.; Speijers, G.; Chiodini, A.; Recker, T.; et al. Impact of food processing and detoxification treatments on mycotoxin contamination. *Mycotoxin Res.* **2016**, *32*, 179–205. [CrossRef]
32. Mannaa, M.; Kim, K.D. Influence of Temperature and Water Activity on Deleterious Fungi and Mycotoxin Production during Grain Storage. *Mycobiology* **2017**, *45*, 240–254. [CrossRef]
33. Tola, M.; Kebede, B. Occurrence, importance and control of mycotoxins: A review. *Cogent Food Agric.* **2016**, *2*. [CrossRef]
34. D'Mello, J.P.F.; Placinta, C.M.; Macdonald, A.M.C. Fusarium mycotoxins: A review of global implications for animal health, welfare and productivity. *Anim. Feed Sci. Technol.* **1999**, *80*, 183–205. [CrossRef]
35. Scheidegger, K.; Payne, G. Unlocking the Secrets Behind Secondary Metabolism: A Review of Aspergillus flavus from Pathogenicity to Functional Genomics. *J. Toxicol. Toxin Rev.* **2003**, *22*, 423–459. [CrossRef]
36. Doughari, J. The Occurrence, Properties and Significance of Citrinin Mycotoxin. *J. Plant Pathol. Microbiol.* **2015**, *6*. [CrossRef]
37. Schneweis, I.; Meyer, K.; Hormansdorfer, S.; Bauer, J. Mycophenolic Acid in Silage. *Appl. Environ. Microbiol.* **2000**, *66*, 3639–3641. [CrossRef] [PubMed]
38. Bennett, J.W.; Klich, M. Mycotoxins. *Clin. Microbiol. Rev.* **2003**, *16*, 497–516. [CrossRef] [PubMed]
39. Pestka, J.J. Deoxynivalenol: Mechanisms of action, human exposure, and toxicological relevance. *Arch. Toxicol.* **2010**, *84*, 663–679. [CrossRef] [PubMed]
40. Maresca, M. From the Gut to the Brain: Journey and Pathophysiological Effects of the Food-Associated Trichothecene Mycotoxin Deoxynivalenol. *Toxins Basel* **2013**, *5*, 784–820. [CrossRef]
41. Sobrova, P.; Adam, V.; Vasatkova, A.; Beklova, M.; Zeman, L.; Kizek, R. Deoxynivalenol and its toxicity. *Interdiscip. Toxicol.* **2010**, *3*, 94. [CrossRef]
42. Pestka, J.J. Deoxynivalenol: Toxicity, mechanisms and animal health risks. *Anim. Feed Sci. Technol.* **2007**, *137*, 283–298. [CrossRef]
43. Rocha, O.; Ansari, K.; Doohan, F.M. Effects of trichothecene mycotoxins on eukaryotic cells: A review. *Food Addit. Contam.* **2005**, *22*, 369–378. [CrossRef] [PubMed]

44. Marin, D.E.; Taranu, I.; Burlacu, R.; Manda, G.; Motiu, M.; Neagoe, I.; Dragomir, C.; Stancu, M.; Calin, L. Effects of zearalenone and its derivatives on porcine immune response. *Toxicol. Vitr.* **2011**, *25*, 1981–1988. [CrossRef] [PubMed]
45. Abid-Essefi, S.; Ouanes, Z.; Hassen, W.; Baudrimont, I.; Creppy, E.; Bacha, H. Cytotoxicity, inhibition of DNA and protein syntheses and oxidative damage in cultured cells exposed to zearalenone. *Toxicol. Vitr.* **2004**, *18*, 467–474. [CrossRef] [PubMed]
46. Fan, W.; Shen, T.; Ding, Q.; Lv, Y.; Li, L.; Huang, K.; Yan, L.; Song, S. Zearalenone induces ROS-mediated mitochondrial damage in porcine IPEC-J2 cells. *J. Biochem. Mol. Toxicol.* **2017**, *31*, e21944. [CrossRef] [PubMed]
47. Hassen, W.; Ayed-Boussema, I.; Oscoz, A.A.; De Cerain Lopez, A.; Bacha, H. The role of oxidative stress in zearalenone-mediated toxicity in Hep G2 cells: Oxidative DNA damage, gluthatione depletion and stress proteins induction. *Toxicology* **2007**, *232*, 294–302. [CrossRef]
48. Liu, M.; Gao, R.; Meng, Q.; Zhang, Y.; Bi, C.; Shan, A. Toxic Effects of Maternal Zearalenone Exposure on Intestinal Oxidative Stress, Barrier Function, Immunological and Morphological Changes in Rats. *PLoS ONE* **2014**, *9*. [CrossRef]
49. Zinedine, A.; Soriano, J.M.; Moltó, J.C.; Mañes, J. Review on the toxicity, occurrence, metabolism, detoxification, regulations and intake of zearalenone: An oestrogenic mycotoxin. *Food Chem. Toxicol.* **2007**, *45*, 1–18. [CrossRef]
50. Alshannaq, A.; Yu, J.-H. Occurrence, Toxicity, and Analysis of Major Mycotoxins in Food. *Int. J. Environ. Res. Public. Health* **2017**, *14*, 632. [CrossRef]
51. Rushing, B.R.; Selim, M.I. Aflatoxin B1: A review on metabolism, toxicity, occurrence in food, occupational exposure, and detoxification methods. *Food Chem. Toxicol.* **2019**, *124*, 81–100. [CrossRef]
52. IARC. *Monographs on the Evaluation of Carcinogenic Risks to Humans, Volume 100 F, Chemical Agents and Related Occupations: This Publication Represents the Views and Expert Opinions of an IARC Working Group on the Evaluation of Carcinogenic Risks to Humans, which Met in Lyon, 20–27 October 2009*; International Agency for Research on Cancer, Weltgesundheitsorganisation, Ed.; IARC: Lyon, France, 2012; ISBN 978-92-832-1323-9.
53. Amstad, P.; Levy, A.; Emerit, I.; Cerutti, P. Evidence for membrane-mediated chromosomal damage by aflatoxin B_1 in human lymphocytes. *Carcinogenesis* **1984**, *5*, 719–723. [CrossRef]
54. Bouslimi, A.; Bouaziz, C.; Ayed-Boussema, I.; Hassen, W.; Bacha, H. Individual and combined effects of ochratoxin A and citrinin on viability and DNA fragmentation in cultured Vero cells and on chromosome aberrations in mice bone marrow cells. *Toxicology* **2008**, *251*, 1–7. [CrossRef] [PubMed]
55. Liu, B.-H.; Yu, F.-Y.; Wu, T.-S.; Li, S.-Y.; Su, M.-C.; Wang, M.-C.; Shih, S.-M. Evaluation of genotoxic risk and oxidative DNA damage in mammalian cells exposed to mycotoxins, patulin and citrinin. *Toxicol. Appl. Pharmacol.* **2003**, *191*, 255–263. [CrossRef]
56. Klaric, M.S.; Zeljezic, D.; Domijan, A.-M.; Peraica, M.; Pepeljnjak, S. Cytotoxicity, genotoxicity and apoptosis induced by ochratoxin A and citrinin in porcine kidney PK15 cells: Effects of single and combined mycotoxins. *Toxicol. Lett.* **2007**, *172*, S56. [CrossRef]
57. Heussner, A.H.; Bingle, L.E.H. Comparative Ochratoxin Toxicity: A Review of the Available Data. *Toxins* **2015**, *7*, 4253–4282. [CrossRef] [PubMed]
58. Marquardt, R.R.; Frohlich, A.A. A Review of Recent Advances in Understanding Ochratoxicosis'12. *J. Anim. Sci.* **1992**, *70*, 3968–3988. [CrossRef] [PubMed]
59. Peraica, M.; Domijan, A.-M.; Matašin, M.; Lucić, A.; Radić, B.; Delaš, F.; Horvat, M.; Bosanac, I.; Balija, M.; Grgičević, D. Variations of ochratoxin A concentration in the blood of healthy populations in some Croatian cities. *Arch. Toxicol.* **2001**, *75*, 410–414. [CrossRef] [PubMed]
60. Fink-Gremmels, J. Conclusions from the workshops on Ochratoxin A in Food: Recent developments and significance, organized by ILSI Europe in Baden (Austria), 29 June–1 July 2005. *Food Addit. Contam.* **2005**, *22*, 1–5. [CrossRef]
61. Grollman, A.P.; Jelaković, B. Role of Environmental Toxins in Endemic (Balkan) Nephropathy. *J. Am. Soc. Nephrol.* **2007**, *18*, 2817–2823. [CrossRef]
62. Akbari, P.; Braber, S.; Varasteh, S.; Alizadeh, A.; Garssen, J.; Fink-Gremmels, J. The intestinal barrier as an emerging target in the toxicological assessment of mycotoxins. *Arch. Toxicol.* **2017**, *91*, 1007–1029. [CrossRef]
63. Kuiper-Goodman, T.; Scott, P.M. Risk assessment of the mycotoxin ochratoxin A. *Biomed. Environ. Sci. BES* **1989**, *2*, 179–248.

64. Adler, M.; Müller, K.; Rached, E.; Dekant, W.; Mally, A. Modulation of key regulators of mitosis linked to chromosomal instability is an early event in ochratoxin A carcinogenicity. *Carcinogenesis* **2009**, *30*, 711–719. [CrossRef] [PubMed]
65. Cui, J.; Xing, L.; Li, Z.; Wu, S.; Wang, J.; Liu, J.; Wang, J.; Yan, X.; Zhang, X. Ochratoxin A induces G2 phase arrest in human gastric epithelium GES-1 cells in vitro. *Toxicol. Lett.* **2010**, *193*, 152–158. [CrossRef] [PubMed]
66. Czakai, K.; Müller, K.; Mosesso, P.; Pepe, G.; Schulze, M.; Gohla, A.; Patnaik, D.; Dekant, W.; Higgins, J.M.G.; Mally, A. Perturbation of Mitosis through Inhibition of Histone Acetyltransferases: The Key to Ochratoxin A Toxicity and Carcinogenicity? *Toxicol. Sci.* **2011**, *122*, 317–329. [CrossRef] [PubMed]
67. Mally, A. Ochratoxin A and Mitotic Disruption: Mode of Action Analysis of Renal Tumor Formation by Ochratoxin A. *Toxicol. Sci.* **2012**, *127*, 315–330. [CrossRef] [PubMed]
68. Mally, A.; Dekant, W. Mycotoxins and the kidney: Modes of action for renal tumor formation by ochratoxin A in rodents. *Mol. Nutr. Food Res.* **2009**, *53*, 467–478. [CrossRef] [PubMed]
69. Rached, E.; Pfeiffer, E.; Dekant, W.; Mally, A. Ochratoxin A: Apoptosis and Aberrant Exit from Mitosis due to Perturbation of Microtubule Dynamics? *Toxicol. Sci.* **2006**, *92*, 78–86. [CrossRef]
70. Wang, Y.; Liu, J.; Cui, J.; Xing, L.; Wang, J.; Yan, X.; Zhang, X. ERK and p38 MAPK signaling pathways are involved in ochratoxin A-induced G2 phase arrest in human gastric epithelium cells. *Toxicol. Lett.* **2012**, *209*, 186–192. [CrossRef]
71. Pfohl-Leszkowicz, A.; Manderville, R.A. An Update on Direct Genotoxicity as a Molecular Mechanism of Ochratoxin A Carcinogenicity. *Chem. Res. Toxicol.* **2012**, *25*, 252–262. [CrossRef]
72. Sorrenti, V.; Di Giacomo, C.; Acquaviva, R.; Barbagallo, I.; Bognanno, M.; Galvano, F. Toxicity of Ochratoxin A and Its Modulation by Antioxidants: A Review. *Toxins* **2013**, *5*, 1742–1766. [CrossRef]
73. Boysen, M.E.; Jacobsson, K.-G.; Schnürer, J. Molecular Identification of Species from the Penicillium roqueforti Group Associated with Spoiled Animal Feed. *Appl. Environ. Microbiol.* **2000**, *66*, 1523–1526. [CrossRef]
74. Driehuis, F. Silage and the safety and quality of dairy foods: A review. *Agric. Food Sci.* **2013**, *22*, 16–34. [CrossRef]
75. Hymery, N.; Mounier, J.; Coton, E. Effect of Penicillium roqueforti mycotoxins on Caco-2 cells: Acute and chronic exposure. *Toxicol. Vitr.* **2018**, *48*, 188–194. [CrossRef] [PubMed]
76. Pereyra, C.; Alonso, V.; Rosa, C.; Chiacchiera, S.; Dalcero, A.; Cavaglieri, L. Gliotoxin natural incidence and toxigenicity of *Aspergillus fumigatus* isolated from corn silage and ready dairy cattle feed. *World Mycotoxin J.* **2008**, *1*, 457–462. [CrossRef]
77. Richard, E.; Heutte, N.; Sage, L.; Pottier, D.; Bouchart, V.; Lebailly, P.; Garon, D. Toxigenic fungi and mycotoxins in mature corn silage. *Food Chem. Toxicol.* **2007**, *45*, 2420–2425. [CrossRef] [PubMed]
78. Storm, I.M.L.D.; Kristensen, N.B.; Raun, B.M.L.; Smedsgaard, J.; Thrane, U. Dynamics in the microbiology of maize silage during whole-season storage. *J. Appl. Microbiol.* **2010**, *109*, 1017–1026. [CrossRef] [PubMed]
79. Gallo, A.; Giuberti, G.; Frisvad, J.C.; Bertuzzi, T.; Nielsen, K.F. Review on Mycotoxin Issues in Ruminants: Occurrence in Forages, Effects of Mycotoxin Ingestion on Health Status and Animal Performance and Practical Strategies to Counteract Their Negative Effects. *Toxins* **2015**, *7*, 3057–3111. [CrossRef]
80. Bentley, R. Mycophenolic Acid: A One Hundred Year Odyssey from Antibiotic to Immunosuppressant. *Chem. Rev.* **2000**, *100*, 3801–3826. [CrossRef]
81. Eugui, E.M.; Almquist, S.J.; Muller, C.D.; Allison, A.C. Lymphocyte-Selective Cytostatic and Immunosuppressive Effects of Mycophenolic Acid in vitro: Role of Deoxyguanosine Nucleotide Depletion. *Scand. J. Immunol.* **1991**, *33*, 161–173. [CrossRef]
82. Cole, R.J.; Cox, R.H. *Handbook of Toxic Fungal Metabolites*; Academic Press: New York, NY, USA, 1981; ISBN 978-0-12-179760-7.
83. Puel, O.; Tadrist, S.; Galtier, P.; Oswald, I.P.; Delaforge, M. Byssochlamys nivea as a Source of Mycophenolic Acid. *Appl. Environ. Microbiol.* **2005**, *71*, 550–553. [CrossRef]
84. Dzidic, A.; Meyer, H.H.D.; Bauer, J.; Pfaffl, M.W. Long-term effects of mycophenolic acid on the immunoglobulin and inflammatory marker-gene expression in sheep white blood cells. *Mycotoxin Res.* **2010**, *26*, 235–240. [CrossRef]
85. Swanson, S.P.; Nicoletti, J.; Rood, H.D.; Buck, W.B.; Cote, L.M.; Yoshizawa, T. Metabolism of three trichothecene ycotoxins, T-2 toxin, diacetoxyscirpenol and deoxynivalenol, by bovne rumen microorganisms. *J. Chromatogr. B. Biomed. Sci. Appl.* **1987**, *414*, 335–342. [CrossRef]

86. Cummings, J.H.; Antoine, J.-M.; Azpiroz, F.; Bourdet-Sicard, R.; Brandtzaeg, P.; Calder, P.C.; Gibson, G.R.; Guarner, F.; Isolauri, E.; Pannemans, D.; et al. PASSCLAIM[1]–Gut health and immunity. *Eur. J. Nutr.* **2004**, *43*, ii118–ii173. [CrossRef] [PubMed]
87. Brandtzaeg, P. The gut as communicator between environment and host: Immunological consequences. *Eur. J. Pharmacol.* **2011**, *668*, S16–S32. [CrossRef] [PubMed]
88. Vancamelbeke, M.; Vermeire, S. The intestinal barrier: A fundamental role in health and disease. *Expert Rev. Gastroenterol. Hepatol.* **2017**, *11*, 821–834. [CrossRef] [PubMed]
89. Bischoff, S.C.; Barbara, G.; Buurman, W.; Ockhuizen, T.; Schulzke, J.-D.; Serino, M.; Tilg, H.; Watson, A.; Wells, J.M. Intestinal permeability—A new target for disease prevention and therapy. *BMC Gastroenterol.* **2014**, *14*. [CrossRef] [PubMed]
90. Sato, T.; Vries, R.G.; Snippert, H.J.; Van de Wetering, M.; Barker, N.; Stange, D.E.; Van Es, J.H.; Abo, A.; Kujala, P.; Peters, P.J.; et al. Single Lgr5 stem cells build crypt-villus structures in vitro without a mesenchymal niche. *Nature* **2009**, *459*, 262–265. [CrossRef]
91. Mueller, C.; Macpherson, A.J. Layers of mutualism with commensal bacteria protect us from intestinal inflammation. *Gut* **2006**, *55*, 276–284. [CrossRef] [PubMed]
92. Groschwitz, K.R.; Hogan, S.P. Intestinal Barrier Function: Molecular Regulation and Disease Pathogenesis. *J. Allergy Clin. Immunol.* **2009**, *124*, 3–22. [CrossRef]
93. Peterson, L.W.; Artis, D. Intestinal epithelial cells: Regulators of barrier function and immune homeostasis. *Nat. Rev. Immunol.* **2014**, *14*, 141–153. [CrossRef]
94. Donaldson, G.P.; Lee, S.M.; Mazmanian, S.K. Gut biogeography of the bacterial microbiota. *Nat. Rev. Microbiol.* **2016**, *14*, 20–32. [CrossRef]
95. Ley, R.E.; Peterson, D.A.; Gordon, J.I. Ecological and Evolutionary Forces Shaping Microbial Diversity in the Human Intestine. *Cell* **2006**, *124*, 837–848. [CrossRef] [PubMed]
96. Schenk, M.; Mueller, C. The mucosal immune system at the gastrointestinal barrier. *Best Pract. Res. Clin. Gastroenterol.* **2008**, *22*, 391–409. [CrossRef] [PubMed]
97. Mukherjee, S.; Hooper, L.V. Antimicrobial Defense of the Intestine. *Immunity* **2015**, *42*, 28–39. [CrossRef] [PubMed]
98. Gill, N.; Wlodarska, M.; Finlay, B.B. The future of mucosal immunology: Studying an integrated system-wide organ. *Nat. Immunol.* **2010**, *11*, 558–560. [CrossRef] [PubMed]
99. Philpott, D.J.; Sorbara, M.T.; Robertson, S.J.; Croitoru, K.; Girardin, S.E. NOD proteins: Regulators of inflammation in health and disease. *Nat. Rev. Immunol.* **2014**, *14*, 9–23. [CrossRef]
100. Song, D.H.; Lee, J.-O. Sensing of microbial molecular patterns by Toll-like receptors. *Immunol. Rev.* **2012**, *250*, 216–229. [CrossRef]
101. Fukushima, K.; Sasaki, I.; Ogawa, H.; Naito, H.; Funayama, Y.; Matsuno, S. Colonization of microflora in mice: Mucosal defense against luminal bacteria. *J. Gastroenterol.* **1999**, *34*, 54–60. [CrossRef]
102. McDole, J.R.; Wheeler, L.W.; McDonald, K.G.; Wang, B.; Konjufca, V.; Knoop, K.A.; Newberry, R.D.; Miller, M.J. Goblet cells deliver luminal antigen to CD103 + dendritic cells in the small intestine. *Nature* **2012**, *483*, 345–349. [CrossRef]
103. McDonald, B.D.; Jabri, B.; Bendelac, A. Diverse developmental pathways of intestinal intraepithelial lymphocytes. *Nat. Rev. Immunol.* **2018**, *18*, 514–525. [CrossRef]
104. Olivares-Villagómez, D.; Van Kaer, L. Intestinal Intraepithelial Lymphocytes: Sentinels of the Mucosal Barrier. *Trends Immunol.* **2018**, *39*, 264–275. [CrossRef]
105. Mowat, A.M.; Agace, W.W. Regional specialization within the intestinal immune system. *Nat. Rev. Immunol.* **2014**, *14*, 667–685. [CrossRef] [PubMed]
106. Hume, D.A.; Perry, V.H.; Gordon, S. The mononuclear phagocyte system of the mouse defined by immunohistochemical localisation of antigen F4/80: Macrophages associated with epithelia. *Anat. Rec.* **1984**, *210*, 503–512. [CrossRef] [PubMed]
107. Lee, S.-H.; Starkey, P.M.; Gordon, S. Quantitative analysis of total macrophage content in adult mouse tissues. Imrnunochemical Studies with Monoclonal Antibody F4/80. *J. Exp. Med.* **1985**, *3*, 475–489. [CrossRef] [PubMed]
108. Smythies, L.E.; Sellers, M.; Clements, R.H.; Mosteller-Barnum, M.; Meng, G.; Benjamin, W.H.; Orenstein, J.M.; Smith, P.D. Human intestinal macrophages display profound inflammatory anergy despite avid phagocytic and bacteriocidal activity. *J. Clin. Investig.* **2005**, *115*, 66–75. [CrossRef] [PubMed]

109. Kumawat, A.K.; Yu, C.; Mann, E.A.; Schridde, A.; Finnemann, S.C.; Mowat, A.M. Expression and characterization of αvβ5 integrin on intestinal macrophages. *Eur. J. Immunol.* **2018**, *48*, 1181–1187. [CrossRef] [PubMed]
110. Schridde, A.; Bain, C.C.; Mayer, J.U.; Montgomery, J.; Pollet, E.; Denecke, B.; Milling, S.W.F.; Jenkins, S.J.; Dalod, M.; Henri, S.; et al. Tissue-specific differentiation of colonic macrophages requires TGFβ receptor-mediated signaling. *Mucosal Immunol.* **2017**, *10*, 1387–1399. [CrossRef]
111. Smith, P.D.; Ochsenbauer-Jambor, C.; Smythies, L.E. Intestinal macrophages: Unique effector cells of the innate immune system. *Immunol. Rev.* **2005**, *206*, 149–159. [CrossRef]
112. Gordon, S. The macrophage. *BioEssays* **1995**, *17*, 977–986. [CrossRef]
113. Müller, A.J.; Kaiser, P.; Dittmar, K.E.J.; Weber, T.C.; Haueter, S.; Endt, K.; Songhet, P.; Zellweger, C.; Kremer, M.; Fehling, H.-J.; et al. Salmonella Gut Invasion Involves TTSS-2-Dependent Epithelial Traversal, Basolateral Exit, and Uptake by Epithelium-Sampling Lamina Propria Phagocytes. *Cell Host Microbe* **2012**, *11*, 19–32. [CrossRef]
114. Montalban-Arques, A.; Chaparro, M.; Gisbert, J.P.; Bernardo, D. The Innate Immune System in the Gastrointestinal Tract: Role of Intraepithelial Lymphocytes and Lamina Propria Innate Lymphoid Cells in Intestinal Inflammation. *Inflamm. Bowel Dis.* **2018**, *24*, 1649–1659. [CrossRef]
115. Artis, D.; Spits, H. The biology of innate lymphoid cells. *Nature* **2015**, *517*, 293–301. [CrossRef] [PubMed]
116. Cella, M.; Fuchs, A.; Vermi, W.; Facchetti, F.; Otero, K.; Lennerz, J.K.M.; Doherty, J.M.; Mills, J.C.; Colonna, M. A human natural killer cell subset provides an innate source of IL-22 for mucosal immunity. *Nature* **2009**, *457*, 722–725. [CrossRef] [PubMed]
117. Satoh-Takayama, N.; Vosshenrich, C.A.J.; Lesjean-Pottier, S.; Sawa, S.; Lochner, M.; Rattis, F.; Mention, J.-J.; Thiam, K.; Cerf-Bensussan, N.; Mandelboim, O.; et al. Microbial Flora Drives Interleukin 22 Production in Intestinal NKp46+ Cells that Provide Innate Mucosal Immune Defense. *Immunity* **2008**, *29*, 958–970. [CrossRef] [PubMed]
118. Zook, E.C.; Kee, B.L. Development of innate lymphoid cells. *Nat. Immunol.* **2016**, *17*, 775–782. [CrossRef] [PubMed]
119. Klose, C.S.N.; Artis, D. Innate lymphoid cells as regulators of immunity, inflammation and tissue homeostasis. *Nat. Immunol.* **2016**, *17*, 765–774. [CrossRef] [PubMed]
120. Hori, S.; Nomura, T.; Sakaguchi, S. Control of Regulatory T Cell Development by the Transcription Factor Foxp3. *Science* **2003**, *299*, 1057–1061. [CrossRef] [PubMed]
121. Makita, S.; Kanai, T.; Oshima, S.; Uraushihara, K.; Totsuka, T.; Sawada, T.; Nakamura, T.; Koganei, K.; Fukushima, T.; Watanabe, M. CD4+CD25bright T Cells in Human Intestinal Lamina Propria as Regulatory Cells. *J. Immunol.* **2004**, *173*, 3119–3130. [CrossRef] [PubMed]
122. Brandtzaeg, P.; Johansen, F.-E. Mucosal B cells: Phenotypic characteristics, transcriptional regulation, and homing properties. *Immunol. Rev.* **2005**, *206*, 32–63. [CrossRef]
123. Macpherson, A.J.; McCoy, K.D.; Johansen, F.-E.; Brandtzaeg, P. The immune geography of IgA induction and function. *Mucosal Immunol.* **2008**, *1*, 11–22. [CrossRef]
124. Reboldi, A.; Cyster, J.G. Peyer's patches: Organizing B-cell responses at the intestinal frontier. *Immunol. Rev.* **2016**, *271*, 230–245. [CrossRef]
125. Jung, H.C.; Eckmann, L.; Yang, S.K.; Panja, A.; Fierer, J.; Morzycka-Wroblewska, E.; Kagnoff, M.F. A Distinct Array of Proinflammatory Cytokines is Expressed in Human Colon Epithelial Cells in Response to Bacterial Invasion. *J. Clin. Investig.* **1995**, *95*, 55–65. Available online: https://www.jci.org/articles/view/117676/pdf (accessed on 6 February 2020). [CrossRef] [PubMed]
126. Johansson, M.E.; Gustafsson, J.K.; Holmén-Larsson, J.; Jabbar, K.S.; Xia, L.; Xu, H.; Ghishan, F.K.; Carvalho, F.A.; Gewirtz, A.T.; Sjövall, H.; et al. Bacteria penetrate the normally impenetrable inner colon mucus layer in both murine colitis models and patients with ulcerative colitis. *Gut* **2014**, *63*, 281–291. [CrossRef] [PubMed]
127. Capaldo, C.T.; Nusrat, A. Cytokine regulation of tight junctions. *Biochim. Biophys. Acta Biomembr.* **2009**, *1788*, 864–871. [CrossRef] [PubMed]
128. McGee, D.W.; Vitkus, S.J.D.; Lee, P. The Effect of Cytokine Stimulation on IL-1 Receptor mRNA Expression by Intestinal Epithelial Cells. *Cell. Immunol.* **1996**, *168*, 276–280. [CrossRef] [PubMed]

129. Langerholc, T.; Maragkoudakis, P.A.; Wollgast, J.; Gradisnik, L.; Cencic, A. Novel and established intestinal cell line models—An indispensable tool in food science and nutrition. *Trends Food Sci. Technol.* **2011**, *22*, S11–S20. [CrossRef]
130. Sambruy, Y.; Ferruzza, S.; Ranaldi, G.; De Angelis, I. Intestinal Cell Culture Models: Applications in Toxicology and Pharmacology. *Cell Biol. Toxicol.* **2001**, *17*, 301–317. [CrossRef] [PubMed]
131. Manda, G.; Mocanu, M.A.; Marin, D.E.; Taranu, I. Dual Effects Exerted in vitro by Micromolar Concentrations of Deoxynivalenol on Undifferentiated Caco-2 Cells. *Toxins* **2015**, *7*, 593–603. [CrossRef] [PubMed]
132. Vandenbroucke, V.; Croubels, S.; Martel, A.; Verbrugghe, E.; Goossens, J.; Van Deun, K.; Boyen, F.; Thompson, A.; Shearer, N.; De Backer, P.; et al. The Mycotoxin Deoxynivalenol Potentiates Intestinal Inflammation by Salmonella Typhimurium in Porcine Ileal Loops. *PLoS ONE* **2011**, *6*. [CrossRef]
133. Lee, M.; Vasioukhin, V. Cell polarity and cancer—Cell and tissue polarity as a non-canonical tumor suppressor. *J. Cell Sci.* **2008**, *121*, 1141–1150. [CrossRef]
134. Hauck, W.; Stanners, C.P. Control of Carcinoembryonic Antigen Gene Family Expression in a Differentiating Colon Carcinoma Cell Line, Caco-2. *Cancer Res.* **1991**, *51*, 3526–3533.
135. Ude, V.C.; Brown, D.M.; Viale, L.; Kanase, N.; Stone, V.; Johnston, H.J. Impact of copper oxide nanomaterials on differentiated and undifferentiated Caco-2 intestinal epithelial cells; assessment of cytotoxicity, barrier integrity, cytokine production and nanomaterial penetration. *Part. Fibre Toxicol.* **2017**, *14*, 31. [CrossRef] [PubMed]
136. Cheng, K.-C.; Li, C.; Uss, A.S. Prediction of oral drug absorption in humans – from cultured cell lines and experimental animals. *Expert Opin. Drug Metab. Toxicol.* **2008**, *4*, 581–590. [CrossRef] [PubMed]
137. Fogh, J.; Trempe, G. New Human Tumor Cell Lines. In *Human Tumor Cells in vitro*; Fogh, J., Ed.; Springer: Boston, MA, USA, 1975; pp. 115–159. ISBN 978-1-4757-1647-4.
138. Lea, T. Caco-2 Cell Line. In *The Impact of Food Bioactives on Health: In Vitro and Ex Vivo Models*; Verhoeckx, K., Cotter, P., López-Expósito, I., Kleiveland, C., Lea, T., Mackie, A., Requena, T., Swiatecka, D., Wichers, H., Eds.; Springer: Cham, Switzerland, 2015; ISBN 978-3-319-15791-7.
139. Pearce, S.C.; Coia, H.G.; Karl, J.P.; Pantoja-Feliciano, I.G.; Zachos, N.C.; Racicot, K. Intestinal in vitro and ex vivo Models to Study Host-Microbiome Interactions and Acute Stressors. *Front. Physiol.* **2018**, *9*. [CrossRef] [PubMed]
140. Ponce de León-Rodríguez, M.C.; Guyot, J.-P.; Laurent-Babot, C. Intestinal in vitro cell culture models and their potential to study the effect of food components on intestinal inflammation. *Crit. Rev. Food Sci. Nutr.* **2019**, *59*, 3648–3666. [CrossRef] [PubMed]
141. Hidalgo, I.J.; Raub, T.J.; Borchardt, R.T. Characterization of the human colon carcinoma cell line (Caco-2) as a model system for intestinal epithelial permeability. *Gastroenterology* **1989**, *96*, 736–749. [CrossRef]
142. Furrie, E.; Macfarlane, S.; Thomson, G.; Macfarlane, G.T. Toll-like receptors-2, -3 and -4 expression patterns on human colon and their regulation by mucosal-associated bacteria. *Immunology* **2005**, *115*, 565–574. [CrossRef] [PubMed]
143. Diesing, A.-K.; Nossol, C.; Panther, P.; Walk, N.; Post, A.; Kluess, J.; Kreutzmann, P.; Dänicke, S.; Rothkötter, H.-J.; Kahlert, S. Mycotoxin deoxynivalenol (DON) mediates biphasic cellular response in intestinal porcine epithelial cell lines IPEC-1 and IPEC-J2. *Toxicol. Lett.* **2011**, *200*, 8–18. [CrossRef]
144. Nossol, C.; Barta-Böszörményi, A.; Kahlert, S.; Zuschratter, W.; Faber-Zuschratter, H.; Reinhardt, N.; Ponsuksili, S.; Wimmers, K.; Diesing, A.-K.; Rothkötter, H.-J. Comparing Two Intestinal Porcine Epithelial Cell Lines (IPECs): Morphological Differentiation, Function and Metabolism. *PLoS ONE* **2015**, *10*. [CrossRef]
145. Koh, S.Y.; George, S.; Brözel, V.; Moxley, R.; Francis, D.; Kaushik, R.S. Porcine intestinal epithelial cell lines as a new in vitro model for studying adherence and pathogenesis of enterotoxigenic Escherichia coli. *Vet. Microbiol.* **2008**, *130*, 191–197. [CrossRef]
146. Bertero, A.; Spicer, L.J.; Caloni, F. Fusarium mycotoxins and in vitro species-specific approach with porcine intestinal and brain in vitro barriers: A review. *Food Chem. Toxicol.* **2018**, *121*, 666–675. [CrossRef]
147. Campbell, J.J.; Davidenko, N.; Caffarel, M.M.; Cameron, R.E.; Watson, C.J. A Multifunctional 3D Co-Culture System for Studies of Mammary Tissue Morphogenesis and Stem Cell Biology. *PLoS ONE* **2011**, *6*. [CrossRef] [PubMed]
148. Bertero, A.; Augustyniak, J.; Buzanska, L.; Caloni, F. Species-specific models in toxicology: In vitro epithelial barriers. *Environ. Toxicol. Pharmacol.* **2019**, *70*. [CrossRef] [PubMed]

149. Tremblay, E.; Auclair, J.; Delvin, E.; Levy, E.; Ménard, D.; Pshezhetsky, A.V.; Rivard, N.; Seidman, E.G.; Sinnett, D.; Vachon, P.H.; et al. Gene expression profiles of normal proliferating and differentiating human intestinal epithelial cells: A comparison with the Caco-2 cell model. *J. Cell. Biochem.* **2006**, *99*, 1175–1186. [CrossRef] [PubMed]

150. Mahler, G.J.; Shuler, M.L.; Glahn, R.P. Characterization of Caco-2 and HT29-MTX cocultures in an in vitro digestion/cell culture model used to predict iron bioavailability. *J. Nutr. Biochem.* **2009**, *20*, 494–502. [CrossRef] [PubMed]

151. Smith, M.-C.; Gheux, A.; Coton, M.; Madec, S.; Hymery, N.; Coton, E. In vitro co-culture models to evaluate acute cytotoxicity of individual and combined mycotoxin exposures on Caco-2, THP-1 and HepaRG human cell lines. *Chem. Biol. Interact.* **2018**, *281*, 51–59. [CrossRef]

152. Akbari, P.; Braber, S.; Gremmels, H.; Koelink, P.J.; Verheijden, K.A.T.; Garssen, J.; Fink-Gremmels, J. Deoxynivalenol: A trigger for intestinal integrity breakdown. *FASEB J.* **2014**, *28*, 2414–2429. [CrossRef]

153. Pierron, A.; Mimoun, S.; Murate, L.S.; Loiseau, N.; Lippi, Y.; Bracarense, A.-P.F.L.; Liaubet, L.; Schatzmayr, G.; Berthiller, F.; Moll, W.-D.; et al. Intestinal toxicity of the masked mycotoxin deoxynivalenol-3-β-d-glucoside. *Arch. Toxicol.* **2016**, *90*, 2037–2046. [CrossRef]

154. Bony, S.; Carcelen, M.; Olivier, L.; Devaux, A. Genotoxicity assessment of deoxynivalenol in the Caco-2 cell line model using the Comet assay. *Toxicol. Lett.* **2006**, *166*, 67–76. [CrossRef]

155. Kouadio, J.H.; Mobio, T.A.; Baudrimont, I.; Moukha, S.; Dano, S.D.; Creppy, E.E. Comparative study of cytotoxicity and oxidative stress induced by deoxynivalenol, zearalenone or fumonisin B1 in human intestinal cell line Caco-2. *Toxicology* **2005**, *213*, 56–65. [CrossRef]

156. Ji, J.; Wang, Q.; Wu, H.; Xia, S.; Guo, H.; Blaženović, I.; Zhang, Y.; Sun, X. Insights into cellular metabolic pathways of the combined toxicity responses of Caco-2 cells exposed to deoxynivalenol, zearalenone and Aflatoxin B1. *Food Chem. Toxicol.* **2019**, *126*, 106–112. [CrossRef]

157. Diesing, A.-K.; Nossol, C.; Dänicke, S.; Walk, N.; Post, A.; Kahlert, S.; Rothkötter, H.-J.; Kluess, J. Vulnerability of Polarised Intestinal Porcine Epithelial Cells to Mycotoxin Deoxynivalenol Depends on the Route of Application. *PLoS ONE* **2011**, *6*. [CrossRef] [PubMed]

158. Goossens, J.; Pasmans, F.; Verbrugghe, E.; Vandenbroucke, V.; De Baere, S.; Meyer, E.; Haesebrouck, F.; De Backer, P.; Croubels, S. Porcine intestinal epithelial barrier disruption by the Fusariummycotoxins deoxynivalenol and T-2 toxin promotes transepithelial passage of doxycycline and paromomycin. *BMC Vet. Res.* **2012**, *8*, 245. [CrossRef] [PubMed]

159. Broekaert, N.; Devreese, M.; Demeyere, K.; Berthiller, F.; Michlmayr, H.; Varga, E.; Adam, G.; Meyer, E.; Croubels, S. Comparative in vitro cytotoxicity of modified deoxynivalenol on porcine intestinal epithelial cells. *Food Chem. Toxicol.* **2016**, *95*, 103–109. [CrossRef] [PubMed]

160. Liao, P.; Liao, M.; Li, L.; Tan, B.; Yin, Y. Effect of deoxynivalenol on apoptosis, barrier function, and expression levels of genes involved in nutrient transport, mitochondrial biogenesis and function in IPEC-J2 cells. *Toxicol. Res.* **2017**, *6*, 866–877. [CrossRef] [PubMed]

161. Wan, L.Y.M.; Turner, P.C.; El-Nezami, H. Individual and combined cytotoxic effects of Fusarium toxins (deoxynivalenol, nivalenol, zearalenone and fumonisins B1) on swine jejunal epithelial cells. *Food Chem. Toxicol.* **2013**, *57*, 276–283. [CrossRef] [PubMed]

162. Wang, X.; Zhang, Y.; Zhao, J.; Cao, L.; Zhu, L.; Huang, Y.; Chen, X.; Rahman, S.U.; Feng, S.; Li, Y.; et al. Deoxynivalenol Induces Inflammatory Injury in IPEC-J2 Cells via NF-κB Signaling Pathway. *Toxins* **2019**, *11*, 733. [CrossRef] [PubMed]

163. Taranu, I.; Braicu, C.; Marin, D.E.; Pistol, G.C.; Motiu, M.; Balacescu, L.; Beridan Neagoe, I.; Burlacu, R. Exposure to zearalenone mycotoxin alters in vitro porcine intestinal epithelial cells by differential gene expression. *Toxicol. Lett.* **2015**, *232*, 310–325. [CrossRef]

164. Marin, D.E.; Motiu, M.; Taranu, I. Food Contaminant Zearalenone and Its Metabolites Affect Cytokine Synthesis and Intestinal Epithelial Integrity of Porcine Cells. *Toxins* **2015**, *7*, 1979–1988. [CrossRef]

165. Zhang, J.; Zheng, N.; Liu, J.; Li, F.D.; Li, S.L.; Wang, J.Q. Aflatoxin B1 and aflatoxin M1 induced cytotoxicity and DNA damage in differentiated and undifferentiated Caco-2 cells. *Food Chem. Toxicol.* **2015**, *83*, 54–60. [CrossRef]

166. Romero, A.; Ares, I.; Ramos, E.; Castellano, V.; Martínez, M.; Martínez-Larrañaga, M.-R.; Anadón, A.; Martínez, M.-A. Mycotoxins modify the barrier function of Caco-2 cells through differential gene expression of specific claudin isoforms: Protective effect of illite mineral clay. *Toxicology* **2016**, *353–354*, 21–33. [CrossRef]

167. Guerra, M.C.; Galvano, F.; Bonsi, L.; Speroni, E.; Costa, S.; Renzulli, C.; Cervellati, R. Cyanidin-3-O-b-glucopyranoside, a natural free-radical scavenger against aflatoxin B1- and ochratoxin A-induced cell damage in a human hepatoma cell line (Hep G2) and a human colonic adenocarcinoma cell line (CaCo-2). *Br. J. Nutr.* **2005**, *94*, 211–220. [CrossRef] [PubMed]
168. Bovdisova, I.; Grabacka, M.; Capcarova, M. Interaction of citrinin and resveratrol and their effect on Caco-2 cell growth. *J. Cent. Eur. Agric.* **2016**, *17*, 1287–1297. [CrossRef]
169. Salah, A.; Bouaziz, C.; Prola, A.; Silva, J.P.D.; Bacha, H.; Abid-Essefi, S.; Lemaire, C. Citrinin induces apoptosis in human HCT116 colon cancer cells through endoplasmic reticulum stress. *J. Toxicol. Environ. Health A* **2017**, *80*, 1230–1241. [CrossRef] [PubMed]
170. Assunção, R.; Pinhão, M.; Loureiro, S.; Alvito, P.; Silva, M.J. A multi-endpoint approach to the combined toxic effects of patulin and ochratoxin a in human intestinal cells. *Toxicol. Lett.* **2019**, *313*, 120–129. [CrossRef] [PubMed]
171. Hanelt, M.; Gareis, M.; Kollarczik, B. Cytotoxicity of mycotoxins evaluated by the MTT-cell culture assay. *Mycopathologia* **1994**, *128*, 167–174. [CrossRef]
172. Schneeberger, K.; Roth, S.; Nieuwenhuis, E.E.S.; Middendorp, S. Intestinal epithelial cell polarity defects in disease: Lessons from microvillus inclusion disease. *Dis. Model. Mech.* **2018**, *11*. [CrossRef]
173. Khamchun, S.; Thongboonkerd, V. Cell cycle shift from G0/G1 to S and G2/M phases is responsible for increased adhesion of calcium oxalate crystals on repairing renal tubular cells at injured site. *Cell Death Discov.* **2018**, *4*, 1–12. [CrossRef]
174. Maresca, M.; Mahfoud, R.; Pfohl-Leszkowicz, A.; Fantini, J. The Mycotoxin Ochratoxin A Alters Intestinal Barrier and Absorption Functions but Has No Effect on Chloride Secretion. *Toxicol. Appl. Pharmacol.* **2001**, *176*, 54–63. [CrossRef]
175. Yang, H.; Chung, D.H.; Kim, Y.B.; Choi, Y.H.; Moon, Y. Ribotoxic mycotoxin deoxynivalenol induces G2/M cell cycle arrest via p21Cip/WAF1 mRNA stabilization in human epithelial cells. *Toxicology* **2008**, *243*, 145–154. [CrossRef]
176. Pucci, B.; Kasten, M.; Giordano, A. Cell Cycle and Apoptosis. *Neoplasia* **2000**, *2*, 291–299. [CrossRef]
177. Bensassi, F.; Gallerne, C.; Sharaf el dein, O.; Hajlaoui, M.R.; Lemaire, C.; Bacha, H. In vitro investigation of toxicological interactions between the fusariotoxins deoxynivalenol and zearalenone. *Toxicon* **2014**, *84*, 1–6. [CrossRef] [PubMed]
178. Odenwald, M.A.; Turner, J.R. Intestinal Permeability Defects: Is It Time to Treat? *Clin. Gastroenterol. Hepatol.* **2013**, *11*, 1075–1083. [CrossRef] [PubMed]
179. Madara, J.L. Regulation of the movement of solutes across tight junctions. *Annu. Rev. Physiol.* **1998**, *60*, 143–159. [CrossRef] [PubMed]
180. Jimison, L.H.; Tria, S.A.; Khodagholy, D.; Gurfinkel, M.; Lanzarini, E.; Hama, A.; Malliaras, G.G.; Owens, R.M. Measurement of Barrier Tissue Integrity with an Organic Electrochemical Transistor. *Adv. Mater.* **2012**, *24*, 5919–5923. [CrossRef] [PubMed]
181. González-Mariscal, L.; Domínguez-Calderón, A.; Raya-Sandino, A.; Ortega-Olvera, J.M.; Vargas-Sierra, O.; Martínez-Revollar, G. Tight junctions and the regulation of gene expression. *Semin. Cell Dev. Biol.* **2014**, *36*, 213–223. [CrossRef]
182. Maresca, M.; Mahfoud, R.; Garmy, N.; Fantini, J. The Mycotoxin Deoxynivalenol Affects Nutrient Absorption in Human Intestinal Epithelial Cells. *J. Nutr.* **2002**, *132*, 2723–2731. [CrossRef]
183. Van De Walle, J.; Sergent, T.; Piront, N.; Toussaint, O.; Schneider, Y.-J.; Larondelle, Y. Deoxynivalenol affects in vitro intestinal epithelial cell barrier integrity through inhibition of protein synthesis. *Toxicol. Appl. Pharmacol.* **2010**, *245*, 291–298. [CrossRef]
184. Pinton, P.; Nougayrède, J.-P.; Del Rio, J.-C.; Moreno, C.; Marin, D.E.; Ferrier, L.; Bracarense, A.-P.; Kolf-Clauw, M.; Oswald, I.P. The food contaminant deoxynivalenol, decreases intestinal barrier permeability and reduces claudin expression. *Toxicol. Appl. Pharmacol.* **2009**, *237*, 41–48. [CrossRef]
185. McLaughlin, J.; Padfield, P.J.; Burt, J.P.H.; O'Neill, C.A. Ochratoxin A increases permeability through tight junctions by removal of specific claudin isoforms. *Am. J. Physiol. Cell Physiol.* **2004**, *287*, C1412–C1417. [CrossRef]
186. Ranaldi, G.; Mancini, E.; Ferruzza, S.; Sambuy, Y.; Perozzi, G. Effects of red wine on ochratoxin A toxicity in intestinal Caco-2/TC7 cells. *Toxicol. Vitr.* **2007**, *21*, 204–210. [CrossRef]

187. Watson, P.M.D.; Paterson, J.C.; Thom, G.; Ginman, U.; Lundquist, S.; Webster, C.I. Modelling the endothelial blood-CNS barriers: A method for the production of robust in vitromodels of the rat blood-brain barrier and blood-spinal cord barrier. *BMC Neurosci.* **2013**, *14*, 59. [CrossRef] [PubMed]
188. Srinivasan, B.; Kolli, A.R.; Esch, M.B.; Abaci, H.E.; Shuler, M.L.; Hickman, J.J. TEER Measurement Techniques for In vitro Barrier Model Systems. *J. Lab. Autom.* **2015**. [CrossRef] [PubMed]
189. Ling, K.-H.; Wan, M.L.Y.; El-Nezami, H.; Wang, M. Protective Capacity of Resveratrol, a Natural Polyphenolic Compound, against Deoxynivalenol-Induced Intestinal Barrier Dysfunction and Bacterial Translocation. *Chem. Res. Toxicol.* **2016**, *29*, 823–833. [CrossRef] [PubMed]
190. Schwanhäusser, B.; Busse, D.; Li, N.; Dittmar, G.; Schuchhardt, J.; Wolf, J.; Chen, W.; Selbach, M. Global quantification of mammalian gene expression control. *Nature* **2011**, *473*, 337–342. [CrossRef] [PubMed]
191. Vogel, C.; De Sousa Abreu, R.; Ko, D.; Le, S.-Y.; Shapiro, B.A.; Burns, S.C.; Sandhu, D.; Boutz, D.R.; Marcotte, E.M.; Penalva, L.O. Sequence signatures and mRNA concentration can explain two-thirds of protein abundance variation in a human cell line. *Mol. Syst. Biol.* **2010**, *6*, 400. [CrossRef] [PubMed]
192. Lambert, D.; Padfield, P.J.; McLaughlin, J.; Cannell, S.; O'Neill, C.A. Ochratoxin A displaces claudins from detergent resistant membrane microdomains. *Biochem. Biophys. Res. Commun.* **2007**, *358*, 632–636. [CrossRef]
193. Pinton, P.; Braicu, C.; Nougayrede, J.-P.; Laffitte, J.; Taranu, I.; Oswald, I.P. Deoxynivalenol Impairs Porcine Intestinal Barrier Function and Decreases the Protein Expression of Claudin-4 through a Mitogen-Activated Protein Kinase-Dependent Mechanism. *J. Nutr.* **2010**, *140*, 1956–1962. [CrossRef]
194. Maresca, M.; Yahi, N.; Younès-Sakr, L.; Boyron, M.; Caporiccio, B.; Fantini, J. Both direct and indirect effects account for the pro-inflammatory activity of enteropathogenic mycotoxins on the human intestinal epithelium: Stimulation of interleukin-8 secretion, potentiation of interleukin-1β effect and increase in the transepithelial passage of commensal bacteria. *Toxicol. Appl. Pharmacol.* **2008**, *228*, 84–92.
195. DeMeo, M.T.; Mutlu, E.A.; Keshavarzian, A.; Tobin, M.C. Intestinal permeation and gastrointestinal disease. *J. Clin. Gastroenterol.* **2002**, *34*, 385–396. [CrossRef]
196. Pastorelli, L.; De Salvo, C.; Mercado, J.R.; Vecchi, M.; Pizarro, T.T. Central Role of the Gut Epithelial Barrier in the Pathogenesis of Chronic Intestinal Inflammation: Lessons Learned from Animal Models and Human Genetics. *Front. Immunol.* **2013**, *4*. [CrossRef]
197. Zhou, H.-R.; Islam, Z.; Pestka, J.J. Induction of Competing Apoptotic and Survival Signaling Pathways in the Macrophage by the Ribotoxic Trichothecene Deoxynivalenol. *Toxicol. Sci.* **2005**, *87*, 113–122. [CrossRef] [PubMed]
198. Pestka, J.J.; Uzarski, R.L.; Islam, Z. Induction of apoptosis and cytokine production in the Jurkat human T cells by deoxynivalenol: Role of mitogen-activated protein kinases and comparison to other 8-ketotrichothecenes. *Toxicology* **2005**, *206*, 207–219. [CrossRef] [PubMed]
199. Oh, S.-Y.; Boermans, H.J.; Swamy, H.V.L.N.; Sharma, B.S.; Karrow, N.A. Immunotoxicity of Penicillium Mycotoxins on Viability and Proliferation of Bovine Macrophage Cell Line (BOMACs). *Open Mycol. J.* **2012**, *6*, 11–16. [CrossRef]
200. Wan, L.-Y.M.; Woo, C.-S.J.; Turner, P.C.; Wan, J.M.-F.; El-Nezami, H. Individual and combined effects of Fusarium toxins on the mRNA expression of pro-inflammatory cytokines in swine jejunal epithelial cells. *Toxicol. Lett.* **2013**, *220*, 238–246. [CrossRef] [PubMed]
201. Van De Walle, J.; Romier, B.; Larondelle, Y.; Schneider, Y.-J. Influence of deoxynivalenol on NF-κB activation and IL-8 secretion in human intestinal Caco-2 cells. *Toxicol. Lett.* **2008**, *177*, 205–214. [CrossRef] [PubMed]
202. Vandenbroucke, V.; Croubels, S.; Verbrugghe, E.; Boyen, F.; Backer, P.D.; Ducatelle, R.; Rychlik, I.; Haesebrouck, F.; Pasmans, F. The mycotoxin deoxynivalenol promotes uptake of Salmonella Typhimurium in porcine macrophages, associated with ERK1/2 induced cytoskeleton reorganization. *Vet. Res.* **2009**, *40*. [CrossRef] [PubMed]
203. Oh, S.-Y.; Mead, P.J.; Sharma, B.S.; Quinton, V.M.; Boermans, H.J.; Smith, T.K.; Swamy, H.V.L.N.; Karrow, N.A. Effect of Penicillium mycotoxins on the cytokine gene expression, reactive oxygen species production, and phagocytosis of bovine macrophage (BoMacs) function. *Toxicol. Vitr.* **2015**, *30*, 446–453. [CrossRef]
204. Devreese, M.; Backer, P.D.; Croubels, S. Different methods to counteract mycotoxin production and its impact on animal health. *Vlaams Diergeneeskd. Tijdschr.* **2013**, *82*, 181–190.
205. Faucet-Marquis, V.; Joannis-Cassan, C.; Hadjeba-Medjdoub, K.; Ballet, N.; Pfohl-Leszkowicz, A. Development of an in vitro method for the prediction of mycotoxin binding on yeast-based products: Case of aflatoxin B1, zearalenone and ochratoxin A. *Appl. Microbiol. Biotechnol.* **2014**, *98*, 7583–7596. [CrossRef]

206. Kabak, B.; Dobson, A.D.W.; Var, I. Strategies to Prevent Mycotoxin Contamination of Food and Animal Feed: A Review. *Crit. Rev. Food Sci. Nutr.* **2006**, *46*, 593–619. [CrossRef]
207. Peng, W.-X.; Marchal, J.L.M.; Van der Poel, A.F.B. Strategies to prevent and reduce mycotoxins for compound feed manufacturing. *Anim. Feed Sci. Technol.* **2018**, *237*, 129–153. [CrossRef]
208. Horky, P.; Skalickova, S.; Baholet, D.; Skladanka, J. Nanoparticles as a Solution for Eliminating the Risk of Mycotoxins. *Nanomaterials* **2018**, *8*, 727. [CrossRef] [PubMed]
209. Abdel-Wahhab, M.A.; Nada, S.A.; Khalil, F.A. Physiological and toxicological responses in rats fed aflatoxin-contaminated diet with or without sorbent materials. *Anim. Feed Sci. Technol.* **2002**, *97*, 209–219. [CrossRef]
210. Avantaggiato, G.; Havenaar, R.; Visconti, A. Assessing the zearalenone-binding activity of adsorbent materials during passage through a dynamic in vitro gastrointestinal model. *Food Chem. Toxicol.* **2003**, *41*, 1283–1290. [CrossRef]
211. Huwig, A.; Freimund, S.; Käppeli, O.; Dutler, H. Mycotoxin detoxication of animal feed by different adsorbents. *Toxicol. Lett.* **2001**, *122*, 179–188. [CrossRef]
212. Ramos, A.-J.; Fink-Gremmels, J.; Hernández, E. Prevention of Toxic Effects of Mycotoxins by Means of Nonnutritive Adsorbent Compounds. *J. Food Prot.* **1996**, *59*, 631–641. [CrossRef] [PubMed]
213. Boudergue, C.; Burel, C.; Dragacci, S.; Favrot, M.-C.; Fremy, J.-M.; Massimi, C.; Prigent, P.; Debongnie, P.; Pussemier, L.; Boudra, H.; et al. Review of mycotoxin-detoxifying agents used as feed additives: Mode of action, efficacy and feed/food safety. *EFSA Supporting Publ.* **2009**, *6*. [CrossRef]
214. Avantaggiato, G.; Solfrizzo, M.; Visconti, A. Recent advances on the use of adsorbent materials for detoxification of Fusarium mycotoxins. *Food Addit. Contam.* **2005**, *22*, 379–388. [CrossRef]
215. Phillips, T.D.; Afriyie-Gyawu, E.; Williams, J.; Huebner, H.; Ankrah, N.-A.; Ofori-Adjei, D.; Jolly, P.; Johnson, N.; Taylor, J.; Marroquin-Cardona, A.; et al. Reducing human exposure to aflatoxin through the use of clay: A review. *Food Addit. Contam. Part A* **2008**, *25*, 134–145. [CrossRef]
216. Karlovsky, P. Biological detoxification of the mycotoxin deoxynivalenol and its use in genetically engineered crops and feed additives. *Appl. Microbiol. Biotechnol.* **2011**, *91*, 491–504. [CrossRef]
217. Döll, S.; Dänicke, S.; Valenta, H.; Flachowsky, G. In vitro studies on the evaluation of mycotoxin detoxifying agents for their efficacy on deoxynivalenol and zearalenone. *Arch. Anim. Nutr.* **2004**, *58*, 311–324. [CrossRef] [PubMed]
218. Kolosova, A.; Stroka, J. Evaluation of the effect of mycotoxin binders in animal feed on the analytical performance of standardised methods for the determination of mycotoxins in feed. *Food Addit. Contam. Part A* **2012**, *29*, 1959–1971. [CrossRef] [PubMed]
219. Jouany, J.P. Methods for preventing, decontaminating and minimizing the toxicity of mycotoxins in feeds. *Anim. Feed Sci. Technol.* **2007**, *137*, 342–362. [CrossRef]
220. Kogan, G.; Kocher, A. Role of yeast cell wall polysaccharides in pig nutrition and health protection. *Livest. Sci.* **2007**, *109*, 161–165. [CrossRef]
221. Pereyra, C.M.; Cavaglieri, L.R.; Chiacchiera, S.M.; Dalcero, A. The corn influence on the adsorption levels of aflatoxin B1 and zearalenone by yeast cell wall. *J. Appl. Microbiol.* **2013**, *114*, 655–662. [CrossRef] [PubMed]
222. Shetty, P.H.; Jespersen, L. Saccharomyces cerevisiae and lactic acid bacteria as potential mycotoxin decontaminating agents. *Trends Food Sci. Technol.* **2006**, *17*, 48–55. [CrossRef]
223. Yiannikouris, A.; André, G.; Buléon, A.; Jeminet, G.; Canet, I.; François, J.; Bertin, G.; Jouany, J.-P. Comprehensive Conformational Study of Key Interactions Involved in Zearalenone Complexation with β-d-Glucans. *Biomacromolecules* **2004**, *5*, 2176–2185. [CrossRef]
224. Yiannikouris, A.; André, G.; Poughon, L.; François, J.; Dussap, C.-G.; Jeminet, G.; Bertin, G.; Jouany, J.-P. Chemical and Conformational Study of the Interactions Involved in Mycotoxin Complexation with β-d-Glucans. *Biomacromolecules* **2006**, *7*, 1147–1155. [CrossRef]
225. Binder, E.M. Managing the risk of mycotoxins in modern feed production. *Anim. Feed Sci. Technol.* **2007**, *133*, 149–166. [CrossRef]
226. Firmin, S.; Gandia, P.; Morgavi, D.P.; Houin, G.; Jouany, J.P.; Bertin, G.; Boudra, H. Modification of aflatoxin B1 and ochratoxin A toxicokinetics in rats administered a yeast cell wall preparation. *Food Addit. Contam. Part A* **2010**, *27*, 1153–1160. [CrossRef]
227. Firmin, S.; Morgavi, D.P.; Yiannikouris, A.; Boudra, H. Effectiveness of modified yeast cell wall extracts to reduce aflatoxin B1 absorption in dairy ewes. *J. Dairy Sci.* **2011**, *94*, 5611–5619. [CrossRef] [PubMed]

228. Yiannikouris, A.; Kettunen, H.; Apajalahti, J.; Pennala, E.; Moran, C.A. Comparison of the sequestering properties of yeast cell wall extract and hydrated sodium calcium aluminosilicate in three in vitro models accounting for the animal physiological bioavailability of zearalenone. *Food Addit. Contam. Part A* **2013**, *30*, 1641–1650. [CrossRef] [PubMed]
229. Shetty, P.H.; Hald, B.; Jespersen, L. Surface binding of aflatoxin B1 by Saccharomyces cerevisiae strains with potential decontaminating abilities in indigenous fermented foods. *Int. J. Food Microbiol.* **2007**, *113*, 41–46. [CrossRef] [PubMed]
230. Ringot, D.; Lerzy, B.; Chaplain, K.; Bonhoure, J.-P.; Auclair, E.; Larondelle, Y. In vitro biosorption of ochratoxin A on the yeast industry by-products: Comparison of isotherm models. *Bioresour. Technol.* **2007**, *98*, 1812–1821. [CrossRef] [PubMed]
231. Sabater-Vilar, M.; Malekinejad, H.; Selman, M.H.J.; Van der Doelen, M.A.M.; Fink-Gremmels, J. In vitro assessment of adsorbents aiming to prevent deoxynivalenol and zearalenone mycotoxicoses. *Mycopathologia* **2007**, *163*, 81. [CrossRef] [PubMed]
232. Joannis-Cassan, C.; Tozlovanu, M.; Hadjeba-Medjdoub, K.; Ballet, N.; Pfohl-Leszkowicz, A. Binding of zearalenone, aflatoxin B1, and ochratoxin A by yeast-based products: A method for quantification of adsorption performance. *J. Food Prot.* **2011**, *74*, 1175–1185. [CrossRef] [PubMed]
233. Gerbaldo, G.A.; Barberis, C.; Pascual, L.; Dalcero, A.; Barberis, L. Antifungal activity of two Lactobacillus strains with potential probiotic properties. *FEMS Microbiol. Lett.* **2012**, *332*, 27–33. [CrossRef]
234. Hahn, I.; Kunz-Vekiru, E.; Twarużek, M.; Grajewski, J.; Krska, R.; Berthiller, F. Aerobic and anaerobic in vitro testing of feed additives claiming to detoxify deoxynivalenol and zearalenone. *Food Addit. Contam. Part A* **2015**, *32*, 922–933. [CrossRef]
235. Cavret, S.; Laurent, N.; Videmann, B.; Mazallon, M.; Lecoeur, S. Assessment of deoxynivalenol (DON) adsorbents and characterisation of their efficacy using complementary in vitro tests. *Food Addit. Contam. Part A* **2010**, *27*, 43–53. [CrossRef]
236. Oh, S.-Y.; Quinton, V.M.; Boermans, H.J.; Swamy, H.V.L.N.; Karrow, N.A. In vitro exposure of Penicillium mycotoxins with or without a modified yeast cell wall extract (mYCW) on bovine macrophages (BoMacs). *Mycotoxin Res.* **2015**, *31*, 167–175. [CrossRef]
237. Avantaggiato, G.; Havenaar, R.; Visconti, A. Evaluation of the intestinal absorption of deoxynivalenol and nivalenol by an in vitro gastrointestinal model, and the binding efficacy of activated carbon and other adsorbent materials. *Food Chem. Toxicol.* **2004**, *42*, 817–824. [CrossRef] [PubMed]
238. Prapapanpong, J.; Udomkusonsri, P.; Mahavorasirikul, W.; Choochuay, S.; Tansakul, N. In vitro studies on gastrointestinal monogastric and avian models to evaluate the binding efficacy of mycotoxin adsorbents by liquid chromatography-tandem mass spectrometry. *J. Adv. Vet. Anim. Res.* **2019**, *6*, 125–132. [CrossRef] [PubMed]
239. Natsch, A.; Gfeller, H.; Emter, R.; Ellis, G. Use of in vitro testing to identify an unexpected skin sensitizing impurity in a commercial product: A case study. *Toxicol. Vitr. Int. J. Publ. Assoc. BIBRA* **2010**, *24*, 411–416. [CrossRef] [PubMed]
240. Trapecar, M.; Cencic, A. Application of Gut Cell Models for Toxicological and Bioactivity Studies of Functional and Novel Foods. *Foods* **2012**, *1*, 40–51. [CrossRef] [PubMed]
241. Zeissig, S.; Bürgel, N.; Günzel, D.; Richter, J.; Mankertz, J.; Wahnschaffe, U.; Kroesen, A.J.; Zeitz, M.; Fromm, M.; Schulzke, J.-D. Changes in expression and distribution of claudin 2, 5 and 8 lead to discontinuous tight junctions and barrier dysfunction in active Crohn's disease. *Gut* **2007**, *56*, 61–72. [CrossRef] [PubMed]
242. Lemke, S.L.; Grant, P.G.; Phillips, T.D. Adsorption of Zearalenone by Organophilic Montmorillonite Clay. *J. Agric. Food Chem.* **1998**, *46*, 3789–3796. [CrossRef]
243. Pan, F.; Han, L.; Zhang, Y.; Yu, Y.; Liu, J. Optimization of Caco-2 and HT29 co-culture in vitro cell models for permeability studies. *Int. J. Food Sci. Nutr.* **2015**, *66*, 680–685. [CrossRef]
244. Borenfreund, E.; Puerner, J.A. Toxicity determined in vitro by morphological alterations and neutral red absorption. *Toxicol. Lett.* **1985**, *24*, 119–124. [CrossRef]
245. Cencič, A.; Langerholc, T. Functional cell models of the gut and their applications in food microbiology—A review. *Int. J. Food Microbiol.* **2010**, *141*, S4–S14. [CrossRef]
246. Suzuki, K.; Oida, T.; Hamada, H.; Hitotsumatsu, O.; Watanabe, M.; Hibi, T.; Yamamoto, H.; Kubota, E.; Kaminogawa, S.; Ishikawa, H. Gut Cryptopatches: Direct Evidence of Extrathymic Anatomical Sites for Intestinal T Lymphopoiesis. *Immunity* **2000**, *13*, 691–702. [CrossRef]

247. Trapecar, M.; Leouffre, T.; Faure, M.; Jensen, H.E.; Granum, P.E.; Cencic, A.; Hardy, S.P. The use of a porcine intestinal cell model system for evaluating the food safety risk of Bacillus cereus probiotics and the implications for assessing enterotoxigenicity. *APMIS* **2011**, *119*, 877–884. [CrossRef] [PubMed]

248. Vamadevan, A.S.; Fukata, M.; Arnold, E.T.; Thomas, L.S.; Hsu, D.; Abreu, M.T. Regulation of Toll-like receptor 4-associated MD-2 in intestinal epithelial cells: A comprehensive analysis. *Innate Immun.* **2010**, *16*, 93–103. [CrossRef] [PubMed]

249. Tavelin, S.; Taipalensuu, J.; Soderberg, L.; Morrison, R.; Chong, S.; Artursson, P. Prediction of the Oral Absorption of Low-Permeability Drugs Using Small Intestine-Like 2/4/A1 Cell Monolayers. *Pharm. Res.* **2003**, *20*, 397–405. [CrossRef] [PubMed]

250. Nakayama, H.; Kitagawa, N.; Otani, T.; Iida, H.; Anan, H.; Inai, T. Ochratoxin A, citrinin and deoxynivalenol decrease claudin-2 expression in mouse rectum CMT93-II cells. *Microscopy* **2018**, *67*, 99–111. [CrossRef] [PubMed]

251. Artursson, P.; Palm, K.; Luthman, K. Caco-2 monolayers in experimental and theoretical predictions of drug transport1PII of original article: S0169-409X(96)00415-2. The article was originally published in Advanced Drug Delivery Reviews 22 (1996) 67–84.1. *Adv. Drug Deliv. Rev.* **2001**, *46*, 27–43. [CrossRef]

252. Klarić, M.Š. Adverse Effects Of Combined Mycotoxins / Štetni Učinci Kombiniranih Mikotoksina. *Arch. Ind. Hyg. Toxicol.* **2012**, *63*, 519–530.

253. Kleiveland, C.R. Co-culture Caco-2/Immune Cells. In *The Impact of Food Bioactives on Health: In Vitro and Ex Vivo Models*; Verhoeckx, K., Cotter, P., López-Expósito, I., Kleiveland, C., Lea, T., Mackie, A., Requena, T., Swiatecka, D., Wichers, H., Eds.; Springer International Publishing: Cham, Switzerland, 2015; pp. 197–205. ISBN 978-3-319-16104-4.

254. Fitzgerald, K.A.; Malhotra, M.; Curtin, C.M.; O' Brien, F.J.; O' Driscoll, C.M. Life in 3D is never flat: 3D models to optimise drug delivery. *J. Control. Release* **2015**, *215*, 39–54. [CrossRef]

255. Goers, L.; Freemont, P.; Polizzi, K.M. Co-culture systems and technologies: Taking synthetic biology to the next level. *J. R. Soc. Interface* **2014**, *11*. [CrossRef]

256. Thomsen, L.B.; Burkhart, A.; Moos, T. A Triple Culture Model of the Blood-Brain Barrier Using Porcine Brain Endothelial cells, Astrocytes and Pericytes. *PLoS ONE* **2015**, *10*. [CrossRef]

257. Cheli, F.; Campagnoli, A.; Dell'Orto, V. Fungal populations and mycotoxins in silages: From occurrence to analysis. *Anim. Feed Sci. Technol.* **2013**, *183*, 1–16. [CrossRef]

258. Richard, E.; Heutte, N.; Bouchart, V.; Garon, D. Evaluation of fungal contamination and mycotoxin production in maize silage. *Anim. Feed Sci. Technol.* **2009**, *148*, 309–320. [CrossRef]

259. Rodrigues, I. A review on the effects of mycotoxins in dairy ruminants. *Anim. Prod. Sci.* **2014**, *54*, 1155–1165. [CrossRef]

260. Malmuthuge, N.; Griebel, P.J.; Guan, L.L. The Gut Microbiome and Its Potential Role in the Development and Function of Newborn Calf Gastrointestinal Tract. *Front. Vet. Sci.* **2015**, *2*. [CrossRef] [PubMed]

261. Kruber, P.; Trump, S.; Behrens, J.; Lehmann, I. T-2 toxin is a cytochrome P450 1A1 inducer and leads to MAPK/p38- but not aryl hydrocarbon receptor-dependent interleukin-8 secretion in the human intestinal epithelial cell line Caco-2. *Toxicology* **2011**, *284*, 34–41. [CrossRef] [PubMed]

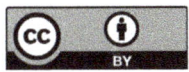

© 2020 by the authors. Licensee MDPI, Basel, Switzerland. This article is an open access article distributed under the terms and conditions of the Creative Commons Attribution (CC BY) license (http://creativecommons.org/licenses/by/4.0/).

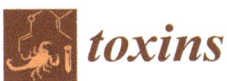

Review

Decontamination of Mycotoxin-Contaminated Feedstuffs and Compound Feed

Radmilo Čolović [1],*, Nikola Puvača [2],*, Federica Cheli [3],*, Giuseppina Avantaggiato [4], Donato Greco [4], Olivera Đuragić [1], Jovana Kos [1] and Luciano Pinotti [3]

[1] Institute of Food Technology, University of Novi Sad, Bulevar cara Lazara, 21000 Novi Sad, Serbia; olivera.djuragic@fins.uns.ac.rs (O.Đ.); jovana.kos@fins.uns.ac.rs (J.K.)
[2] Department of Engineering Management in Biotechnology, Faculty of Economics and Engineering Management in Novi Sad, University Business Academy in Novi Sad, Cvećarska, 21000 Novi Sad, Serbia
[3] Department of Health, Animal Science and Food Safety, University of Milan, Via Trentacoste, 20134 Milan, Italy; luciano.pinotti@unimi.it
[4] Institute of Sciences of Food Production (ISPA), National Research Council (CNR), Via Amendola, 70126 Bari, Italy; giuseppina.avantaggiato@ispa.cnr.it (G.A.); greco_donato@libero.it (D.G.)
* Correspondence: radmilo.colovic@fins.uns.ac.rs (R.Č.); nikola.puvaca@fimek.edu.rs (N.P.); federica.cheli@unimi.it (F.C.)

Received: 8 August 2019; Accepted: 23 October 2019; Published: 25 October 2019

Abstract: Mycotoxins are known worldwide as fungus-produced toxins that adulterate a wide heterogeneity of raw feed ingredients and final products. Consumption of mycotoxins-contaminated feed causes a plethora of harmful responses from acute toxicity to many persistent health disorders with lethal outcomes; such as mycotoxicosis when ingested by animals. Therefore, the main task for feed producers is to minimize the concentration of mycotoxin by applying different strategies aimed at minimizing the risk of mycotoxin effects on animals and human health. Once mycotoxins enter the production chain it is hard to eliminate or inactivate them. This paper examines the most recent findings on different processes and strategies for the reduction of toxicity of mycotoxins in animals. The review gives detailed information about the decontamination approaches to mitigate mycotoxin contamination of feedstuffs and compound feed, which could be implemented in practice.

Keywords: mycotoxins; reduction; grain cleaning; thermal processing; chemicals; adsorbents

Key Contribution: This article reviews the latest results on how different procedures and policies can be applied to reduce the toxicity of mycotoxins in animals.

1. Introduction

Modern feed mills produce a wide range of products on a daily basis, regardless of whether they have one or several processing lines. Formulated diets are often composed of more than 20 ingredients and each of the ingredients is carefully selected based on the nutritional quality, safety, price, and availability [1]. Safe ingredients are important for the production of safe animal feed, which is in turn important for animal health, production of safe animal products for human consumption, and for the environment. To ensure security in the agro-food chain, the feed mills are obliged to control all raw materials and products for the presence of possible contaminants as well as to test numerous samples on a daily basis [2]. Mycotoxins are a major contaminant of feed ingredients and products. Since these secondary metabolites of molds are toxic, feed producers have to ensure that concentrations of these contaminants do not exceed maximum allowed values for a specific mycotoxin. The occurrence of mycotoxin is a significant global challenge, accompanied by rising animal and human health hazards and huge financial losses in the food and feed production industries [3,4].

Different methods are used to decontaminate mycotoxin-contaminated commodities or to reduce the exposure to mycotoxins, but not all approaches are appropriate for feed and compound feed manufacturers. An efficient method for the reduction of mycotoxins should be able to remove or inactivate the mycotoxins without producing toxic residues and affecting the technological properties, nutritive value, and palatability of products [5]. Modern feed production is mainly done on a large scale, and proposed strategies should also be capable of being implemented on a large scale as well [6]. Due to the high cost of raw materials, which contribute up to 70% of the costs of compound feed, feed production costs are optimized, and only relatively simple and/or inexpensive strategies are acceptable for mycotoxin removal [7].

Essential oils are biological technologies for the decontamination of mycotoxins in feedstuffs. The oils present secondary metabolites extracted from plants and consist primarily of monoterpenes and sesquiterpenes and phenylpropanoids, compounds responsible for the oil's organoleptic characteristics [8]. Fungi metabolize and synthesize many organic compounds with bad properties during their life cycle [9].

Many physical, chemical and biological technologies have been suggested with the aim of reducing unavoidable and unpredictable mycotoxin contamination and many have shown excellent effectiveness. This article reviews the latest results on various procedures and strategies used to reduce mycotoxin contamination in the feedstuffs and compound feed, as well as to reduce the toxicity of mycotoxins in animals.

2. Grain Cleaning

Grains are normally received in bulk from receiving hoppers of feed mills. Since the unloading area is the largest source for dust emissions, and since there is an explosion risk, this is the place where the dust control equipment is installed. Also, mills are often equipped with vibratory screens, or other grain cleaning equipment, which removes oversized or undersized material [10]. These processing steps are introduced to remove foreign material, such as stalks, paper, wood scraps, etc., but they have also shown to be effective in mycotoxin removal. The mycotoxin concentration can be decreased by removing kernels with mold growth, crushed kernels and dust [11].

Cereals, which are a major part of animal diets, are often received in a feed mill in grain form. Depending on the climate conditions in the location where the crops are grown, cereals might be a favorable substrate for mycotoxigenic fungal species. These ingredients have high inclusion rates in animal compound feed, and if contaminated, could be a source of contamination of the final products [12,13]. Therefore, the focus of numerous studies was the investigation of procedures for decontamination of cereal grains [14–20].

Not all parts of the grain kernels are susceptible to fungal contamination. The outer parts of grains, such as germ and pericarp, have a higher tendency to be contaminated by mycotoxins than the endosperm [21,22]. The data from the literature confirms that the milling process redirects the mycotoxins into inedible byproducts, but these byproducts are commonly used as animal feed, such as bran, feed flour, polishings, etc. [23,24]. Also, dehulling, scouring or other processes where a part of the grain is removed are not typical for the animal feed production process. When the whole grains are used in the feed mill, the most commonly used grinding equipment is a hammer mill, roller mill, pulverizer, disk mill, etc. All of these machines grind a whole cereal grain without subsequent fractionation and possible redirection of mycotoxins [25].

Dust removal can be efficient in removing mycotoxins. As shown by different studies, mycotoxins are often accumulated in the grain dust, and exposure to it can have toxic effects on animals and humans [26,27]. Efficient dust collection systems and separation systems can be efficient in mycotoxin redirection into fine fractions which are excluded from the raw materials or final products. Different dust separation systems might be implemented in the feed mill. Some of the installed options have the possibility to adjust the cutting point for the separation of fine particles in wider ranges of particle sizes. Vidosavljević et al. [28] have applied gravitational cascade zig-zag classifier for dust removal, and have been able to reach the level of aflatoxin reduction higher than 90% in the coarse fraction. Higher airspeed might be more efficient in mycotoxin removal, but they also increase the yield of the fine fraction which is considered a waste product [28]. In addition, separation systems can also be used for the removal of broken kernels. Broken kernels might be a potential source of mycotoxin contamination since they have a higher mycotoxin level than whole kernels. Screening and gravity are used more frequently than air separation/classification for the separation of broken kernels and coarse impurities separation. Dry cleaning of grain surface may also lead to a reduction of molds and mycotoxins. For example, it has been demonstrated that deoxynivalenol content can be reduced up to 84%, while the aflatoxin level was reduced by approximately 62% by the use of polypropylene bristle brushes for polishing of grain surface without damage of pericarp [28]. The increase in the retention time of contaminated material in the cleaning device and cleaning intensity increases the effectiveness of mycotoxin removal [28,29]. However, these processing steps are not commonly used in the processing line in order to avoid potential bottlenecks.

In cases where the size of contaminated kernels is similar to the size of whole kernels, typical separation technologies based on a difference in a mass or density are not very efficient in the removal of infected material [29]. Since these infected grains can be visually differentiated from the healthy grains, their separation from the intact commodity can be effective in mycotoxin reduction. It has been reported that even manual sorting can be effective in aflatoxin, deoxynivalenol, and fumonisin reduction by up to 80%, 83.6%, and 84%, respectively [28,30]. Taking into account that the average feed mill capacity is approx. 50,000 tons per year, it is clear why it is not possible to implement manual sorting at a large scale. On the other hand, optical sorting has been successfully implemented at a large scale in the feed industry for the removal of infected kernels based on color difference. Within the optical sorting machines, grain streams are directed along by optical sensors and the grains different in color were removed by a jet of pressurized air from the stream. By removing infected grains, it is also possible to reduce mycotoxin content by more than 80% [14,31].

Other physical treatments that have shown to be effective in mycotoxin decontamination are flotation in various solutions, cold plasma, gamma-radiation, microwave heating, etc. They are not commonly used by the feed industry due to different reasons, such as high investment cost, high operational costs, unavailable processing units on a large scale required by the feed producers, etc.

3. Thermal Processing

In general, mycotoxins are mainly stable compounds under conditions of thermal processes that are most commonly used in food and feed production [11,32]. The following factors of thermal processing are the most important for the degradation and reduction of mycotoxins in food and feed: type of mycotoxin, the initial mycotoxin concentration, temperature, time of exposure to high temperature, the degree of heat penetration, pH, moisture content, etc. [32]. If raw materials are contaminated with some regulated and/or non-regulated mycotoxins there is a great possibility that final products will also contain those mycotoxins, since they are not completely destroyed during the applied thermal process. Different processes of thermal food and feed treatment that can have different impacts on mycotoxins include extrusion, cooking, frying, baking, canning, crumbling, pelleting, roasting, flaking, nixtamalization, alkaline cooking, etc. [11]. Only a few of the listed processes, such as crumbling, pelleting and extrusion are commonly used in compound feed preparation as well as in feed production. Even though these processes can significantly reduce the mycotoxin concentration, their implementation usually does not lead to the complete elimination of mycotoxins. Among the thermal treatments, the utilization of high-temperature processes demonstrated the greatest potential for mycotoxins reduction [11]. Kabak [32] examined the effect of different extrusion parameters on the reduction of some regulated mycotoxins. He concluded that the application of extrusion at a temperature higher than 150 °C have a significant impact on the reduction of zearalenone and fumonisins, while the same conditions led to moderate reduction of aflatoxins and deoxynivalenol. The extrusion process with temperatures at around 160 °C or higher, in combination with glucose, demonstrated the greatest degree of reduction of fumonisins. For example, after the extrusion of corn grits with 10% added glucose, initial fumonisin B_1 concentration was reduced by 75–85%. In addition to fumonisin reduction, the applied extrusion process resulted in the formation of high amounts of N-(1-deoxy-d-fructos-1-yl)-Fumonisin B_1, and in small amounts of hydrolyzed fumonisin B_1 and N-(Carboxymethyl)—Fumonisin B_1. Fumonisins contaminated corn grits extruded with glucose demonstrated lower toxicity during feeding trial toxicity tests in rats [33]. However, it is important to note that the process for the production of animal feed includes mixing different batches of different raw ingredients. Therefore, creating a new complex feed mixture represents a great risk since each raw ingredient has its own initial contamination with an entirely new risk profile for the majority of mycotoxins [34]. Roasting and extrusion processing, reaching temperatures of 150 °C or more, could contribute to the reduction of contaminated batches [15,18,28]. In this complex scenario, further investigation related to the fate of various mycotoxins during thermal feed processing, as well as their overall loss in toxicity in different feed matrixes is clearly required in order to define the best thermal processes for mycotoxins reductions on one hand, and to avoid losses of feed nutritional quality on the other hand. However, the application of high temperatures in feed processes can have variable effects on mycotoxins, from significant to slight reduction.

4. Chemical Agents

In spite of all positive sides of available chemical treatments for decontamination of mycotoxin contaminated feedstuffs and compound feed, their limitations are also present, since the products handled must be safe from the chemicals used and the nutritional value of the products should not be altered or deteriorated [15]. Not all agents are efficient to the same degree against mycotoxins, but science is still making efforts to find a broad variety of chemicals that will be effective on a higher scale against a larger number of mycotoxins [16]. Nowadays, there are several chemicals agents used for mycotoxin contaminations mycotoxin decontaminations and can be divided into categories such as alkaline (Ammonia gas NH_4OH; Sodium hydroxide $NaOH$; Calcium hydroxide $Ca(OH)_2$), acids (Acetic acid C_2H_3OH; Phosphoric acid H_3PO_4; Formic acid CH_2O_2; Propionic acid CH_3CH_2COOH; Sorbic acid $C_6H_8O_2$; Sodium hypochlorite $NaClO$), reducing agents (Sodium bisulfite $NaHSO_3$; Sugars: D-glucose or D-fructose), oxidising reagents (Ozone O_3; Hydrogen peroxide H_2O_2), and many others such as chlorinating agents, salts and miscellaneous reagents [15,17].

Cereals treatment with ammonia gas is known as the method of ammoniation, which gained great attention in detoxification of aflatoxin and ochratoxin, and have been used for decontamination in several countries [16,17]. However, the efficacy of ammoniation varies on the type of mycotoxin. The efficiency of applied NH_4OH on laboratory animals with the purpose of lowering concentrations of fumonisins did not show any promising results since there was no decrease in toxicity when ammonia fumonisin B_1 was supplied to livestock despite a decrease in fumonisin B_1 concentration. In the last several years in developed countries, ammoniation has been successfully used in maize grain decontaminations, in particular, to reduce the amount of contamination of aflatoxins in feed [14,18]. Ammoniation is usually the most effective against aflatoxin B_1, with the remaining side product of aflatoxin D_1, which is far less toxic than the aflatoxin B_1. In addition, the positive effects of ammoniation in feedstuffs and compound feed detoxification could be compared to the high cost of applied methodology, and more the ineffectiveness of the method against other mycotoxins. Nevertheless, this method can lead to food quality decrease and deterioration due to involved excessive ammonia levels in the food [35]. Calcium hydroxide was used to decontaminate feeds contaminated with T-2 toxin and diacetoxyscirpenol. Under the aforementioned alkaline conditions, mycotoxin structure can certainly be changed [19].

Feedstuffs and compound feed treatment with strong acids could destroy the biological activity of aflatoxin B_1 Thus converting aflatoxin B1 to a compound which is hemiacetal or a hemiketal compound the results from the addition of an alcohol to an aldehyde or a ketone, which are formed when a second alkoxy group has been added to the structure, respectively [36]. HCl treatment (pH 2) showed a 19.3%

reduction in aflatoxin B_1 concentrations within 24 h. Formic, propionic and sorbic acids show their positive influence when it comes to the degradation of ochratoxin A with concentrations ranging from 0.25 to 1.0% after exposure to this particular acid during the time which is no longer of 24 h. Sodium hypochlorite can be used successfully in the destruction of ochratoxin A as a pale greenish-yellow dilute solution commonly known as liquid bleach or simply bleach [37].

Reducing agents such as sodium bisulfite have the affinity to react with aflatoxins and trichothecenes. Their mechanism of action includes the formation of sulphonate derivatives while peroxide and heat enhance the destruction of aflatoxin B_1 by sodium bisulfite [38]. Besides aflatoxin B_1 and trichothecenes, reducing agents decreased the levels of deoxynivalenol as well. The conversion of sodium bisulfite from deoxynivalenol to deoxynivalenol-sulfonate, which is less toxic than deoxynivalenol, has been recorded as an efficient instrument to overcome the depressive impacts of deoxynivalenol on feed consumption in certain species and farm animal categories. Temperatures at approximately 65 °C for 48 h can block the primary amino group of fumonisin B_1 and prevent toxicity of cell tissue cultures of farm and laboratory animals caused by the presence of fumonisin in feed, but only in the presence of D-glucose or D-fructose sugar reduction [39].

Oxidizing agents such as ozone and hydrogen peroxide were used to decontaminate mycotoxin contaminated raw feed and compound feed [40]. In addition to feed and compound feed, ozone treatment has been used with very high success over the years to decontaminate food products. Many of the chemical methods mentioned above could be used to reduce mycotoxin levels in feed and compound foods with a high percentage of efficacy, but it could not be neglected that these chemicals could potentially activate changes in the nutritional, physical and sensory properties of treated materials [41]. Protection against aflatoxin B_1 in poultry has been proven in the research where it has been shown that chemically oxidizing agents react with a wide range of different functional groups, where aflatoxin B1 contaminated corn was treated with electrochemically produced ozone. Other research has also proved the positive effects of the ozone when a contaminated cereal with ochratoxin A was treated [42]. Ozone possesses the ability to reduce mycotoxin contamination and improve microbiological status. When 10% of hydrogen peroxide (H_2O_2) was used to decontaminate zearalenone contaminated grains during a period of 16 h at a temperature of 80 °C, a degradation of 84% was recorded. The elevated degree of contamination of feedstuffs by these microorganisms has resulted in significant losses to enterprises as these microorganisms generate mycotoxins on a massive scale, in addition to the decay of the raw materials. *Aspergillus carbonarius* and *Aspergillus niger* produce ochratoxin A trough their secondary metabolism [43].

The use of both physical or chemical processes outlined earlier to decontaminate feed and compound feed is restricted by very high expenses and some nutrient quality losses. Scientists have reached the concept of detoxifying mycotoxins through biological conversion, which can be described as the degradation or enzymatic conversion of mycotoxins into less toxic compounds.

5. Feed Additives for the Prevention of Mycotoxin Effects

Feed additives are mixed with contaminated diet to minimize the effect of mycotoxins on the animal prior to intake or during digestion [44,45].

The use of feed additives or supplements that decrease animal exposure to mycotoxins can be viewed as a means of enhancing animal welfare. These feed supplements are referred to as the substances blended into feed (e.g., mineral clay, micro-organism, yeast cell wall), adsorbing or detoxifying mycotoxins in the digestive tract of animals (biological detoxification) [46]. These additives have received increasing attention from the feed industry and numerous products have been developed and some of them have already been tested on animals and marketed.

European Regulation (EC) No 1831/2003 of 22 September 2003 on animal feed additives has been revised and the category of technological feed additives includes a special functional group [47]. That is a group which is described as "substances that can suppress or decrease the absorption of food through mycotoxins, encourage the excretion of mycotoxins or alter their mode of action", under

Commission Regulation (EC) No 386/2009 of 12 May 2009 [48]. It should be pointed out that the use of such products does not mean that the animal feed exceeding the established maximum limits may be used. Their use should rather improve the quality of the feed which is lawfully on the market, providing an additional guarantee for the protection of animal and public health. Therefore, after adding an additive, these additives may not be used as compatible in non-conforming camouflage consignments. Following a request for technical assistance, in July 2010, the European Food Safety Authority (EFSA) through its Panel on Additives and Products or Substances used in Animal Feed (FEEDAP) issued a statement where it detailed the additional information that would be required to perform an assessment of safety and efficacy of this new group of additives [49]. This statement lists only the requirements which are not common in relation to the rest of technological additives. In 2012, EFSA published several guidelines on its website pertaining to the marketing of several feed additives and safety measures [50]. This guidance document follows the structure and definitions of Regulation (EC) No 1831/2003 and it is intended to assist the applicant in the preparation and the presentation of its application, as foreseen in Article 7.6 of Regulation (EC) No 1831/2003 [48].

Various materials have been tested as mycotoxin-detoxifying agents in order to avoid deleterious impacts of mycotoxins on livestock (mainly poultry and swine). They work either in adsorption or in the bonding or transformation of mycotoxins to their surfaces (biotransformation), depending on their mode of action. Biotransformation of mycotoxins can be caused by the addition of enzymes or micro-organisms generating such enzymes [46].

Mycotoxin binders are nutritionally inert adsorbents that reduce mycotoxin absorption from the gastrointestinal tract by integrating them into contaminated feed, thereby preventing and decreasing mycotoxicosis and transportation of mycotoxins into animal products [46]. The adsorbent materials are designed to behave like a "chemical sponge", preventing the blood and target organ absorption and later distribution of mycotoxins. The effectiveness of adsorbent on mycotoxin seems to depend on the chemical structure. The main feature is the physical adsorbent structure, i.e., the total distribution of load and load, the dimensions of pores and the available surface. On the other side, adsorbing mycotoxins also have a major part to play, such as polarity, solubility, form and load distribution. The stability of the sorbent toxin bond and the efficacy over a broad pH range are important criteria for the assessment of possible mycotoxin binders because a product has to be implemented on the entire gastrointestinal tract [51]. The feed composition can also have a major impact on adsorption effectiveness [51]. Potential absorbent materials include activated carbon, aluminosilicates (bentonite, zeolite, phyllosilicates, etc.), complex indigestible carbohydrates (cellulose, polysaccharides in the cell walls of yeast and bacteria such as glucomannans, peptidoglycans, and others), and synthetic polymers such as cholestyramine and polyvinylpyrrolidone and derivatives [20,45,46,52–54]. Many studies have shown that the formation of stable connections of these adsorbent products has a strong affinity with mycotoxins. These are found in a number of fluid systems, such as beer, wine, milk, and peanut oil.

Activated carbon is a widely used adsorption material that has an outstanding adsorption ability with a wide surface region. It is recommended for multiple digestive toxins as a general toxic adsorbing agent and is frequently suggested (The Merck Veterinary Manual, Eighth Edition, Merck & Co., Inc., Whitehouse Station, NJ) [55]. Activated carbon effectiveness depends on the source materials, the surface area and the distribution of the pores on the adsorption characteristics of the activated carbon. The surface features of activated carbons are greatly altered by preparation techniques and chemical treatments. The contrasting findings regarding the capacity of activated carbon for mycotoxin binding can explain different adsorbing characteristics of different carbonaceous materials [51]. Activated carbon adsorbs most mycotoxins effectively in water, whereas animals are less or not affected by mycotoxicosis. For aflatoxin B_1 and ochratoxin A adsorption, the highest capacity for in vitro activated carbon was noted whereas deoxynivalenol adsorption was lower. The efficacy of activated carbon has been demonstrated in vivo and in vitro by vibrant gastrointestinal models for deoxynivalenol, nivalenol, zearalenone, aflatoxin, ochratoxin A, diacetoxyscirpenol and T-2 toxins [44,53,56–60]. Responses to charcoal in cows, broilers, turkey poults, rats and mink suggest that charcoal may not be as effective in binding aflatoxin as the clay-based binders. The biomarker assay in rats did not confirm the in vivo efficacy of activated carbon to bind fumonisin [52,61]. Also, research conducted with weaning pigs showed that they were not effectively protected against the adverse effects of consuming fumonisin B_1 by adding activated carbon to contaminated feed [62]. Finally, although having a potential for acute exposure to a number of mycotoxins, activated carbon is a non-specific sequester with large variability in efficacy, which reduces possibilities for its practical application.

Mycotoxin binders are the largest and most complicated class of silicate minerals [63–67]. There are two major sub-classes in this group, phyllosilicate, and tectosilicate [68,69]. The phyllosilicate sub-class mineral clays include significant adsorbents such as the montmorillonite/smectite group, the kaolinite group and the illite (or clay-mica) group [51]. Montmorillonite is a predominantly layered, oxygen-coordinated, phyllosilicate consisting of octahedral aluminum and tetrahedral silicon layers. The bentonite is usually impure smectite clay. The tectosilicates include important and highly studied zeolites. Zeolites consist of SiO_4 and AlO_4 tetrahedrons having a cage-like structure that is infinite in three dimensions. In such minerals, some tetravalent silicones are replaced by trivalent aluminum, which results in inorganic cations, such as sodium, calcium and potassium ions, that have a lack of a positive charge. Clay minerals, primarily montmorillonite, have been used in the early 1970s to reduce aflatoxin toxicity [70]. There is ample literature on this subject, mainly in the field of in vitro water studies [53,63,64,66,71], and animal feed trials [20,72–74]. The use of smectite in human nutrition was also tested for its safety as well as the efficacy in the decrease of aflatoxin biomarkers [64,75–77]. In Europe, bentonite is allowed as a feed additive for all animal species, as well as for mitigation of mycotoxin contamination for ruminants, swine, and poultry (1m558). It is also used for control of radionuclide contamination and as an anticaking agent (1m558i). The chemisorption of aflatoxin to smectites involves the formation of a complex by the β-keto-lactone or bilactone system of aflatoxin with uncoordinated metal ions in the mineral. Aflatoxin B_1 is able to be attached on the surface of the mineral particle and in its interlayers. A huge difference in the effectiveness of bentonites in sequestration of aflatoxin B_1 was shown in several in vitro studies [51]. These studies indicated that aflatoxin B_1 bentonite adsorption efficacy may rely on the physical, chemical and mineralogical characteristics of the smectite, including clay contents, the capacities of the cation exchange (CECs), the interlayer cation hydrate radius, distributions of particle size and the specific surface area. Notwithstanding these findings, an important correlation has not been well created between smectites minero-chemical and physicochemical characteristics and aflatoxin B_1 adsorption. Therefore, there is still no predictive model of aflatoxin B_1 adsorption by the bentonite as the crystal-chemical variation in the smectite group is complex. Recently, the study by D'Ascanio et al. [67] showed a strong correlation between aflatoxin adsorption parameters and the geological origin of samples. In adsorbing toxin at distinct pH values, sedimentary bentonites were considerably better than hydrothermal bentonites [51]. The extent of aflatoxin B_1-adsorption was negative and linear with the extent of desorption. Mineralogical and physicochemical analyses confirmed that some physical and chemical properties of bentonites correlate linearly with AFB_1 adsorption. However, these studies cannot be deemed to be conclusive since it is still hard to depict the link between properties of these mineral adsorbents and aflatoxin B_1 adsorption/desorption. Due to the complexity of interactions and factors that can affect the adsorption of the aflatoxins by smectites, further research is required to describe the mechanisms of adsorption [51].

However, bentonite cannot be used as a binder for all mycotoxins due to their limited binding effects. Several in vivo studies have previously shown that aluminosilicates do not significantly adsorb other mycotoxins, such as cyclopiazonic acid and ergotamine, zearalenone, deoxynivalenol, T-2 toxin, ochratoxin A and others. The selective chemisorption of bentonites for aflatoxins can be overcome by chemical modifications. These include changes in the surface characteristics, resulting in enhanced hydrophobicity when structural load balancing cations are exchanged with molecular heavyweight amines [66,78]. Several in vitro studies showed the binding efficacy of modified montmorillonite and clinoptilolite against zearalenone and ochratoxin A [20]. Aflatoxin B_1 was adsorbed with non-modified zeolites. However, the in vivo ineffectiveness of these binders in sequestering a large spectrum of mycotoxins has been recently observed in piglets [79], and some of those clay forms were pointed out to the potential toxicity [80,81].

Recently, questions have been raised about the nanotechnology solution of mycotoxin risk [82]. One of the most promising methods is the use of carbon-based nanomaterials. Graphene has shown a huge surface and a high mycotoxin binding capacity. Polymeric nanoparticles have also been drawn to attention; they may replace adsorbents or contain a substance that would improve the organism's health status. Modified nanodiamonds synthesized by detonation were proposed as intestinal adsorbent of aflatoxins [83]. Highly advanced surfaces, and the existence on the surface of nanoparticles of multiple functional chemical-active groups, hydrocarbon fragments, and metal micro impurities, establish their elevated affinity to biomolecular sorption. The findings of in vitro experiments, showing that nanodiamonds adsorb aflatoxin B_1 from aqueous solutions at different pH, were confirmed by in vivo experiments with rats [83]. In order to confirm the effectivity and safety of this adsorbent on animal species, further studies including well-designed in vitro trials are needed. The practical and economic feasibility aspects should also be taken into account [82].

The formation of bonds between polymers, such as cholestyramine, divinylbenzene-styrene and polyvinylpyrrolidone, and mycotoxins were confirmed in vitro and in vivo [52]. Cholestyramine is a binding resin that has proven to bind bile acids in the gastrointestinal tract and decrease low-density lipoproteins and cholesterol. It has been shown that cholestyramine is an efficient binder for ochratoxin A, fumonisins and zearalenone in vitro [52,57,61]. Efficacy of cholestyramine in the dietary concentration of 2% on top of compound feed was confirmed in experiments with feed contaminated by zearalenone and by the biomarker assay in vivo in laboratory animals for fumonisins [52,57,61]. Cholestyramine efficacy for detoxification of zearalenone was also confirmed during other studies on laboratory animals [84]. A polyvinylpyrrolidone, a synthetic water-soluble polymer, was researched as a binder for mycotoxins as well [85]. It was shown that polyvinylpyrrolidone is able to bind aflatoxin B_1 and zearalenone, while it did not alleviate the toxicity of deoxynivalenol in pigs. It should be noted that the high costs of polymers are a limiting factor for its practical applications.

The mycotoxin-sequestering capacity of different high-fiber feedstuffs, such as hays (e.g., alfalfa hay) or straws (e.g., wheat straw), was recognized a long time ago, but there are principally practical experiences, e.g., in equine nutrition, without scientific assessment. The positive effect of alfalfa fiber was first proved against zearalenone in laboratory animals and pigs and also against T-2 toxicosis in laboratory animals, respectively [86–89]. However, it should also be mentioned that, besides its positive effects, alfalfa fiber is a potential source of *Fusarium* contamination, and its high inclusion rates (15–25%) required in the diet may cause digestive-physiological disturbances. Micronized wheat fiber has recently been found effective in decreasing the accumulation of ochratoxin A in laboratory animals' liver and kidney tissues. When used at an inclusion level of 20 kg/t, it significantly increased the excretion of ochratoxin A via the feces [90,91]. Recently, Avantaggiato et al. [92] showed that a red-grape pomace (pulp and skin) can sequester distinct mycotoxins quickly and simultaneously. Aflatoxin B_1, followed by zearalenone, ochratoxin A and fumonisin B_1, was the most affected mycotoxin. In pigs, using a urinary biomarker method the effectiveness of grape pomace in secreting mycotoxins has been confirmed [79]. Aflatoxin B_1 (67%) and zearalenone (69%) considerably lowered the urinary mycotoxin biomarker of the grape pomace. Taking these outcomes into consideration, the authors indicated that the use of grape pomace as a large-spectrum adsorbent material has its potential. Greco et al. [93] recorded evidence on the capacity of food plants and by-products other than grape pomace and wheat fibers to absorb mycotoxins. The research results are highly innovative and prove that a wide range of mycotoxins is also available in some dietary fibers. Aflatoxin B_1, zearalenone, and ochratoxin A were most of the adsorbed mycotoxins. Adsorption of aflatoxin B_1, zearalenone, and ochratoxin A was not impacted by pH, and the adsorbed fraction was not released when acid-to-neutral pH increased. Mycotoxin fumonisin B_1 has been adsorbed to a lesser level in this research and its adsorption has been affected by a medium's pH.

Polymeric humic materials comprise several binding sites and are being incorporated into humans as a compound to minimize bacterial endotoxins absorption and systemic accessibility. A high-quality humic acid derivative, called oxyhumate, has been reported to have the mycotoxin-sequestering capacity and recommended for use against aflatoxicosis based on in vivo studies in chickens [94]. The excellent connection capability of humic substances with zearalenone was an exciting finding, as assessed in vitro research [60]. These compounds should, therefore, be further tested in vivo.

The other groups of fiber components are the cell wall components of the yeast *Saccharomyces cerevisiae*, the mannan-oligosaccharides (MOS) or their esterified form with β-D-glucan (esterified glucomannan), which showed the considerable binding ability for several mycotoxins in vivo. *Saccharomyces cerevisiae* and lactic acid bacteria are the two most important food fermentation microorganisms that have proven to bind various mycotoxins [20,54,95]. The reversible and strain and dose-dependent phenomenon of mycotoxin binding of some chosen lactic acid bacteria was outlined and did not influence the viability of the lactic acid bacteria. It should be noted that there may be a relationship between lactic acid bacteria and the accumulation of mycotoxins through two particular procedures like binding and biosynthesis inhibition. There could, therefore, be a high value for the reduction of mycotoxin exposure for lactic acid cultures with a strong anti-fungal, anti-mycotoxigenic and mycotoxin potential [96].

Fungal conidia can bind mycotoxin individually or together (between 29 and 60%), particularly zearalenone and ochratoxin A [97]. *Saccharomyces cerevisiae* live yeast was shown to reduce the detrimental effects of aflatoxin in broiler diets [20,34,95,98,99]. The aflatoxin protective effect of live yeast was confirmed in rats, but thermolyzed yeast was shown ineffective. The potential to bind several mycotoxins was shown as fibrous material from the cell wall of the yeast. It has been shown that esterified glucomannan polymer obtained from the yeast cell wall separately and in combination binds aflatoxin, ochratoxin and toxin T-2. Additions of 0.5 or 1.0 kg/t doses of esterified glucomannan to aflatoxin-contaminated diets resulted in broiler chicks, with dose-dependent reactions. Similarly, in relation to aflatoxin-contaminated diets of dairy cows, esterified glucan polymer considerably decreased residues of aflatoxin in milk. The esterified glucan polymer may have the capability to bind several mycotoxins. A glucan polymer-bound both T-2 toxin and zearalenone in vitro, and it was protective against depression in antioxidant activities resulting from T-2 toxin consumed by growing quail. A glucan polymer product has protected swine, broilers, and hens against some of the detrimental effects of multiple mycotoxins, while another glucan polymer product did not alleviate the toxic effects on mink consuming diets contaminated with fumonisin B_1, ochratoxin A, moniliformin and zearalenone [98,99]. These polysaccharides, in addition to binding mycotoxins, also provide other functions to regulate the damage of mycotoxins in animal organs, including modulation of immune operations and binding gastrointestinal pathogens [100–102]. It should also be noticed that many trials are carried out using commercial products which may not consist exclusively of glucomannans, but contain tiny quantities of aluminosilicates that are specifically added to bind aflatoxins.

Numerous studies and several comprehensive reviews as above demonstrate the increasing interest in the use of mycotoxin-detoxifying agents as technological feed additives.

The best way to evaluate mycotoxin binders is with in vivo experiments. Naturally, in vivo models are perfect and hard to conduct in theory. It is complicated, costly, and time-consuming to collect the definitive data. Individual bioassays with the same strain, age, body weight, and dietary type should take place in vivo research to achieve coherent outcomes. Differences in farm conditions and types, health, development, and maturity of animals may also have an effect on outcomes. Binders with varying rates of incorporation, distinct mycotoxins, animal species, age, gender, and environment should be assessed as well. Moreover, according to the EU Guideline 2001/79/EC on additives for use in animal nutrition [50], the in vivo efficacy of binders should be proven by using an experimental design justified according to the claim for the use of the additive, and by using specific biological markers such as tissue residues or changes in biochemical parameters [103]. The chosen biomarker for exposure should be specific for each mycotoxin and target species, closely related to exposure and easy to detect with sensitive analytical methods validated for the matrix used [3]. EFSA has proposed different biomarkers for exposure to aflatoxin B_1, deoxynivalenol, zearalenone, ochratoxin A, and fumonisins. To date, the majority of the research on the effectiveness of mycotoxin binders has only been done on the feed consumption and measurements of performance. Few in vivo research papers have explored potential side impacts on animal performance or the health of these agents.

6. Biological Detoxification and Biotransformation

The application of microorganisms or enzyme systems to contaminated feeds can detoxify mycotoxins by metabolism or degradation in their gastrointestinal tract. This process is an irreversible and environmentally friendly method of detoxification, as it does not leave toxic residues or unwanted by-products. A large number of detoxifying studies were performed in the 1980s and 1990s on ochratoxin A, trichothecenes and zearalenone [32,46,98,104–106]. While initial in vitro reports of the microbial mycotoxins detoxification can be dated back to the 1960s, until now, only a few organically transforming agents mainly microorganisms were tested in vivo for their efficacy.

Aflatoxin degradation in laboratory conditions has been investigated in numerous cases over the years [107–110], but there is currently no biological system for the entire commercial sphere to be used. Interesting results have been obtained for *Nocardia corynebacteroides* application. This soil bacterium is supposed to remove aflatoxins B, G, and M_1 from a variety of food products, including milk, oil, peanut butter, peanuts, and maize, without leaving any toxic by-products. It has been shown to be effective in the irreversible removal of aflatoxin B_1 from aflatoxin-contaminated compound feed for broiler chicken nutrition [111].

In the last 20 years, many tests on trichothecenes with cows' rumen, gastrointestinal experimental or soil in the laboratory were conducted in vitro. Microbial biodegradation of trichothecenes via various pathways such as oxygenation, de-epoxidation, epimerization, and glucosylation has been elucidated [106]. Rumen fluid is selected due to knowledge of the fact that ruminants are very resistant to the toxic effects of mycotoxins, such as deoxynivalenol and trichothecenes. Deoxynivalenol's 12,13-epoxy-ring and T-2 toxin seem to be a part of the toxicity molecule. The mycotoxins are less toxic when opening up this ring. The *Eubacterium* sp. strain BBSH 797 has been developed into a commercial product for detoxifying trichothecenes in animal feed [98,105]. There are few studies on the transformation of toxins of T-2 and HT-2. Certain metabolites had been de-acetylated and de-epoxidized T-2. Some microorganisms could transform T-2 into HT-2, but detoxification has not been recorded.

Some bacteria, molds, yeasts, and plants can transform ochratoxin A into a less toxic compound which has been confirmed in many scientific reports [51,112,113]. These changes lead to phenylalanine formation [32,46,98,104–106,114]. *Aspergillus*, *Rhyzopus* and *Penicillium* spp. are particularly effective for ochratoxin A removal [113]. As a biologic controller in wine, *Aureobasidium pullulans* prevents the accumulation of ochratoxin A in the grape and decreases the symptoms of *Aspergillosis*. Plants, such as wheat and maize, or fungi, such as *P. ostreatus*, are capable of removing ochratoxin A but no transformation products have been identified [115]. Moreover, a new yeast strain that can degrade ochratoxin A and zearalenone was isolated and characterized. This strain was called *Trichosporon mycotoxinivorants* because of its property for degrading these mycotoxins. A feeding trial, which tested the efficacy of *T. mycotoxinivorans* to suppress ochratoxicosis, proved that the dietary inclusion of this yeast blocks ochratoxin A induced immune suppression in broiler chicks. *T. mycotoxinivorans* have been recognized as the principal transformation product of zearalenone. The structure of the metabolite, ZOM-1 is characterized by the opening in the group of ketones in C6 of the macrocyclic ring of zearalenone [116]. Even at concentrations 1000-fold higher that zearalenone, the ZOM-1 did not show estrogen activity in a sensitive yeast bioassay and did not interact with the human estrogen receptor in the competitive in vitro binding experiment [116].

Fumonisin B_1's main amine is responsible for its toxicity. Thus, this molecule's deamination would significantly decrease its toxicity. Very few biodegradation studies for fumonisin B_1 have been conducted. The main microorganism capable of degrading fumonisin B_1 is the black yeast, *Exophiala spinifera*. The transformation of fumonisin B_1 into amino polyol AP_1 is performed by an extracellular carboxylesterase. This enzyme has been cloned and proven effective in transgenic maize since the plant became fumonisin resistant [117]. Two genes that cause fumonisin B_1 degradation by the bacterium *Sphingopyxis* sp. in the latest study have been recognized, isolated and expressed in heterological terms. The researchers found that the successive effect of these gene-encoded enzymes to detoxify fumonisin B_1 [118]. It is important to mention that molecular oxygen is not necessary for the operation of the mentioned enzymes. The results of this study, therefore, provide the foundation for the development of an enzyme detoxification process for fumonisin B_1 in animal feed.

Although numerous papers on biological transformation by microorganisms of mycotoxins are present, they were limited in their use for feed detoxifying. This may result from a lack of understanding about the conversion process, the toxicity of the products being transformed, the impact of conversion responses on nutritional values for feed and animal safety. Biological agents used as feed additives should generally degrade mycotoxins into non-toxic metabolites under various environmental conditions. They must be safe and stable in the gastrointestinal tract of animals. To date, few micro-organisms meet these needs.

Dietary manipulations include improved dietary ingredients, dietary supplementation or additives with toxicity-protective characteristics or the addition of no-nutrient sequestrants to reduce mycotoxin bioavailability, in order to decrease mycotoxin induced intake [20,44,52].

The control of multiple metabolic route ways has an influence on protection from stress, which may be attributed to the sensitive equilibrium between antioxidants and pro-oxidants. Diet antioxidants like vitamin E, carotenoids and selenium can regulate this equilibrium [119–122]. On the other side, this antioxidant/prooxidant equilibrium has an adverse effect on dietary stress variables. In this regard, mycotoxins are regarded as one of the main stress variables in feed [121,123–125]. In fact, enhanced supplementation for antioxidants can safeguard against mycotoxins' poisonous behavior. The antioxidant characteristics of selenium and retinol, ascorbic acid, tocopherol, and their precursors are known to operate as free radical scavengers and to safeguard mycotoxin from membrane harm [126]. Certain antioxidants, selenium, and vitamins can also induce or boost liver and other tissue detoxication mechanisms, thereby increasing mycotoxin detoxification. Food elements in coffee, strawberries, tea, pepper, raisins, turmeric, tonka beans, garlic, chocolate, and onions achieved attractive outcomes. Furthermore, certain medicinal herbs and plant extracts could possibly protect them from aflatoxin B_1, fumonisin B_1, and ochratoxin A [121,127–129]. However, there is much less information on other mycotoxins, primarily from in-vitro research and focusing on aflatoxin B_1. For the assessment of their practical benefits further feeding studies with antioxidants and vitamins with farm animals are necessary. The choice of the most appropriate nutritional methods requires knowledge of the type of antioxidants in the diet, their bioavailability and food sources, and the exact intake required to achieve these protective effects. In addition, a mixture of natural antioxidants (e.g., medicinal plant extracts, essential oils, herbs, spices, some vitamins, etc.) with feed additives that act as detoxifiers of mycotoxins could be a further step in the fight against mycotoxicosis in animal production.

A similar tendency in research was noticed with regards to the usage of ozone in laboratory test animals for the prevention of zearalenone estrogenic effects [130]. Trichothecenes' biological activities were also altered by oxidation, with ozone most probably attacking trichothecenes' double bond. Recently, essential oils, natural-based or natural identical, have been tested for their efficacy to reduce ochratoxin A contamination in feed [8,131,132]. Ochratoxin A is found in various kinds of feed such as cereals, coffee, beans and foods such as dried fruits, grapes, wines, and their derivatives [39]. Nephrotoxic, cancer-genic, immunotoxic, teratogenic and genotoxic activities become noticeable when animals ingest contaminated feed [112]. In Puvača et al.'s [114] in vitro research, the influence of tea tree essential oil (*Melaleuca alternifolia*) on ochratoxin A fungal synthesis has been verified. The essential oil's (7.5; 15.0 and 30.0 µg/mL) decontamination potential was assessed on the growth of ochratoxin A producer (*Aspergillus niger*). The production of ochratoxin A in the presence of the essential oil depended on the incubation temperature, 20 and 30 °C. The values obtained from 20 °C showed a reduction in ochratoxin A synthesis by A. niger ranging from 53.87% to 96.22% while 18.36% to 72.85% at 30 °C. Based on the obtained results Puvača et al. [114] concluded that essential tea tree oil could serve as a prospective biocontrol agent for contamination of ochratoxin A in feed and compound feed.

7. Conclusions

In conclusion, levels of particular mycotoxins in feeds have been reduced, but, so far, no single technique has been established that is equally efficient against the broad variety of mycotoxins that can co-occur in various commodities. Furthermore, procedures of detoxication that appear to be efficient in vitro will not necessarily maintain their effectiveness in an in vivo test. Therefore, further research on the stability of toxins in the whole "field to fork" chain is required in order to have general recommendations for the reduction of these adverse contaminants and to avoid re-contamination. Research on mycotoxins in feeds and their potential interactions should be carried out simultaneously, and the solutions concerning how the toxicological importance of such interactions could be evaluated and practically used. There is increasing business interest in the use of feed additives to avoid mycotoxin absorption and the toxic impacts on farm animals. There are also new products on the market available and some of them have been in wide use for several years. The efficacy of the additives for the distinct mycotoxins and livestock must be proved, e.g., by means of peer-checked research. It is recommended that cell lines or artificial models be used in the simulation instead of living experimental animals, questioning the animal's welfare.

Author Contributions: R.Č., N.P., F.C., L.P., and O.Ð. together initiated, designed, and drafted the manuscript. J.K., G.A. and D.G. contributed to the literature collection, each section, and overall design. All the authors have equally contributed and revised the manuscript. All authors read and approved the final manuscript.

Funding: "The study has been funded by the project "SUSTAINABLE ANIMAL NUTRITION" funded by the Italian Ministry of Foreign Affairs and International Cooperation in the frame of the executive program of Scientific and Technological Cooperation between the Italian Republic and the Republic of Serbia for the years 2019–2021—SIGNIFICANT RESEARCH".

Acknowledgments: Authors would like to express their gratitude to European Union's Horizon 2020 Research and innovation program under Grant Agreement No. 678781 (MycoKey).

Conflicts of Interest: The authors declare no conflict of interest.

References

1. Burton, E.; Gatcliffe, J.; O'Neill, H.M.; Scholey, D. *Which Feedstuffs Will Be Used in the Future*; Sustainable Poultry Production in Europe; CABI: São Paulo, Brazil, 2016; ISBN 978-1-78064-530-8.
2. Park, B. 15 International regulatory issues on animal feed additives: Impacts on consumer safety and related-industry. *J. Anim. Sci.* **2018**, *96*, 1–2. [CrossRef]
3. EFSA Panel on Contaminants in the Food Chain (CONTAM). Scientific Opinion on the risks for animal and public health related to the presence of T-2 and HT-2 toxin in food and feed. *EFSA J.* **2011**, *9*, 2481. [CrossRef]
4. Pinotti, L.; Ottoboni, M.; Giromini, C.; Dell'Orto, V.; Cheli, F. Mycotoxin Contamination in the EU Feed Supply Chain: A Focus on Cereal Byproducts. *Toxins* **2016**, *8*, 45. [CrossRef] [PubMed]
5. Pankaj, S.K.; Shi, H.; Keener, K.M. A review of novel physical and chemical decontamination technologies for aflatoxin in food. *Trends Food Sci. Technol.* **2018**, *71*, 73–83. [CrossRef]
6. Zhu, Y.; Hassan, Y.; Lepp, D.; Shao, S.; Zhou, T. Strategies and Methodologies for Developing Microbial Detoxification Systems to Mitigate Mycotoxins. *Toxins* **2017**, *9*, 130. [CrossRef]
7. Huss, A.; Cochrane, R.; Muckey, M.; Jones, C. Animal Feed Mill Biosecurity. In *Food and Feed Safety Systems and Analysis*; Elsevier: Amsterdam, The Netherlands, 2018; pp. 63–81. ISBN 978-0-12-811835-1.
8. Puvača, N.; Čabarkapa, I.; Bursić, V.; Petrović, A.; Aćimović, M. Antimicrobial, antioxidant and acaricidal properties of tea tree (Melaleuca alternifolia). *J. Agron. Technol. Eng. Manag.* **2018**, *1*, 29–38.
9. Puvača, N.; Čabarkapa, I.; Petrović, A.; Bursić, V.; Prodanović, R.; Soleša, D.; Lević, J. Tea tree (*Melaleuca alternifolia*) and its essential oil: Antimicrobial, antioxidant and acaricidal effects in poultry production. *Worlds Poult. Sci. J.* **2019**, *75*, 235–246. [CrossRef]

10. Schofield, E.K. *Feed Manufacturing Technology*; American Feed Industry Association, Inc.: Arlington, VA, USA, 2005.
11. Bullerman, L.B.; Bianchini, A. Stability of mycotoxins during food processing. *Int. J. Food Microbiol.* **2007**, *119*, 140–146. [CrossRef]
12. Svihus, B.; Uhlen, A.K.; Harstad, O.M. Effect of starch granule structure, associated components and processing on nutritive value of cereal starch: A review. *Anim. Feed Sci. Technol.* **2005**, *122*, 303–320. [CrossRef]
13. Juan, C.; Covarelli, L.; Beccari, G.; Colasante, V.; Mañes, J. Simultaneous analysis of twenty-six mycotoxins in durum wheat grain from Italy. *Food Control* **2016**, *62*, 322–329. [CrossRef]
14. Karlovsky, P.; Suman, M.; Berthiller, F.; De Meester, J.; Eisenbrand, G.; Perrin, I.; Oswald, I.P.; Speijers, G.; Chiodini, A.; Recker, T.; et al. Impact of food processing and detoxification treatments on mycotoxin contamination. *Mycotoxin Res.* **2016**, *32*, 179–205. [CrossRef] [PubMed]
15. Awad, W.A.; Ghareeb, K.; Böhm, J.; Zentek, J. Decontamination and detoxification strategies for the *Fusarium* mycotoxin deoxynivalenol in animal feed and the effectiveness of microbial biodegradation. *Food Addit. Contam. Part A* **2010**, *27*, 510–520. [CrossRef] [PubMed]
16. Puvača, N.; Ljubojević, D.; Živkov Baloš, M.; Đuragić, O.; Bursić, V.; Vuković, G.; Prodanović, R.; Bošković, J. Occurance of Mycotoxins and Mycotoxicosis in Poultry. *Concepts Dairy Vet. Sci.* **2018**, *2*. [CrossRef]
17. Kabak, B.; Dobson, A.D.W.; Var, I. Strategies to Prevent Mycotoxin Contamination of Food and Animal Feed: A Review. *Crit. Rev. Food Sci. Nutr.* **2006**, *46*, 593–619. [CrossRef]
18. Jalili, M. A Review on Aflatoxins Reduction in Food. *Iran. J. Health Saf. Environ.* **2016**, *3*, 445–459.
19. Hojnik, N.; Cvelbar, U.; Tavčar-Kalcher, G.; Walsh, J.; Križaj, I. Mycotoxin Decontamination of Food: Cold Atmospheric Pressure Plasma versus "Classic" Decontamination. *Toxins* **2017**, *9*, 151. [CrossRef]
20. Vila-Donat, P.; Marín, S.; Sanchis, V.; Ramos, A.J. A review of the mycotoxin adsorbing agents, with an emphasis on their multi-binding capacity, for animal feed decontamination. *Food Chem. Toxicol.* **2018**, *114*, 246–259. [CrossRef]
21. Tibola, C.S.; Fernandes, J.M.C.; Guarienti, E.M. Effect of cleaning, sorting and milling processes in wheat mycotoxin content. *Food Control* **2016**, *60*, 174–179. [CrossRef]
22. Zhao, Y.; Ambrose, R.P.K. Structural characteristics of sorghum kernel: Effects of temperature. *Int. J. Food Prop.* **2017**, *20*, 2630–2638. [CrossRef]
23. Janić Hajnal, E.; Mastilović, J.; Bagi, F.; Orčić, D.; Budakov, D.; Kos, J.; Savić, Z. Effect of Wheat Milling Process on the Distribution of Alternaria Toxins. *Toxins* **2019**, *11*, 139. [CrossRef]
24. Vanara, F.; Scarpino, V.; Blandino, M. Fumonisin Distribution in Maize Dry-Milling Products and By-Products: Impact of Two Industrial Degermination Systems. *Toxins* **2018**, *10*, 357. [CrossRef] [PubMed]
25. Thomas, M.; Hendriks, W.H.; van der Poel, A.F.B. Size distribution analysis of wheat, maize and soybeans and energy efficiency using different methods for coarse grinding. *Anim. Feed Sci. Technol.* **2018**, *240*, 11–21. [CrossRef]
26. Niculita-Hirzel, H.; Hantier, G.; Storti, F.; Plateel, G.; Roger, T. Frequent Occupational Exposure to Fusarium Mycotoxins of Workers in the Swiss Grain Industry. *Toxins* **2016**, *8*, 370. [CrossRef] [PubMed]
27. Sanders, M.; McPartlin, D.; Moran, K.; Guo, Y.; Eeckhout, M.; O'Kennedy, R.; De Saeger, S.; Maragos, C. Comparison of Enzyme-Linked Immunosorbent Assay, Surface Plasmon Resonance and Biolayer Interferometry for Screening of Deoxynivalenol in Wheat and Wheat Dust. *Toxins* **2016**, *8*, 103. [CrossRef] [PubMed]
28. Vidosavljević, S.; Kos, J.; Banjac, V.; Janić Hajnal, E.; Dragojlović, D.; Đuragić, O.; Čolović, R. Simple technologies for removal of mycotoxins in feed. In Proceedings of the Feed Technology; University of Novi Sad, Institute of Food Technology: Novi Sad, Serbia, 2018; Volume 18, pp. 81–88.
29. Čolović, R.; Vukmirović, Đ.; Pezo, L.; Kos, J.; Čolović, D.; Bagi, F.; Memiši, N. Corn Grain Brushing for Deoxynivalenol Reduction. *Ital. J. Food Sci.* **2018**, *31*. [CrossRef]
30. Park, D.L. Effect of Processing on Aflatoxin. In *Mycotoxins and Food Safety*; DeVries, J.W., Trucksess, M.W., Jackson, L.S., Eds.; Springer: Boston, MA, USA, 2002; Volume 504, pp. 173–179. ISBN 978-1-4613-5166-5.
31. Pearson, T.C.; Wicklow, D.T.; Pasikatan, M.C. Reduction of Aflatoxin and Fumonisin Contamination in Yellow Corn by High-Speed Dual-Wavelength Sorting. *Cereal Chem. J.* **2004**, *81*, 490–498. [CrossRef]
32. Kabak, B. The fate of mycotoxins during thermal food processing. *J. Sci. Food Agric.* **2009**, *89*, 549–554. [CrossRef]

33. Lu, Z.; Dantzer, W.R.; Hopmans, E.C.; Prisk, V.; Cunnick, J.E.; Murphy, P.A.; Hendrich, S. Reaction with Fructose Detoxifies Fumonisin B_1 while Stimulating Liver-Associated Natural Killer Cell Activity in Rats. *J. Agric. Food Chem.* **1997**, *45*, 803–809. [CrossRef]
34. Santos Pereira, C.; Cunha, S.C.; Fernandes, J.O. Prevalent Mycotoxins in Animal Feed: Occurrence and Analytical Methods. *Toxins* **2019**, *11*, 290. [CrossRef]
35. Negash, D. A Review of Aflatoxin: Occurrence, Prevention, and Gaps in Both Food and Feed Safety. *J. Nutr. Health Food Eng.* **2018**, *8*, 190–197. [CrossRef]
36. Luo, X.; Wang, R.; Wang, L.; Li, Y.; Wang, Y.; Chen, Z. Detoxification of aflatoxin in corn flour by ozone: Detoxification of aflatoxin in corn flour by ozone. *J. Sci. Food Agric.* **2014**, *94*, 2253–2258. [CrossRef] [PubMed]
37. Phillips, T.D.; Clement, B.A.; Kubena, L.F.; Harvey, R.B. Detection and detoxification of aflatoxins: Prevention of aflatoxicosis and aflatoxin residues with hydrated sodium calcium aluminosilicate. *Vet. Hum. Toxicol.* **1990**, *32*, 15–19. [PubMed]
38. Hasan, M.I.; Walsh, J.L. Numerical investigation of the spatiotemporal distribution of chemical species in an atmospheric surface barrier-discharge. *J. Appl. Phys.* **2016**, *119*, 203302. [CrossRef]
39. Hathout, A.S.; Aly, S.E. Biological detoxification of mycotoxins: A review. *Ann. Microbiol.* **2014**, *64*, 905–919. [CrossRef]
40. Weltmann, K.-D.; von Woedtke, T. Plasma medicine—Current state of research and medical application. *Plasma Phys. Control. Fusion* **2017**, *59*, 014031. [CrossRef]
41. Scholtz, V.; Pazlarova, J.; Souskova, H.; Khun, J.; Julak, J. Nonthermal plasma—A tool for decontamination and disinfection. *Biotechnol. Adv.* **2015**, *33*, 1108–1119. [CrossRef]
42. Machala, Z.; Chládeková, L.; Pelach, M. Plasma agents in bio-decontamination by dc discharges in atmospheric air. *J. Phys. Appl. Phys.* **2010**, *43*, 222001. [CrossRef]
43. De Saeger, S.; Logrieco, A. Report from the 1st MYCOKEY International Conference Global Mycotoxin Reduction in the Food and Feed Chain Held in Ghent, Belgium, 11–14 September 2017. *Toxins* **2017**, *9*, 276. [CrossRef]
44. Avantaggiato, G.; Visconti, A. Mycotoxin Issues in farm animals and strategies to reduce mycotoxins in animal feeds. In *Recent Advances in Animal Nutrition-2009*; Nottingham University Press: Nottingham, UK, 2010; pp. 149–189. ISBN 978-1-907284-65-6.
45. Kolosova, A.; Stroka, J. Substances for reduction of the contamination of feed by mycotoxins: A review. *World Mycotoxin J.* **2011**, *4*, 225–256. [CrossRef]
46. Boudergue, C.; Burel, C.; Dragacci, S.; Favrot, M.-C.; Fremy, J.-M.; Massimi, C.; Prigent, P.; Debongnie, P.; Pussemier, L.; Boudra, H.; et al. Review of mycotoxin-detoxifying agents used as feed additives: Mode of action, efficacy and feed/food safety. *EFSA Support. Publ.* **2009**, *6*, 22E. [CrossRef]
47. EUR-Lex-02002L0032-20131227-EN-EUR-Lex. Available online: https://eur-lex.europa.eu/eli/dir/2002/32/2013-12-27 (accessed on 8 August 2019).
48. Publication Office of the European Union. CELEX1, Commission Regulation (EC) No 386/2009 of 12 May 2009 amending Regulation (EC) No 1831/2003 of the European Parliament and of the Council as Regards the Establishment of a New Functional Group of Feed Additives (Text with EEA relevance). Available online: https://publications.europa.eu/en/publication-detail/-/publication/d4eb22d2-78f2-45c5-813e-b77f85ebb2fe (accessed on 8 August 2019).
49. Statement on Guidelines for 'Substances for Reduction of the Contamination of Feed by Mycotoxins'. Available online: https://www.efsa.europa.eu/en/efsajournal/pub/1693 (accessed on 8 August 2019).
50. Guidance on Technological Additives. Available online: https://www.efsa.europa.eu/en/efsajournal/pub/2528 (accessed on 8 August 2019).
51. De Mil, T.; Devreese, M.; De Baere, S.; Van Ranst, E.; Eeckhout, M.; De Backer, P.; Croubels, S. Characterization of 27 Mycotoxin Binders and the Relation with in Vitro Zearalenone Adsorption at a Single Concentration. *Toxins* **2015**, *7*, 21–33. [CrossRef] [PubMed]
52. Avantaggiato, G.; Solfrizzo, M.; Visconti, A. Recent advances on the use of adsorbent materials for detoxification of *Fusarium* mycotoxins. *Food Addit. Contam.* **2005**, *22*, 379–388. [CrossRef] [PubMed]
53. Ramos, A.J.; Hernández, E. In vitro aflatoxin adsorption by means of a montmorillonite silicate. A study of adsorption isotherms. *Anim. Feed Sci. Technol.* **1996**, *62*, 263–269. [CrossRef]
54. Peng, W.-X.; Marchal, J.L.M.; van der Poel, A.F.B. Strategies to prevent and reduce mycotoxins for compound feed manufacturing. *Anim. Feed Sci. Technol.* **2018**, *237*, 129–153. [CrossRef]

55. Huwig, A.; Freimund, S.; Käppeli, O.; Dutler, H. Mycotoxin detoxication of animal feed by different adsorbents. *Toxicol. Lett.* **2001**, *122*, 179–188. [CrossRef]
56. Avantaggiato, G.; Havenaar, R.; Visconti, A. Evaluation of the intestinal absorption of deoxynivalenol and nivalenol by an in vitro gastrointestinal model, and the binding efficacy of activated carbon and other adsorbent materials. *Food Chem. Toxicol.* **2004**, *42*, 817–824. [CrossRef] [PubMed]
57. Avantaggiato, G.; Havenaar, R.; Visconti, A. Assessing the zearalenone-binding activity of adsorbent materials during passage through a dynamic in vitro gastrointestinal model. *Food Chem. Toxicol. Int. J. Publ. Br. Ind. Biol. Res. Assoc.* **2003**, *41*, 1283–1290. [CrossRef]
58. Diaz, D.; Smith, T. Mycotoxin Sequestering Agents: Practical Tools for the Neutralization of Mycotoxins. In *Mycotoxin Blue Book*; Context Products: Leicestershire, UK, 2005; pp. 323–340.
59. Mézes, M.; Balogh, K.; Tóth, K. Preventive and therapeutic methods against the toxic effects of mycotoxins—A review. *Acta Vet. Hung.* **2010**, *58*, 1–17. [CrossRef]
60. Sabater-Vilar, M.; Malekinejad, H.; Selman, M.H.J.; van der Doelen, M.A.M.; Fink-Gremmels, J. In vitro assessment of adsorbents aiming to prevent deoxynivalenol and zearalenone mycotoxicoses. *Mycopathologia* **2007**, *163*, 81–90. [CrossRef]
61. Solfrizzo, M.; Visconti, A.; Avantaggiato, G.; Torres, A.; Chulze, S. In vitro and in vivo studies to assess the effectiveness of cholestyramine as a binding agent for fumonisins. *Mycopathologia* **2001**, *151*, 147–153. [CrossRef]
62. Piva, A.; Casadei, G.; Pagliuca, G.; Cabassi, E.; Galvano, F.; Solfrizzo, M.; Riley, R.T.; Diaz, D.E. Activated carbon does not prevent the toxicity of culture material containing fumonisin B1 when fed to weanling piglets. *J. Anim. Sci.* **2005**, *83*, 1939–1947. [CrossRef] [PubMed]
63. Phillips, T.D.; Sarr, A.B.; Grant, P.G. Selective chemisorption and detoxification of aflatoxins by phyllosilicate clay. *Nat. Toxins* **1995**, *3*, 204–213; discussion 221. [CrossRef] [PubMed]
64. Phillips, T.D.; Afriyie-Gyawu, E.; Williams, J.; Huebner, H.; Ankrah, N.-A.; Ofori-Adjei, D.; Jolly, P.; Johnson, N.; Taylor, J.; Marroquin-Cardona, A.; et al. Reducing human exposure to aflatoxin through the use of clay: A review. *Food Addit. Contam. Part A* **2008**, *25*, 134–145. [CrossRef] [PubMed]
65. Avantaggiato, G.; Havenaar, R.; Visconti, A. Assessment of the Multi-mycotoxin-Binding Efficacy of a Carbon/Aluminosilicate-Based Product in an in Vitro Gastrointestinal Model. *J. Agric. Food Chem.* **2007**, *55*, 4810–4819. [CrossRef]
66. Li, Y.; Tian, G.; Dong, G.; Bai, S.; Han, X.; Liang, J.; Meng, J.; Zhang, H. Research progress on the raw and modified montmorillonites as adsorbents for mycotoxins: A review. *Appl. Clay Sci.* **2018**, *163*, 299–311. [CrossRef]
67. D'Ascanio, V.; Greco, D.; Menicagli, E.; Santovito, E.; Catucci, L.; Logrieco, A.F.; Avantaggiato, G. The role of geological origin of smectites and of their physico-chemical properties on aflatoxin adsorption. *Appl. Clay Sci.* **2019**, *181*, 105209. [CrossRef]
68. WHO Bentonite, Kaolin and Selected Clay Minerals. Available online: https://apps.who.int/iris/handle/10665/43102 (accessed on 8 August 2019).
69. Bergaya, F.; Lagaly, G. Chapter 1 General Introduction: Clays, Clay Minerals, and Clay Science. In *Developments in Clay Science*; Handbook of Clay Science; Bergaya, F., Theng, B.K.G., Lagaly, G., Eds.; Elsevier: Amsterdam, The Netherlands, 2006; Volume 1, pp. 1–18.
70. Masimango, N.; Remacle, J.; Ramaut, J.L. The role of adsorption in the elimination of aflatoxin B1 from contaminated media. *Eur. J. Appl. Microbiol. Biotechnol.* **1978**, *6*, 101–105. [CrossRef]
71. Chaturvedi, V.B.; Singh, K.S.; Agnihotri, A.K. In vitro aflatoxin adsorption capacity of some indigenous aflatoxin adsorbents. *Indian J. Anim. Sci.* **2002**, *72*, 257–260.
72. Phillips, T.D.; Kubena, L.F.; Harvey, R.B.; Taylor, D.R.; Heidelbaugh, N.D. Hydrated Sodium Calcium Aluminosilicate: A High Affinity Sorbent for Aflatoxin. *Poult. Sci.* **1988**, *67*, 243–247. [CrossRef]
73. Márquez, R.N.M.; De Hernandez, I.T. Aflatoxin adsorbent capacity of two Mexican aluminosilicates in experimentally contaminated chick diets. *Food Addit. Contam.* **1995**, *12*, 431–433. [CrossRef]
74. Desheng, Q.; Fan, L.; Yanhu, Y.; Niya, Z. Adsorption of aflatoxin B1 on montmorillonite. *Poult. Sci.* **2005**, *84*, 959–961. [CrossRef] [PubMed]
75. Afriyie-Gyawu, E.; Ankrah, N.-A.; Huebner, H.J.; Ofosuhene, M.; Kumi, J.; Johnson, N.M.; Tang, L.; Xu, L.; Jolly, P.E.; Ellis, W.O.; et al. NovaSil clay intervention in Ghanaians at high risk for aflatoxicosis. I. Study design and clinical outcomes. *Food Addit. Contam. Part A* **2008**, *25*, 76–87. [CrossRef] [PubMed]

76. Wang, P.; Afriyie-gyawu, E.; Tang, Y.; Johnson, N.M.; Xu, L.; Tang, L.; Huebner, H.J.; Ankrah, N.-A.; Ofori-adjei, D.; Ellis, W.; et al. NovaSil clay intervention in Ghanaians at high risk for aflatoxicosis: II. Reduction in biomarkers of aflatoxin exposure in blood and urine. *Food Addit. Contam. Part A* **2008**, *25*, 622–634. [CrossRef] [PubMed]
77. Wang, J.-S.; Luo, H.; Billam, M.; Wang, Z.; Guan, H.; Tang, L.; Goldston, T.; Afriyie-Gyawu, E.; Lovett, C.; Griswold, J.; et al. Short-term safety evaluation of processed calcium montmorillonite clay (NovaSil) in humans. *Food Addit. Contam.* **2005**, *22*, 270–279. [CrossRef]
78. Wang, G.; Miao, Y.; Sun, Z.; Zheng, S. Simultaneous adsorption of aflatoxin B 1 and zearalenone by mono- and di-alkyl cationic surfactants modified montmorillonites. *J. Colloid Interface Sci.* **2018**, *511*, 67–76. [CrossRef] [PubMed]
79. Gambacorta, L.; Pinton, P.; Avantaggiato, G.; Oswald, I.P.; Solfrizzo, M. Grape Pomace, an Agricultural Byproduct Reducing Mycotoxin Absorption: In Vivo Assessment in Pig Using Urinary Biomarkers. *J. Agric. Food Chem.* **2016**, *64*, 6762–6771. [CrossRef] [PubMed]
80. Lemke, S.L.; Mayura, K.; Reeves, W.R.; Wang, N.; Fickey, C.; Phillips, T.D. Investigation of Organophilic Montmorillonite Clay Inclusion in Zearalenone-Contaminated Diets Using the Mouse Uterine Weight Bioassay. *J. Toxicol. Environ. Health A* **2001**, *62*, 243–258. [CrossRef]
81. Marroquín-Cardona, A.; Deng, Y.; Taylor, J.F.; Hallmark, C.T.; Johnson, N.M.; Phillips, T.D. In vitro and in vivo characterization of mycotoxin-binding additives used for animal feeds in Mexico. *Food Addit. Contam. Part A* **2009**, *26*, 733–743. [CrossRef]
82. Horky, P.; Skalickova, S.; Baholet, D.; Skladanka, J. Nanoparticles as a Solution for Eliminating the Risk of Mycotoxins. *Nanomaterials* **2018**, *8*, 727. [CrossRef]
83. Mogilnaya, O.; Puzyr, A.; Baron, A.; Bondar, V. Hematological Parameters and the State of Liver Cells of Rats After Oral Administration of Aflatoxin B1 Alone and Together with Nanodiamonds. *Nanoscale Res. Lett.* **2010**, *5*, 908–912. [CrossRef]
84. Underhill, K.L.; Rotter, B.A.; Thompson, B.K.; Prelusky, D.B.; Trenholm, H.L. Effectiveness of Cholestyramine in the Detoxification of Zearalenone as Determined in Mice. Available online: https://eurekamag.com/research/002/606/002606081.php (accessed on 8 August 2019).
85. Alegakis, A.K.; Tsatsakis, A.M.; Shtilman, M.I.; Lysovenko, D.L.; Vlachonikolis, I.G. Deactivation of mycotoxins. I. An in vitro study of zearalenone adsorption on new polymeric adsorbents. *J. Environ. Sci. Health Part B* **1999**, *34*, 633–644. [CrossRef] [PubMed]
86. Smith, T.K. Influence of Dietary Fiber, Protein and Zeolite on Zearalenone Toxicosis in Rats and Swine. *J. Anim. Sci.* **1980**, *50*, 278–285. [CrossRef] [PubMed]
87. James, L.J.; Smith, T.K. Effect of Dietary Alfalfa on Zearalenone Toxicity and Metabolism in Rats and Swine. *J. Anim. Sci.* **1982**, *55*, 110–118. [CrossRef] [PubMed]
88. Carson, M.S.; Smith, T.K. Effect of Feeding Alfalfa and Refined Plant Fibers on the Toxicity and Metabolism of T-2 Toxin in Rats. *J. Nutr.* **1983**, *113*, 304–313. [CrossRef] [PubMed]
89. Stangroom, K.E.; Smith, T.K. Effect of whole and fractionated dietary alfalfa meal on zearalenone toxicosis and metabolism in rats and swine. *Can. J. Physiol. Pharmacol.* **1984**, *62*, 1219–1224. [CrossRef] [PubMed]
90. Aoudia, N.; Tangni, E.K.; Larondelle, Y. Distribution of ochratoxin A in plasma and tissues of rats fed a naturally contaminated diet amended with micronized wheat fibres: Effectiveness of mycotoxin sequestering activity. *Food Chem. Toxicol.* **2008**, *46*, 871–878. [CrossRef]
91. Aoudia, N.; Callu, P.; Grosjean, F.; Larondelle, Y. Effectiveness of mycotoxin sequestration activity of micronized wheat fibres on distribution of ochratoxin A in plasma, liver and kidney of piglets fed a naturally contaminated diet. *Food Chem. Toxicol.* **2009**, *47*, 1485–1489. [CrossRef]
92. Avantaggiato, G.; Greco, D.; Damascelli, A.; Solfrizzo, M.; Visconti, A. Assessment of Multi-mycotoxin Adsorption Efficacy of Grape Pomace. *J. Agric. Food Chem.* **2014**, *62*, 497–507. [CrossRef]
93. Greco, D.; D'Ascanio, V.; Santovito, E.; Logrieco, A.F.; Avantaggiato, G. Comparative efficacy of agricultural by-products in sequestering mycotoxins: Multi-mycotoxin adsorption efficacy of agricultural by-products. *J. Sci. Food Agric.* **2019**, *99*, 1623–1634. [CrossRef]
94. Van Rensburg, C.J.; Van Rensburg, C.E.J.; Van Ryssen, J.B.J.; Casey, N.H.; Rottinghaus, G.E. In Vitro and In Vivo Assessment of Humic Acid as an Aflatoxin Binder in Broiler Chickens. *Poult. Sci.* **2006**, *85*, 1576–1583. [CrossRef]

95. Luo, Y.; Liu, X.; Li, J. Updating techniques on controlling mycotoxins—A review. *Food Control* **2018**, *89*, 123–132. [CrossRef]
96. Dalié, D.K.D.; Deschamps, A.M.; Richard-Forget, F. Lactic acid bacteria—Potential for control of mould growth and mycotoxins: A review. *Food Control* **2010**, *21*, 370–380. [CrossRef]
97. Jard, G.; Liboz, T.; Mathieu, F.; Guyonvarc'h, A.; Lebrihi, A. Adsorption of zearalenone by Aspergillus japonicus conidia: New trends for biological decontamination in animal feed. *World Mycotoxin J.* **2009**, *2*, 391–397. [CrossRef]
98. Binder, E.M. Managing the risk of mycotoxins in modern feed production. *Anim. Feed Sci. Technol.* **2007**, *133*, 149–166. [CrossRef]
99. Jouany, J.P. Methods for preventing, decontaminating and minimizing the toxicity of mycotoxins in feeds. *Anim. Feed Sci. Technol.* **2007**, *137*, 342–362. [CrossRef]
100. Santovito, E.; Greco, D.; Logrieco, A.F.; Avantaggiato, G. Eubiotics for Food Security at Farm Level: Yeast Cell Wall Products and Their Antimicrobial Potential against Pathogenic Bacteria. *Foodborne Pathog. Dis.* **2018**, *15*, 531–537. [CrossRef]
101. Santovito, E.; Greco, D.; D'Ascanio, V.; Marquis, V.; Raspoet, R.; Logrieco, A.F.; Avantaggiato, G. Equilibrium Isotherm Approach to Measure the Capability of Yeast Cell Wall to Adsorb *Clostridium perfringens*. *Foodborne Pathog. Dis.* **2019**, *16*. [CrossRef]
102. Santovito, E.; Greco, D.; Marquis, V.; Raspoet, R.; D'Ascanio, V.; Logrieco, A.F.; Avantaggiato, G. Antimicrobial Activity of Yeast Cell Wall Products against Clostridium perfringens. *Foodborne Pathog. Dis.* **2019**, *16*. [CrossRef]
103. Lauwers, M.; Croubels, S.; Letor, B.; Gougoulias, C.; Devreese, M. Biomarkers for Exposure as a Tool for Efficacy Testing of a Mycotoxin Detoxifier in Broiler Chickens and Pigs. *Toxins* **2019**, *11*, 187. [CrossRef]
104. Wu, Q.; Jezkova, A.; Yuan, Z.; Pavlikova, L.; Dohnal, V.; Kuca, K. Biological degradation of aflatoxins. *Drug Metab. Rev.* **2009**, *41*, 1–7. [CrossRef]
105. Schatzmayr, G.; Zehner, F.; Täubel, M.; Schatzmayr, D.; Klimitsch, A.; Loibner, A.P.; Binder, E.M. Microbiologicals for deactivating mycotoxins. *Mol. Nutr. Food Res.* **2006**, *50*, 543–551. [CrossRef] [PubMed]
106. Hassan, Y.I.; Zhou, T. Promising Detoxification Strategies to Mitigate Mycotoxins in Food and Feed. *Toxins* **2018**, *10*, 116. [CrossRef] [PubMed]
107. Afsharmanesh, H.; Perez-Garcia, A.; Zeriouh, H.; Ahmadzadeh, M.; Romero, D. Aflatoxin degradation by Bacillus subtilis UTB1 is based on production of an oxidoreductase involved in bacilysin biosynthesis. *Food Control* **2018**, *94*, 48–55. [CrossRef]
108. Farzaneh, M.; Shi, Z.-Q.; Ghassempour, A.; Sedaghat, N.; Ahmadzadeh, M.; Mirabolfathy, M.; Javan-Nikkhah, M. Aflatoxin B1 degradation by Bacillus subtilis UTBSP1 isolated from pistachio nuts of Iran. *Food Control* **2012**, *23*, 100–106. [CrossRef]
109. Sarlak, Z.; Rouhi, M.; Mohammadi, R.; Khaksar, R.; Mortazavian, A.M.; Sohrabvandi, S.; Garavand, F. Probiotic biological strategies to decontaminate aflatoxin M1 in a traditional Iranian fermented milk drink (Doogh). *Food Control* **2017**, *71*, 152–159. [CrossRef]
110. Xia, X.; Zhang, Y.; Li, M.; Garba, B.; Zhang, Q.; Wang, Y.; Zhang, H.; Li, P. Isolation and characterization of a Bacillus subtilis strain with aflatoxin B1 biodegradation capability. *Food Control* **2017**, *75*, 92–98. [CrossRef]
111. Tejada-Castañeda, Z.I.; Ávila-Gonzalez, E.; Casaubon-Huguenin, M.T.; Cervantes-Olivares, R.A.; Vásquez-Peláez, C.; Hernández-Baumgarten, E.M.; Moreno-Martínez, E. Biodetoxification of Aflatoxin-Contaminated Chick Feed. *Poult. Sci.* **2008**, *87*, 1569–1576. [CrossRef]
112. Zain, M.E. Impact of mycotoxins on humans and animals. *J. Saudi Chem. Soc.* **2011**, *15*, 129–144. [CrossRef]
113. Abrunhosa, L.; Paterson, R.; Venâncio, A. Biodegradation of Ochratoxin A for Food and Feed Decontamination. *Toxins* **2010**, *2*, 1078–1099. [CrossRef]
114. Puvača, N.; Bursić, V.; Petrović, A.; Prodanović, R.; Kharud, M.M.; Obućinski, D.; Vuković, G.; Marić, M. Influence of tea tree essential oil on the synthesis of mycotoxins: Ochratoxin A. *Maced. J. Anim. Sci.* **2019**, *9*, 25–29.
115. Vanhoutte, I.; Audenaert, K.; De Gelder, L. Biodegradation of Mycotoxins: Tales from Known and Unexplored Worlds. *Front. Microbiol.* **2016**, *7*, 561. [CrossRef] [PubMed]

116. Vekiru, E.; Hametner, C.; Mitterbauer, R.; Rechthaler, J.; Adam, G.; Schatzmayr, G.; Krska, R.; Schuhmacher, R. Cleavage of Zearalenone by Trichosporon mycotoxinivorans to a Novel Nonestrogenic Metabolite. *Appl. Environ. Microbiol.* **2010**, *76*, 2353–2359. [CrossRef] [PubMed]
117. Duvick, J. Prospects for reducing fumonisin contamination of maize through genetic modification. *Environ. Health Perspect.* **2001**, *109*, 337–342. [PubMed]
118. Heinl, S.; Hartinger, D.; Thamhesl, M.; Vekiru, E.; Krska, R.; Schatzmayr, G.; Moll, W.-D.; Grabherr, R. Degradation of fumonisin B1 by the consecutive action of two bacterial enzymes. *J. Biotechnol.* **2010**, *145*, 120–129. [CrossRef] [PubMed]
119. Reuter, S.; Gupta, S.C.; Chaturvedi, M.M.; Aggarwal, B.B. Oxidative stress, inflammation, and cancer: How are they linked? *Free Radic. Biol. Med.* **2010**, *49*, 1603–1616. [CrossRef]
120. Zuo, L.; Zhou, T.; Pannell, B.K.; Ziegler, A.C.; Best, T.M. Biological and physiological role of reactive oxygen species—The good, the bad and the ugly. *Acta Physiol.* **2015**, *214*, 329–348. [CrossRef]
121. Da Silva, E.O.; Bracarense, A.P.F.L.; Oswald, I.P. Mycotoxins and oxidative stress: Where are we? *World Mycotoxin J.* **2018**, *11*, 113–134. [CrossRef]
122. Ren, Z.; He, H.; Fan, Y.; Chen, C.; Zuo, Z.; Deng, J. Research Progress on the Toxic Antagonism of Selenium Against Mycotoxins. *Biol. Trace Elem. Res.* **2019**, *190*, 273–280. [CrossRef]
123. Adhikari, M.; Negi, B.; Kaushik, N.; Adhikari, A.; Al-Khedhairy, A.A.; Kaushik, N.K.; Choi, E.H. T-2 mycotoxin: Toxicological effects and decontamination strategies. *Oncotarget* **2017**, *8*, 33933–33952. [CrossRef]
124. Wang, X.; Martínez, M.-A.; Cheng, G.; Liu, Z.; Huang, L.; Dai, M.; Chen, D.; Martínez-Larrañaga, M.-R.; Anadón, A.; Yuan, Z. The critical role of oxidative stress in the toxicity and metabolism of quinoxaline 1,4-di-N-oxides in vitro and in vivo. *Drug Metab. Rev.* **2016**, *48*, 159–182. [CrossRef]
125. JECFA. *Safety Evaluation of Certain Contaminants in Food*, 19th ed.; WHO Food Additives Series; World Health Organization and Food and Agriculture Organization of the United Nations: Geneva, Switzerland, 2018; ISBN 978-92-4-166074-7.
126. Sorrenti, V.; Di Giacomo, C.; Acquaviva, R.; Barbagallo, I.; Bognanno, M.; Galvano, F. Toxicity of Ochratoxin A and Its Modulation by Antioxidants: A Review. *Toxins* **2013**, *5*, 1742–1766. [CrossRef] [PubMed]
127. Mohajeri, M.; Behnam, B.; Cicero, A.F.G.; Sahebkar, A. Protective effects of curcumin against aflatoxicosis: A comprehensive review. *J. Cell. Physiol.* **2018**, *233*, 3552–3577. [CrossRef] [PubMed]
128. Tabeshpour, J.; Mehri, S.; Shaebani Behbahani, F.; Hosseinzadeh, H. Protective effects of Vitis vinifera (grapes) and one of its biologically active constituents, resveratrol, against natural and chemical toxicities: A comprehensive review: Protective effect of grape. *Phytother. Res.* **2018**, *32*, 2164–2190. [CrossRef] [PubMed]
129. Hedayati, N.; Naeini, M.B.; Nezami, A.; Hosseinzadeh, H.; Wallace Hayes, A.; Hosseini, S.; Imenshahidi, M.; Karimi, G. Protective effect of lycopene against chemical and natural toxins: A review: Lycopene against chemical and natural toxins. *BioFactors* **2019**, *45*, 5–23. [CrossRef]
130. Niemira, B.A. Cold Plasma Decontamination of Foods. *Annu. Rev. Food Sci. Technol.* **2012**, *3*, 125–142. [CrossRef]
131. Park, S.Y.; Ha, S.-D. Application of cold oxygen plasma for the reduction of *Cladosporium cladosporioides* and *Penicillium citrinum* on the surface of dried filefish (*Stephanolepis cirrhifer*) fillets. *Int. J. Food Sci. Technol.* **2015**, *50*, 966–973. [CrossRef]
132. Obućinski, D.; Prodanović, R.; Ljubojević Pelić, D.; Puvača, N. Improving competitiveness and sustainable approach to management in animal husbandry. *J. Agron. Technol. Eng. Manag.* **2019**, *2*, 228–234.

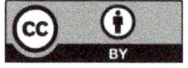

© 2019 by the authors. Licensee MDPI, Basel, Switzerland. This article is an open access article distributed under the terms and conditions of the Creative Commons Attribution (CC BY) license (http://creativecommons.org/licenses/by/4.0/).

MDPI
St. Alban-Anlage 66
4052 Basel
Switzerland
Tel. +41 61 683 77 34
Fax +41 61 302 89 18
www.mdpi.com

Toxins Editorial Office
E-mail: toxins@mdpi.com
www.mdpi.com/journal/toxins

www.ingramcontent.com/pod-product-compliance
Lightning Source LLC
LaVergne TN
LVHW070734100526
838202LV00013B/1229